Strategy and Statistics in Clinical Trials

Strategy and Statistics in Clinical Trials

A Non-Statistician's Guide to Thinking, Designing, and Executing

Joseph Tal

AMSTERDAM • BOSTON • HEIDELBERG • LONDON
NEW YORK • OXFORD • PARIS • SAN DIEGO
SAN FRANCISCO • SINGAPORE • SYDNEY • TOKYO
Academic Press is an imprint of Elsevier

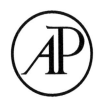

Academic Press is an imprint of Elsevier
225 Wyman Street, Waltham, MA 02451, USA
The Boulevard, Langford Lane, Kidlington, Oxford, OX5 1GB, UK

Library of Congress Cataloging-in-Publication Data
Tal, Joseph.
   Strategy and statistics in clinical trials : a non-statisticians guide to thinking, designing, and executing / Joseph Tal.
      p. cm.
   ISBN 978-0-12-386909-8
1.   Clinical trials–Statistical methods. I. Title.
   R853.C55T35 2011
   615.5072'4–dc22   2011009725

British Library Cataloguing-in-Publication Data
A catalogue record for this book is available from the British Library.

For information on all Academic Press publications
visit our website at www.elsevierdirect.com

Printed and bound by CPI Group (UK) Ltd, Croydon, CR0 4YY

Table of Contents

INTRODUCTION: THINKING, DESIGNING, EXECUTING vii

CHAPTER 1   Clinical Development and Statistics:
            The General View 1

CHAPTER 2   Questions For Planning Trials 17

CHAPTER 3   Medical Product Attributes 25

CHAPTER 4   Setting Research Objectives 35

CHAPTER 5   Statistical Thinking 53

CHAPTER 6   Estimation 67

CHAPTER 7   From Description to Testing: A Beginning 77

CHAPTER 8   Statistical Significance, Explanation,
            and Prediction 91

CHAPTER 9   Exploratory and Confirmatory Clinical Trials 111

CHAPTER 10 One, Two, Three Testing: Hypothesis Testing
            and Multiplicity 135

CHAPTER 11 Elements of Clinical Trial Design I:
            Putting It Together 155

CHAPTER 12 Elements of Clinical Trial Design II 179

CHAPTER 13 Endpoints 203

CHAPTER 14 Sample Size 229

CHAPTER 15 Concluding Remarks 245

GLOSSARY 249
INDEX 261

Introduction: Thinking, Designing, Executing

On those fleeting occasions when I regain my sense of wonder, I marvel at the complexity of things in general. During my own short lifetime we have put a man on the moon and observed ancient organisms on deep ocean floors. Computers and cell phones have become near necessities, and even inexpensive cars do not often break down (a minor miracle to my reminiscing mind). Being adaptable, we have become accustomed to the most elaborate of devices. And we take them for granted as one might have a kitchen knife some hundreds of years ago.

Life sciences have not lagged behind. We have mapped the basic structures of life and increasingly have come to understand the human body and the substances circulating in it. Using this knowledge, we have developed products that can alter and regulate both mind and body. To be sure, there is still much to be done, and hopefully there always will be. But we have achieved a great deal already.

Now and again I talk with people outside my field and find it both fascinating and frustrating. Fascinating because there are so many incredible developments out there, and frustrating because it is nary impossible for me to know enough to truly appreciate them. Our world has become so complex that it is difficult for any one individual to have little more than a single area of expertise. And even this can only be had with a great deal of effort. While I might wish it otherwise—and I do—this is the way it is. But more disconcerting is that specialization often impedes the work of people who *should be* working together: professionals from disparate fields who must team up to get things done.

My own area is statistics. Within it, I specialize in biostatistics. Specializing even further, I have gained some expertise in my discipline's methods in clinical trials. And when I return to Earth from my contemplative heights, I find there is often great disorder in these trials. At times it seems to me a wonder they even work at all. Clinical studies are planned and executed by dozens of people both within and without the organization. In great measure their success depends on the good graces of harried physicians and volunteering subjects who are often very infirm. A single trial may be conducted across many centers, countries, and even continents, making its management that much more difficult. And studies often take years to complete, during which time anything can happen and generally does.

So like most complicated ventures, success depends on numerous processes and professionals with varied expertise. A partial list of specialties includes finance, clinical, regulatory, marketing, toxicology, biology, physics, materials engineering, software engineering, medical monitoring, analytic chemistry, and information technology. And yes, statistics. If we cannot coordinate effectively between these specialties, our trials will be suboptimal at best.

Paradoxically, our complex products demand both added specialization within fields and ever more dialogue between them. So while we ask our people to know more about less, we increasingly require that they communicate with others in the same predicament. And as specialization deepens, interactions between experts become more difficult.

Simply put, for a clinical trial to work people must talk to one another. And while it is impossible for any to fully understand all others, each must know enough for the dialogue to be useful. This then brings me to my book's objective.

Statistics—be they more complex or less—are involved in virtually every clinical trial. The discipline provides essential input in the planning stage on issues like trial design, choice of endpoints, and sample size. And it supplies the language for communicating outcomes using simple statistics like mean and median, and more sophisticated tests for inferring conclusions. This is my work, and I like it. And in medical research, statistics is important work. But just because it is, I do not expect others to take year-long courses in it. Indeed, among those who already have, many are perfectly happy to leave this year behind them.

For a large number of clinical trial professionals my discipline is a black box they are content to leave as is. But this must not be if we are to design, conduct, and report trials effectively. In the chapters that follow I aim to cast some light into this box.

This book explains clinical trial statistics in the simplest language I can manage. There is very little formal mathematics in it and almost no formulas. More importantly, I place the discipline in the wider context of clinical trials—the inevitable constraints of time and money, and limitations associated with clinical practice. I also relate trial design and analysis to its intended audience—to those needing the information it provides, such as regulators, scientists, physicians, corporate managers, investors, and others.

The book is a practical guide. It is based on years of applied experience, much of it my own. In it I present numerous examples from pharmaceuticals, devices, and other products. Crucially, I describe how statisticians must consider a trial's overall needs and reconcile to them. And I show how at times it must be the other way around. Be that as it may, a clinical trial cannot maximize any one discipline's preferences. But it *can* optimize—and it must.

For nonstatisticians this book provides strategies for productive dialogue with those who are; it describes the statistician's approach to clinical trials and the basic tools at the statistician's disposal. For statistical professionals this is a "how-to" guide for interacting with the many others working on clinical studies. In this book I describe—for the benefit of statisticians and nonstatisticians alike—the numerous considerations involved in clinical studies and their effect on a trial's statistics.

Competence and native intelligence will get you a long way in most every field. But little apart from experience can give you *experience*. Well, I present here what I believe to be the next best thing: other people's experience. I describe the central topics of clinical trial statistics with real-world examples, recounting clinical tales and their morals. I have to the best of my ability written a book to facilitate communication between the field I have chosen and those I have not.

CHAPTER 1

Clinical Development and Statistics: The General View

CONTENTS

- Allerton's Palsy: an example in early drug development
- Preclinical development: scientific and statistical contributions
- Statistical input into trial design:
  - sample size
  - trial length
  - recruitment

INTRODUCTION

When putting together a clinical trial, each discipline involved brings its own particular and peculiar view to the table. Some of these are complementary, while others combine less seamlessly. Still others will pull in different directions. It is your job to find the best way to profit from this kaleidoscope of views—to merge the varying approaches to produce a solid study.

Clinical trials are a multidisciplinary effort. Now this is a very general statement and is true of many professional endeavors. Besides, you have long known it to be true. So instead of keeping to generalities, let me begin with a hypothetical, though typical, example from pharmaceuticals. In it I will describe some of the central issues that arise when planning a clinical study and focus on the biostatistician's role in them.

I do not intend to be exhaustive here. It is virtually impossible to cover all relevant issues and, more to the point, it is impractical. My aim is to provide an idea of statistics' contribution to planning a clinical trial. This will be enough to keep me occupied for a while.

ALLERTON'S PALSY

Allerton's Palsy (ALP), whether discovered by him or on him, is a **neurodegenerative** disorder primarily affecting physical function. In about 10% of cases there is internal organ involvement, and there is some question whether these cases constitute a distinct disorder. Be that as it may, ALP is primarily a disease in which the immune system misidentifies a part of the brain as foreign and attacks it—that is, an **autoimmune disease**. The brain cells (**neurons**) attacked by ALP degenerate over time. This usually leads to serious disability and in some cases to death. The **natural history** of the disease—the individual path it takes—is highly variable. Some with ALP show little change in physical functioning over decades, while others will deteriorate within a few years. Most commonly, the disease progresses slowly at first and accelerates over time.

Diagnosis of ALP is difficult so the number of reported cases is unreliable. The onset of the disease is usually between the ages of 30 and 45, though much later onsets have also been documented. ALP is more common in men than women, with an estimated male-to-female ratio of 3:1.

Your Company has developed CTC-11, a molecule designed to protect brain cells at risk from the disorder. As such, your compound aims to provide **neuroprotection** in ALP. Virtually all early studies with CTC-11 have been encouraging: **In vitro** testing demonstrated significant reductions in cell death, whereby animal neuron cultures treated and exposed to a toxic environment displayed a much smaller rate of cell death than those untreated. Other **preclinical** studies showed that the molecule delays onset of the disease in rats. In animals that had already developed ALP, CTC-11 slowed progression of the disease relative to those not treated. Preclinical testing also indicated that in the **animal models** tested, the molecule is safe. Finally, two early **Phase I clinical trials** in healthy volunteers showed that even high doses of CTC-11 produced only minor side effects, such as headaches and transient rashes.

So it seems you have in hand a potentially safe and effective drug for ALP—a chronic disease that currently has only marginally effective treatments and no cure. But it is still early and there are many issues to be considered before moving on to the first clinical study in humans with the disease. In the following sections I examine a sampling of these issues and articulate some typical questions that arise. And for each, I describe the statistical input required for providing answers.

Science

In vitro testing is about as far from the clinic and its patients as you can get. Success at this stage is supportive of **efficacy** in humans but is often little more than that. The positive results observed in animals provide you with stronger support; after all, the molecule has now been tested in a living organism.

But here too the evidence is fragile. First, results in animals frequently do not replicate in humans or only partially replicate. Second, and more important, ALP is a human disease that does not naturally occur in any other species. Unfortunately, the animal models developed to study ALP have yet to be fully **validated**-scientists are unsure whether they mimic the human form of the disease well enough to serve as suitable models for it. So the best you can now say is that CTC-11 has effectively treated animals that have been caused to develop an ALP-like disorder. But has your drug actually treated *ALP*? Well, you would like to think so. Yet you will not know until the molecule is tested in humans with the disease.

Despite all the caveats, there is no denying that your results have been good so far. In fact, some of your outcomes in animals could even be termed impressive. And since you cannot do much better than you have, it is only natural that you want to know what CTC-11 can do for humans with ALP.

Thus your continuing efforts with CTC-11 are scientifically important and may end up helping some very ill people. If successful, they will likely contribute to your Company's coffers and, with a bit of goodwill, to your own modest ones as well. Finally, a successful effort will almost certainly get you that lunch with Aunt Augusta promised in a moment of weakness—the one contingent on your "finally doing something useful with your life."

Your Division Head has asked you to prepare a presentation for management, which is now ready to decide on the molecule's future. Management, she says, would like a summary of the results obtained thus far. She gives you about a week for it. You work late hours and a weekend to convert the large amount of information generated to date into a presentation that even management can understand. You contemplate incorporating something about the importance of the project to patients and a word or two about market potential as well. But you are an R&D manager and your boss has made it clear that the presentation should deal with scientific findings only. "Stick to the facts as you know them," she says, and you wonder which version of the Bible they will have you swear on.

The presentation is done. After more than three hours of endless chatter (only a small part of it your own), it is over. Slightly sweating still, you leave the room and close the door behind you. The air in the hallway feels surprisingly fresh compared to what passed for oxygen in the conference room. You take the stairway down and do not even notice the receptionist's benevolent smile as you wait for the automatic door at the entrance to open. You go through the door and out, and for a while your mind is empty.

Walking to your office you think back to those long hours in the lab—the many frustrations and few rewards. And you ponder the time it took to prepare the presentation with every sentence and chart in its proper place. Did anyone notice? You certainly hope so.

Clutching the laptop as if it were your only friend, you wonder if it all comes down to this: three exhausting hours and a PowerPoint file. Of course you know that a management presentation alone will not determine the fate of a development program. But that is how it feels.

Well, you have done your best and believe you have made a good scientific case for the molecule. Your Division Head backed you throughout the meeting, as did a couple of VPs. The CEO appeared positive, but he has this way of nodding his head that makes you think he would have preferred to shake it instead. You simply do not know. Regardless, other than one wearisome VP nearing retirement, no one was outright negative. And now they must decide whether the scientific evidence supports the substantial investment needed for testing CTC-11 in patients with ALP.

Statistical Input

The preclinical studies were likely conducted with the statistician's help in data analysis and have his stamp of approval. With any luck he was also involved in designing these studies, which was almost certainly the case in Phase I.

But all this is behind you. The evidence from these early experiments is in its final form, and just about all that could be learned has been learned. It is now left for others to decide if R&D has presented sufficient evidence for CTC-11 to justify the cost of moving forward.

Still, the statistician might have helped you prepare your presentation by pointing out which numbers are best presented and how. He may also have suggested a graph or two and some color-coordinated charts. But beyond what he has already done in CTC-11's development, there is little of substance for him to do now. In short, the statistician's input into the scientific aspects of results *after* they have been obtained and analyzed is limited.

There is, however, an exception that typically occurs in **due-diligence**, where individuals consider investing in a particular R&D venture. These potential investors may seek a statistician's evaluation of the *quality* of the evidence obtained—the degree to which the results presented were produced by well-designed and correctly analyzed studies. Clearly, well-designed studies provide more reliable conclusions than sloppy ones, and correct statistical analyses are more apt to yield an accurate picture than incorrect ones.

Trial Sample Size

After numerous management meetings and a discussion with the board, the Company has decided to go ahead with the molecule. Public Relations have come out with a press release emphasizing the favorable results obtained to date and stating that the "Company is excited about pursuing further development of CTC-11, a promising drug for Allerton's Palsy." The drug, states the press release, "will enter a **Phase IIa clinical trial** in the first quarter next year," and there is some hint in the release of a pivotal **Phase III clinical trial** to come. But you are so euphoric with the current decision that the mention of Phase III makes little difference. Besides, you have learned enough about press releases to know they are not meant for you. When doing science, it is better you read Excel sheets than broadsheets.

So the Company will pursue further development of CTC-11. However, as always, you will be testing the molecule with limited resources. At this stage the budget is for a 6-month trial with about 150 subjects; half will receive CTC-11 (**Treatment group**) and half will receive **Standard-of-Care (Control group)**. Will this be enough?

Statistical Input

Many compounds do not go directly from Phase I into full-fledged trials like the one proposed. A smaller pilot study is probably more common and, under the circumstances, perhaps more advisable. In fact, you have no idea where the number 150 came from and suspect it had more to do with budgets and stock prices than with the development program's needs. Regardless, this is what you have been given and it is substantial. But "substantial" does not necessarily mean "sufficient," the relationship between the two depending on the case at hand.

Numbers—as large or small as they may seem at first—cannot be evaluated without a context. A 9-year-old child selling lemonade in front of her family's garage might feel that taking in $30 on a single Sunday makes her the class tycoon. But offer her the same in a toy store and she might complain of underfunding (and, frighteningly, might use these very words).

Be that as it may, this is what you have and you must make the best of it. Still, you are not going to take the numbers proposed as set in stone, and one of your first questions is whether they will provide your development program with the information needed. Specifically, will this study produce enough data for making an informed decision on taking CTC-11 into the next level of testing?

The statistician's role here is central. He will likely begin with straightforward **power analyses**, which here relate to calculations determining the number of subjects needed for demonstrating the drug's efficacy.[1]

---

[1] This is assuming the drug is effective. If a drug is ineffective, no sample size will make it otherwise. Thus, the goal of power analysis is to compute a sample size that will provide statistically significant results given a product that is assumed (or known) to have a particular level of efficacy.

In a future chapter we will deal with power analysis in greater detail. For the moment let us point out that to do these analyses a statistician needs several pieces of information. The most important of these is an estimate of the drug's **effect size** relative to Control. For example, stating that CTC-11 is superior to Control by about 10% is saying that the drug's effect size is about 10%.[2]

The statistician will get these estimates from clinicians and others in the organization. But he should also review results obtained to date within the Company and read some scientific publications on the subject. To do this he will need assistance from life-scientists, without whose help he will have difficulty extracting the required information from medical publications.

This is but one example of professionals from different fields needing to interact in trial planning. In this book I will note many more. So while statisticians need not have deep knowledge of biology or chemistry or medicine, they should be sufficiently conversant in these disciplines to conduct intelligent discussions with those who are. And the same goes for life-scientists, who would do well to be conversant in statistics.

Once acquired, the statistician will incorporate this information into his power analyses. These will yield sample sizes that will be more useful than those proposed primarily on financial considerations. If management's proposal and the power analyses produce very different sample sizes, you will (alas) have another opportunity for multidisciplinary interaction.

A DIFFICULTY WITHIN A PROBLEM

You have asked the statistician to compute the required sample size that will ensure your trial is a success: the number of subjects that will provide sufficient information for making future decisions on CTC-11. The statistician, in turn, has asked *you* for information; he has requested that you estimate the effect of the drug relative to Control. On the face of it, this is a silly request. After all, you are planning to conduct a trial precisely to discover this effect, so how can you be expected to know it *before* conducting your trial? To tell the truth, you cannot know it. But you *can* come up with an intelligent guess and have no choice but to do so. Indeed, estimating an effect size for the purpose of planning a trial of which the purpose is to estimate effect size arises often. We shall deal with it later, but for the moment let me assure you it is not as problematic as it sounds.

When determining sample size, the statistician will do well to talk with physicians and marketing personnel regarding the kind of CTC-11 efficacy needed for the drug to sell. Incorporating this information into power analyses will provide the Company with data on how valuable (or not) trials of varying sizes are likely to be from the standpoint of assessing market need.

---

[2] Quantification of effects—effect sizes—come in a variety of forms, percent being one of several.

The statistician should also expand his exploration to alternative study designs—not just the initially proposed six-month study of 150 subjects in two **arms**. Some of these designs will require fewer resources, while others will require more. He might, for example, examine a scenario where the larger trial is replaced with a smaller **pilot study** of 10 to 30 subjects. This sort of study could provide a more realistic estimate of the drug's effect in humans—an estimate that is now lacking. Once the pilot study is done, there will be more reliable information for planning the larger trial.

The larger the trial, the more informative the data obtained from it. But, as Goldilocks demonstrated years ago, strength does not necessarily reside in numbers; if a smaller trial can provide us with the required information, we should prefer it to a larger one. Conversely, if the larger study has little potential to provide the required data and an even larger trial is needed, you would do well to forgo the former and request more resources.

So a small pilot may be just what the statistician ordered. But this pilot will come at a price: A two-stage approach—a pilot and subsequent, larger trial—will slow down the development process. Moreover, given the fixed budget, any pilot will come at the expense of resources earmarked for the second stage. Here too there is more than one option. For example, you can design a standalone pilot and reassess development strategy after its completion. Alternatively, you can design the larger study with an early stopping point for **interim analysis**—an early check of the results. Once interim results are in, the information can be used to modify the remainder of the trial if needed.

These two approaches—one that specifies two studies and another that implies a single, two-stage study—can have very different implications for the Company. They differ in costs, logistics, time, flexibility, and numerous other parameters. The choice between them should be considered carefully.

For the moment let us simply state that the statistician's role is central when discussing trial sample size—the number of subjects that should be recruited for it. At the same time, it is very important for those requesting sample size estimates to actively involve statisticians in discussions dealing with a wider range of topics as well—for example, the drug's potential clinical effects and alternatives to the initially proposed design. And given that it takes at least two to trial, it is critical that the statistician be open-minded enough to step out of his equation-laden armor and become cognizant of these issues.

In sum, the fact that a relatively large sample size has been proposed for this early trial does not necessarily imply that it will provide the information needed. Together with your colleagues in R&D, logistics, statistics, and elsewhere, you should discuss all realistic alternatives: There can be two trials instead of one, one two-stage trial, as well as trials with more than two arms or less, a longer trial or a shorter one, and so on.

Now all this may seem a bit complicated, and it can be. At the same time you should keep in mind that because your budget is limited, the universe of possibilities is restricted as well; covering all, or nearly all, study design possibilities given fixed resources is definitely doable.

Trial Length

Virtually all published studies investigating treatment for ALP evaluated effects of anti-inflammatory agents, both steroidal and not. Where positive results were obtained (albeit modest ones), they appeared between three weeks and four months into the trial. But CTC-11's hypothesized **mechanism of action** is neuroprotection; it is meant to shield brain cells from processes leading to degeneration and death. **Neuroprotective** activity is most useful in the long term, with its short-term effects likely to be more subtle than those of anti-inflammatory agents. As a result, your new drug may even prove *inferior* to existing treatments in alleviating short-term symptoms, such as pain and fatigue.

So you reason that your best bet for success may be demonstrating CTC-11's effect on Disease Progression rather than short-term alleviation of symptoms. Of course, in any study conducted, you will also collect data on symptom relief. It is just that you feel that longer-term measures will highlight CTC-11's benefit more than short-term ones.

By definition, **endpoints** associated with Disease Progression measure change over time. In chronic diseases these endpoints generally reflect the deterioration that occurs with varying rates, depending on the specific disease, individual patient, quality of treatment, and other factors. One measure of Disease Progression in ALP is the Mannheim Working Group Lower Limb Reflex Response Scale (MLRS). The measure consists of multiple items, most based on a physician's exam of foot and knee reflexes and several reported by the patient. The MLRS is relatively **reliable** and has shown at least moderate relationships with other important disease parameters.

Based on a review of scientific literature you conclude that meaningful declines in MLRS in ALP typically take at least nine months to appear; they are rarely observed in six months or less. This is especially true for patients in early stages of ALP, where progression is slower than at later stages. And your initial trial is intended for early-stage ALP patients.

Based on these data and CTC-11's mechanism of action you believe that a longer trial will increase your chances for success. Consequently, you feel that the MLRS—a measure sensitive to Disease Progression—should be the most important efficacy endpoint in your trial. It will be the study's **Primary Efficacy Endpoint**.

Now it might seem that I have moved away from sample size and study design and entered a discussion of endpoints in a clinical trial—in other words, that I am now dealing with parameters, such as MLRS, that will ultimately determine whether one drug is better than another. This is indeed a very important discussion, but I have *not* entered it despite clear indications to the contrary.

Deciding on a trial's endpoints, particularly the central ones, is critical and will be dealt with in time. But in this section I focus on trial length and will ignore the issue of endpoint selection to the best of my ability.

A MORAL

In clinical trials, as in life in general, just about everything is connected to everything else. So it is that you wish to limit your discussions to trial length and find yourself slipping ever so naturally into sample size computation and endpoint selection. For many of us, it would be nice if both life and science were to proceed in an orderly fashion. There would, as the Greeks taught us, be a "beginning," "middle," and "end" to everything. But the Greeks were strong on mythology, and this concept of orderly progression is often only tenuously related to reality.

Issues and events generally do not advance in the uniform and orderly fashion we would like. And even scientists have questioned the established order. Thus, for example, where evolution was once thought to proceed slowly and at a relatively even pace, this no longer is the consensus. Oddly, artists have found themselves in a similar seafaring vessel. Thus, a good many artists in the last century created works of which the point was that neither time nor space is arranged in a particularly orderly fashion.

The division of larger concepts into smaller, more manageable ones is often artificial. But I will make an effort at order regardless. It is how we learn best and, at this stage, we are learning. At the same time, I suggest you keep in mind that the process of planning a clinical trial typically involves at least as much disorder as order. And the confusion ebbs and flows as we design and execute the trial while dealing with finances, logistics, people, and unexpected events that arise to produce ever more fascinating forms of disorder.

Now let us get back to the trial. Summarizing thus far, you are contemplating a study showing CTC-11's effect on Disease Progression, feeling this is where the drug's greatest advantage is. And you believe MLRS is the best measure for demonstrating it.

But MLRS can only pick up relatively large changes in Disease Progression, and these take more than the six months currently planned for your trial. So if you want to show meaningful Treatment-Control differences on this particular endpoint, you will need a longer trial, which will present its own problems. Longer trials require more resources than shorter ones and are more difficult to get right: The logistics are more complex, larger numbers of patients are lost along the way, and the number of unpleasant surprises popping up will be larger as well. Moreover, a 9- or 12-month trial will delay the Company's development program and, with it, your long-awaited lunch date with Aunt Augusta. On top of all of this there is a price to pay—literally. Given a fixed budget, extending the trial must come at the expense of something else. And this "something else" is probably important for the trial's success as well.

So deciding if you should place your chips on, say, a 12-month study is no trivial matter; any decision you make comes complete with a matching set of risks and rewards. And if you tend toward the longer study, you will need to do some creative budgeting and decide which aspects of the shorter trial to forgo so that resources are freed to finance the extended study.

Statistical Input

One obvious way to cut costs in a clinical trial is reducing its **sample size**; if you are going to conduct a 12-month instead of a 6-month trial, do it with fewer subjects. There are other options as well. For example, you might consider eliminating some expenses like imaging with MRI. You can also go back to management to make the case for more resources. But in this particular section I shall limit myself to discussing the relationship between trial length and sample size.

In principle, the more subjects in a trial, the greater its likelihood for showing meaningful results. An additional principle is that the greater the difference between Treatment and Control, the greater your chance for success as well.

Lengthening the trial and reducing sample size may actually turn out to your advantage. But this will only happen if the increased Treatment-Control difference expected in the 12-month trial will more than offset the study's weakening by reducing sample size. Unfortunately, at this stage of the game you cannot know whether or not this will be the case. In fact, you will not *truly* know until after completing the trial. So what do you do? Well, you do the best you can.

So you are now in the position of having to make a decision under conditions of uncertainty. Put more plainly, you will need to do some gambling here—with patient numbers, Company resources, and your own career. But before going ahead and rolling the dice, you should collect as much information as you can—information that will enable optimizing your risk-taking. Even gambling must be approached wisely—actually, *especially* gambling.

There are two issues here, one of which is clearly statistical, and we shall begin with it: As noted, reducing the number of subjects in a clinical trial will, all else held equal, decrease its chances for success; having fewer subjects in your study as opposed to more will reduce the trial's **statistical power**—its ability to convincingly demonstrate that Treatment is superior to Control.

But all else is not held equal here, since by extending the trial you expect to increase the drug's effect relative to Control, which will increase your study's likelihood for success. So in deciding on a 12-month rather than a 6-month study, you are faced with a tradeoff: The 12-month trial may provide you with a larger clinical effect (good) but compel a smaller sample (bad), while the 6-month trail will allow for a larger sample (good) but may yield a smaller effect (bad).

Keep in mind that this is rarely a zero-sum game; you cannot expect that the same budget distributed differently will provide similar chances for success. For example, a longer trial might necessitate a cut of 10% in the number of subjects while yielding a 15% increase in the Treatment-Control difference. Putting these two together is unlikely to balance your overall power; you might end up with more or with less and cannot know which by simply thinking about it.

All sorts of strange and interesting outcomes can result when doing these kinds of cost-benefit analyses. And some will make you happier than others. Indeed, even experienced clinicians and statisticians are not very good at intuiting these tradeoffs' outcomes. Thus, the relative advantages and disadvantages of longer and shorter studies cannot be resolved by theoretical discussion. Analyses must be conducted, and many of these will be done by the statistician.

Unfortunately, your information about these two sides of the tradeoff is not equal: Reducing sample size will *assuredly* reduce power, while the increase in clinical effect of a longer trial is, at this stage, conjecture. Faced with certain loss and possible gain you might tend to the conservative and go with the certainty. And if you are very unsure about CTC-11's long-term advantage in ALP, this is precisely what you should do. After all, it makes little sense to gamble on a highly uncertain increase in clinical effect with the certainty of reduced power. But we are dealing with biological systems here, and the issues are rarely clear cut. It is more than likely that you are neither completely sure nor completely unsure regarding the drug's effect over time. Indeed, you are probably located in the proverbial "somewhere in between." And if this is where you are firmly placed, and it troubles you deeply, you might do well to see a therapist. And once you've done that, make an appointment with the statistician as well.

Given the reasoning presented thus far, you know something about the "certainty index" attached to your two options. Write this down and save it. But there is still much more to be considered, so let us move on.

For starters, you should ask the following questions: "What is the minimum increase in CTC-11's effect in a 12-month trial relative to a 6-month trial that will offset the loss in sample size?" Now this is something that a statistician knows how to compute. But she will need a few values to do it with and will ask you for them. Some of these can be known and others will be "intelligent guesses" at best.

The first number the statistician will want is the sample size your budget will allow for the 6-month trial. This is known and was originally set at about 150. The second number she will ask for is how many subjects you can expect to recruit for a 12-month trial given the fixed budget provided. This number can also be computed relatively easily. What you need to determine is the cost-per-subject in a 12-month trial[3] and divide your total budget by it. The difference between the number obtained and 150 is the reduction in sample size expected in the longer trial.

The statistician will then ask you for numbers that you can only obtain by intelligent conjecture. The first of these relates to the effect size you expect will emerge from the shorter trial, and the second relates to the expected, larger effect size that will emerge in the longer trial.

As an aside, quantifying effect size is not trivial and the statistician can help you with this as well. For the moment, let us assume that you know how to quantify effect sizes.

Summarizing thus far, to reach an informed decision on a longer versus a shorter trial, the statistician will need the following four quantities:

- Number of subjects in a 6-month trial.
- Number of subjects in a 12-month trial.
- Expected effect of CTC-11 relative to Control in a 6-month trial.
- Expected effect of CTC-11 relative to Control in a 12-month trial.

Using the four values for input and conducting statistical computations called power analyses, the statistician will tell you whether the loss of sample size of the longer trial will be worth your while.

But you are not home free yet. This is due to the nature of the information you gave the statistician and on which the computations were based. Recall that calculating 6-month and 12-month sample sizes was straightforward and based on known quantities: total budget for the project, cost-per-subject in the 6-month trial, and cost-per-subject in the 12-month trial. However, the "expected effect of CTC-11 relative to Control" quantities were "intelligent estimates."

Discussions on trial length revolve around two major issues, only one of which is statistical. Well, we are now with the nonstatistical issue. Specifically, to obtain expected effect sizes in the two trials considered, you need to estimate the relationship between trial length and the effect of CTC-11. This is a clinical matter and will therefore require discussion with those who are experts in this area. On the upside, it is now your turn to ask for the numbers rather than to provide them.

So you now go to your clinical people and ask them to estimate the difference in effect size between 6-month and 12-month trials. They have their tools to do this, which may include earlier results in animal models, knowledge of

---

[3] Cost-per-subject in this case refers to total cost that includes all trial expenses, including payment to physicians, cost of drugs and laboratory tests, data handling, and so on.

biological mechanisms, scientific literature, hunches, and more. Since this is a book about statistics, I will leave it for them to explain how they do what they do. I will, however, enumerate the particular pieces of information you and the statistician will require from them:

1. An estimated range of effect size differences between 6-month and 12-month trials: For example, after due consideration your scientists might tell you that "a 12-month trial is likely to show an increase of 10% to 25% in effect size relative to a 6-month trial."
2. Some indication of certainty attached to the range given: The scientists might, for example, say that "we are fairly certain a 12-month trial will achieve about a 15% increase relative to a 6-month trial. A larger increase is possible but unlikely."

At this stage of the game this is about the best that you can hope for. And it is not bad at all. Having obtained this information, you go back to the statistician with it.

Initially, the statistician may have conducted a power analysis based on specific numbers. For example, he might have told you the following:

- A trial with 150 subjects and 10% CTC-11 superiority over Control has a 75% chance for success.
- A trial with 70 subjects and 20% CTC-11 superiority over Control has a 68% chance for success.

Now that you have a range of effects, you can do better. More specifically, the statistician can now compute your trial's chance for success under different assumptions of effects and sample sizes.

There is no decision yet, but there will be one soon. And you now have at your disposal a great deal of useful information—information that will maximize your likelihood for making the correct decision.

Recruitment

AP is a relatively rare disease with a known **prevalence** of about 45,000 in the United States and 60,000 in Europe. Diagnosis is problematic, and there are many documented cases of mistaken diagnosis. Thus, the true numbers are likely higher—according to some estimates, by as much as a third. These are certainly important data for marketing, but you are not there yet. In fact, you are not even close. Currently you are concerned with patients with a definite diagnosis of ALP, since it is from these patients you will recruit for your upcoming study.

Whether you plan for a 6-month or 12-month trial, the quicker you finish the study, the quicker you will move forward with CTC-11. Firmly believing you have a winner, you are keen to get beyond this early phase and into those that take you closer to market. Truth be told, you are a bit *too* keen, since it will take years regardless. Still, you prefer it be fewer years than more, and the rate at which you recruit patients will have a great deal to do with how many.

Statistical Input

Recruitment in clinical trials is a wide-ranging topic that touches upon many aspects of the study: There are the types of patients to be recruited, the physicians and hospitals involved, costs, logistics, **monitoring**, and so on. In this section I will, to the degree possible, limit my discussion to the statistician's potential involvement in this issue.

CTC-11 is intended for individuals suffering from ALP, which, like every group of people, is heterogeneous. There are male and female, young and old, otherwise healthy and not, and the list goes on. As in all clinical trials, you will need to specify precisely the characteristics of patients who are eligible for your study. This is done via **inclusion criteria** and **exclusion criteria** that are delineated in the clinical trial **protocol**. You may, for example, wish to include only subjects between the ages of 18 and 70 and exclude those who have another serious illness.

Most inclusion and exclusion criteria are determined by clinical rationale, but there may be other considerations as well. Regardless of how these criteria are determined, they will affect your recruitment rate. At the most basic level, setting liberal criteria for entry into the trial will make for quicker recruitment than setting more restrictive criteria.

It would appear that a statistician has little to contribute to the discussion of inclusion/exclusion criteria, and this is generally true—but not entirely true. The statistician's first contribution might be to state the obvious, which is the following: "Make sure that the patients you recruit for the trial are similar to those who will be treated with CTC-11 if and when the drug reaches the market." In statistical parlance, this means making sure that those participating in your trial will constitute a **representative sample** of the **population** for whom you intend the drug: the **intended use population**.

Now this suggestion seems sufficiently self-evident that you would know it without the statistician's help. At the same time it is always nice to have someone around who makes sure you do not forget the obvious. While samples and populations may not be uppermost in your thoughts, they are the statistician's bread and butter. But there is another reason to involve the statistician here, and it relates to the fact that even self-evident principles are not universally applicable.

Recall that the planned clinical trial is the first in individuals who have the disease. Your goal then is to demonstrate that the drug is potentially useful—that it is feasible—and that further development is worthwhile. This is not necessarily the same as demonstrating efficacy of CTC-11 in a "representative sample" of those for whom you intend the drug. Your most urgent goal is showing "some sort of efficacy."

Now it stands to reason that given the specific characteristics of a planned trial, such as its length and endpoints, some types of ALP sufferers might be more likely to benefit from CTC-11 than others. To take but one example, Disease Progression in ALP is generally slow at first and accelerates with time. Thus, a newly diagnosed case may show little deterioration within the first year whether on an effective or ineffective drug. Consequently, you may wish to exclude early-stage cases from a feasibility trial; only in later phases of drug development, when both your samples are larger and time periods longer, will you include such patients. In short, the current trial should be planned to maximize your chances for positive results, even at the expense of other parameters (such as having a representative sample).

Once again we are in "tradeoff territory" in that excluding early-stage ALP patients will not only yield a nonrepresentative sample, but it will also slow recruitment. And aside from being inconvenient, slower recruitment will make for a longer, more expensive trial and may require cuts elsewhere—for example, in sample size. Does this sound familiar? It should. Once more you are faced with cost-benefit analysis and, as before, you will need to weigh various options and their effects on the likelihood of your trial's success. For this you will do well to involve the statistician, who can provide you with probabilities for success under different trial configurations.

SOME CONCLUDING THOUGHTS

I have presented an example of early drug development that in many ways is typical of such efforts. There are questions relating to trial length and size, patient type and recruitment, and many others not mentioned. As can be expected, statistics has roles of varying importance in each of these. For example, the statistician has relatively little to contribute when outcomes have already been obtained and analyzed. Yet, even here his role varies, depending on need. On the other hand, his contribution to determining a trial's sample size is central. And when discussing a study's length and population, his role is not as central but can be important nonetheless.

You may have also noticed that much of the information sought from the statistician in the trial planning stage has to do with determination of the study's sample size. Hence, it would seem that, at least at this stage of the proceedings, statistics has a one-track mind. Well, yes and no.

There is little question that determination of sample size is one of the statistician's major roles in study planning. It is a role he plays often and should know how to play well. But he also has additional responsibilities early on, such as assisting in trial design: determining number of arms, selecting endpoints, advising on length, and assisting on procedures for **randomization and blinding**. These and others will be discussed as we go along. Moreover there will be additional areas requiring statistics that are not directly related to human testing and so will be noted in passing only (like now). These, for example, might include the following:

- Assisting analytical chemists to ensure quality of both **drug substance** and **drug product**.
- Developing sampling plans for chemicals produced in-house and those bought from suppliers.
- Estimating a drug's overall shelf life under different storage conditions varying by temperature and humidity.

At the same time, I do have to admit that the statistician's bag of tricks, like that of virtually every profession, is limited. Indeed, once you have learned a few of the tricks in it, you might justifiably claim to *know* statistics. Still, the distance between *knowing* and *doing* is great. Correct application of statistical methodology to the wide variety of situations that arise in clinical trials may be as much an art as a science. And I hope to have offended neither artist nor scientist here.

CHAPTER 2

Questions For Planning Trials

CONTENTS

- Trial design: multidisciplinary considerations
- Developing a diagnostic kit
- Intended use and trial design
- Essential questions for planning a study

INTRODUCTION

In Chapter 1, I described a situation in which management asks you to justify a molecule's further development. You then prepare a presentation on the scientific merits of the product. Having heard the presentation, management decides to allocate resources for a first trial in humans with the disease. It is only then that you begin to fret about the upcoming study's design. Or is it?

MORAL OF THE SAME

I said before that "everything is connected to everything else"—that most every issue in clinical trials cannot be considered in isolation from others. Well, I will now belabor the point. It is *that* important. One can only hope that having made it twice, I shall henceforth desist (doubtful).

To the point belabored: Scientific justification for a medical product is crucial. Yet, this sort of evidence by itself cannot and should not determine whether to develop a product. To take an obvious example, a company's resources must be considered as well. If the money is not there, the trial will go begging irrespective of the scientific merit for it. Moreover,

potential costs and benefits must be weighed in the context of an organization's overall **pipeline**—the other products it is currently developing and *their* needs and potential returns.

Management has now heard that CTC-11 is a scientifically promising molecule and thinks favorably of it. But it also knows that Allerton's Palsy is relatively rare, so the molecule's potential market is small. What should a company do when choosing between a product with, say, more scientific promise than another but with less market potential? In addition, market potential itself is difficult to estimate in that it depends on numerous factors in addition to disease

Continued

MORAL OF THE SAME—CONT'D

prevalence. For example, knowledge of existing and potential treatments and their costs is crucial. Also important is the **natural history** of the disease. For example, chronic illnesses typically require much more treatment over a patient's lifetime than acute ones. Also important is patent status of current treatments, informing on how soon cheaper generic treatments may be available.

Then there are politics to be considered. When one project gets more resources, others will get fewer. This is likely to make some people unhappy. And unhappy people can be problematic for an organization, particularly if they are important people.

Focusing on the scientific aspects of CTC-11 implies management's decision would be independent of the drug's overall **development plan**. Well, it cannot be. In deciding whether to go ahead with an early-stage trial, management must also consider the steps required beyond this initial trial. And while development plans are imperfect tools, surprises being the rule in the development process, companies must start their planning somewhere. So, in fact, you were probably designing (theoretical) future trials long before you heard management's decision on the first. No clinical trial can be considered in isolation.

I thus suggest that when reading this book you also be aware of what is *not* mentioned. Indeed, I propose that you exercise your clinical trial mind by raising issues beyond those discussed and seeking solutions for them. It is a worthwhile exercise. In routine product development you will be asked to provide many answers and to juggle multiple factors throughout. So if you have ever dreamed of joining the circus, welcome.

I began Chapter 1 with a scientific presentation to management because one needs to start somewhere. I could have just as easily chosen another point in the development process. But while "the beginning" is to some degree an arbitrary concept, there *are* better places to start than others. And the question of sample size—that most associated with my own profession—is typically *not* one of these.

Over the years I have been asked for sample size estimates very early on in the trial planning process. More often than not I find that these requests had come much earlier than relevant. While I cannot be sure why this is, I have my suspicions. First, estimating the number of subjects needed for a trial goes a long way in estimating overall length and cost. Thus, it is certainly reasonable for anyone thinking about a study to want to know something about the efforts required early on. Additionally, there may be some expectation that the statistician and his mathematically driven profession will provide some definite answer at a stage where so few are to be had. Or perhaps it is simply a matter of involving another individual from beyond the pale when no handy answers are available in one's immediate professional circle.

Be that as it may, R&D in the industry typically raise the issue of sample size long before there can be a meaningful answer for it. You see, I can only compute the number of subjects needed after knowing something about the product, the trial's design, endpoints, and expected effects. And obtaining all of these usually requires a great deal of preliminary study and discussion.

Still, being asked the question early on gives me the opportunity to stick my nose into nonstatistical issues as well. I like this. More importantly, if you involve the statistician in issues apparently unrelated to the discipline, you will soon find some related nonetheless. Examples abound, and a few will find their way into this book.

This chapter is about asking questions. Specifically, it is about how questions beget answers that lead to more questions and answers that ultimately yield enough information for designing an intelligent study. I articulate some of these questions and answers in the context of a hypothetical development process. Some of the issues I raise will be specific to the project at hand and, in this sense, of limited use. But this is the way it is; general principles are essential but cannot cover all those aspects you will need to deal with when designing a specific trial. There is no substitute for experience, and being exposed to a variety of examples will make the next one that much easier to deal with. At the same time, by the end of this chapter I will get to those questions that you *must* ask before all others.

WHERE DO I BEGIN?

One of the first questions you typically ask is *"What can my product actually do?"* Now you cannot expect to answer this definitively until you have completed development, gone to market, and received some feedback from it. And even then you may be a bit confused, since medical products usually perform differently in the real world than they do in the more controlled environment of clinical trials. Indeed, a truly accurate answer to this question may only be had after the product has been on the market for some time and used by large numbers of patients. But this should not be an excuse to avoid estimating your product's performance at an early stage. After all, if you do not expect *something*, you would not consider developing it in the first place. In the hypothetical example that follows I explore where this question leads you in the context of planning a study for a diagnostic kit.

KINITIS

Company scientists believe they have discovered a marker for Kinitis, a disorder of the kidney of which the symptoms are typically mild to nonexistent. Prevalence of Kinitis in Western countries is about 1 in 8,000, with men and women about equally likely to suffer from it. Most with the disorder do not know they have it and, given the mild symptoms, are likely never to know. However, some Kinitis cases deteriorate to the point of loss of kidney function and, in rare instances, complete failure. This alone is reason enough for wanting to detect the disorder early on.

Kidney Specific Antigen (KSA) is present at low levels in the blood of most healthy individuals. Yet, researchers also noticed that it tends to be much higher in those with Kinitis. Acting on this information, your Company has developed and patented a diagnostic kit for measuring KSA in serum.

A formal, controlled study has yet to be done. But based on anecdotal evidence, the biology of the kidney, and the hypothesized mechanism of the disease, scientists believe they can detect Kinitis. Moreover, they believe they may also be able to use their test to assess risk for the disorder in those who do not have it. Specifically, they believe that those with high levels of KSA are likely to have Kinitis, and those with low levels do not. And they suspect that those in between do not have the disease but are at greater risk for it. But for now this is mere conjecture. You have yet to sufficiently characterize the KSA-Kinitis relationship, let alone defined "high," "medium," and "low" values on the marker.

Current diagnosis of the disease is difficult and initially involves ruling out disorders that are more easily detected. Definitive diagnosis of Kinitis requires a relatively risky invasive test. Imaging techniques are currently being developed for diagnosing the disease, but at the time of writing this book they are relatively inaccurate and prohibitively expensive. Hence, a simple blood test for the presence of Kinitis would certainly be welcome

On top of all this, no reliable method for assessing *risk* for the disease exists. Instead, there are some general guidelines relating to age and family history: Older people and those with first-degree relatives who contracted particularly severe variants of the disorder are considered at higher risk than the general population. These individuals are told to undergo more frequent testing for (the imperfect) indicators of Kinitis. If the results are positive, the invasive test may be appropriate, depending on the risks and benefits for specific patients. Clearly a marker that could assess *risk* for the condition would be very helpful and would rationalize testing—in other words, it would enable the efficient determination of who should be tested and how often. Thus, the ability to identify individuals at risk has the potential for both saving lives and invasive procedures.

In sum, you have a blood test with the potential for evaluating the presence and/or risk of Kinitis and wish to conduct a clinical trial for it. This is a good start, and you naturally begin with the question "What can my product do?" This is a fine question. Still, you must get more specific and, in this context, parse the requirement for information into the following two questions:

- "How accurate is my product at diagnosing Kinitis?"
- "How accurate is my product at assessing risk for the disease?"

Having asked these questions and in possession of anecdotal data only, you are now pretty well stuck. Other than some very rough estimates from pathology and the few blood tests actually done, you have little to go on. This is fine. You have articulated your questions and have some idea where you are headed.

At about this stage I usually get my first phone call. "We're developing a diagnostic kit," I'm told. "Could you sign a nondisclosure agreement (NDA) so we can get more specific?" I agree, of course (after all, this is what I do for a living), and the conversation picks up again after I have signed the NDA.

"You see," my new client says, "we have an assay for diagnosing Kinitis and need to evaluate its accuracy. We'd like to know how many subjects we need for a study." At this stage my answer is usually one variant or another of "Hold on." I then go on to explain that several critical issues must be addressed *before* considering the mechanics of the trial itself.

The preceding two questions have led you to a fork in the road. Yet, before choosing one branch or the other, you should be asking some other questions. One of these is *"Is my diagnostic kit in anything resembling its final form?"* For example, it may very well be that you have developed an early version of the kit of which the results are unstable—results that come up worryingly different even when testing the same blood. This could happen for any number of reasons, including differences between kit batches, insufficiently precise production, differences in testing between laboratories, and so on. Whatever the reason, a kit that cannot provide **repeatable** results cannot yield accurate results even if the marker it measures is highly associated with the disorder of interest. When this is the case you should first be perfecting the diagnostic kit and assessing its stability. In other words, you should be planning a trial assessing **repeatability** and **reproducibility** (R&R) rather than a clinical trial evaluating the kit's diagnostic accuracy.

We are now in a chicken-and-egg-Catch-22 (CEC22) type stage. If KSA is not an effective marker for Kinitis, you do not want to waste your time and money perfecting the diagnostic kit for it. And if your kit is unstable, you will not be able to know if KSA is effective. Thus, you find yourself in the position of having to invest time and money to perfect a kit so that you can assess whether it should have been perfected in the first place. This leads to the question *"How much should I invest in R&R at this stage?"*

In this context, an R&R study evaluates the degree to which your test provides similar results when assessing the same blood under different conditions—for example, by using kits produced in different batches and/or applied in different laboratories and/or used by different technicians and/or testing bloods from different types of patients. You then analyze your results with an eye to understanding the reason for any instability that arises and take corrective action.

Now, R&R studies are typically much less expensive than clinical trials. Still, they can be costly because they involve producing kits and obtaining blood samples that may be relatively rare. As in all research, you can go for a small study, a large one, or any point between. Well, what should you do?

There is no simple answer. Clearly, it would be nice to have a perfected kit before testing it more extensively. But if perfecting requires exorbitant resources, perhaps something less than perfect can do well enough. And what, you ask, is "well enough"? It seems then that we are as far as ever from "How many subjects do I need for my clinical trial?" Yet, we *are* on our way.

Getting back to the moral of this particular story, you should avoid going into a clinical trial with a product that is expected to undergo meaningful changes. If you do, the estimates you obtain for it will be inaccurate and may lead to erroneous decisions regarding further development.

There are, of course, those times when you have no choice. For example, if you do not show some immediate success, you will lose funding altogether and the project will grind to a halt. Life is like that. And when this happens you can only do your best, which is weigh the risks and rewards and make your investors and researchers aware of them.

For the sake of moving forward, let us assume that your kit is beyond early development—that for now your assay is about as good as it can be. There may be changes in the future, but what you have in hand is sufficient for an early clinical study of efficacy.

So you are once again planning a clinical study, which brings you back to the fork in the road mentioned. And this means asking at least a few more questions, one of which is the seemingly naive *"What is my trial's goal?"* In this context there are at least two options:

1. Testing the presence of Kinitis.
2. Testing the risk for Kinitis.

Choosing the first option—assessing your test's ability to indicate the presence or absence of the disorder only—is certainly the simpler of the two. You might, for example, choose subjects who have already undergone the invasive test and have a definite diagnosis of positive or negative. You then test your assay on these individuals and assess your product's accuracy in discriminating between those who have the disease and those who do not. This is a reasonable, early-stage approach. Yet, as is often the case, things are not as simple as they seem, and you will need to answer another basic question: *"Who is my product intended for?"*

If your product is meant for screening a wider population, the proposed trial is lacking, since it only examines your kit's performance in those who have already undergone the invasive test. This is likely to be a relatively narrow segment of the population—a segment of which the members are at greater risk for Kinitis than your intended use population. This, in turn, will lead to your obtaining **biased estimates** of your kit's accuracy in the intended use population.

So it turns out the trial that is simplest logistically will not provide you with a good estimate of the kit's accuracy in the general population. Dealing with this is a complex issue and beyond the scope of this book. My point, however, is not, and it is this: To the degree possible, your clinical trial should reflect your product's performance in the intended use population. For reasons of cost and convenience you might loosen this requirement at an early stage, and this is fine. But all the while you must be aware of what you are gaining and what you are losing by doing this.

Since at present you wish to show *some* feasibility, it is sufficient to demonstrate reasonable accuracy in an **enriched population**—in a group whose prevalence of the disease is much higher than in the intended use population. If the results are less than satisfactory in this narrow group, your product is probably useless in any case. Thus, this type of trial can lead to a products' complete rejection or qualified acceptance. And you have decided that the possibility of "qualified acceptance" is acceptable given the trial's relatively small expense.

Your second option is conducting a trial to test for both diagnosis *and* risk. This is a much more problematic option that leads to a number of additional questions:

- *"Who is my product intended for?"* This is the same question as the previous one but with different implications. Here you are asking whether you wish to (a) test those already identified at risk and confirming or disconfirming or (b) also test those not currently identified at risk. The first group is much smaller and, as before, makes the trial's logistics simpler and less costly. On the other hand, the second option is nearer to your intended use for the product and will better indicate its market potential in general.
- *"How do I evaluate the accuracy of my kit for assessing risk?"* Other than a few general, and only marginally accurate, guidelines, there is no **gold-standard**, or acceptable standard, for measuring risk. So now you have at least two options:
  a. Use today's guidelines as standard regardless and compare yourself to them. In this instance you would include in your study individuals identified as at risk and those who are not and assess whether your test can discriminate between them. However, if your results are weak, you will not know whether this is due to your kit's inaccuracy or to the fact that today's guidelines imperfectly identified those at risk.
  b. A much more informative trial would involve a long enough follow-up to evaluate whether those you identified as at risk actually develop the disorder. Planning this sort of trial would lead to the question *"How long must my follow-up period be to enable assessing whether a person does or does not develop the disease?"* Unless the answer to this option is "a short period of time," this is not a realistic, early-stage option.

Keep in mind that your first order of business is demonstrating that your kit has *some* potential to be useful. And this is most easily done with subjects who have already been diagnosed. Once you have demonstrated some sort of accuracy, you can move on to more complicated trials intended to answer more difficult questions. There may be other options as well, and I suggest you come up with one or two of them yourself.

THE ESSENTIALS

In this chapter I could have brought up many more examples and articulated many more questions. Indeed, I shall do this as we proceed; it is part and parcel of the process. For the moment I wish only to address the issue of Q&A in general and hope to make the point sufficiently to move on. For me, "moving on" actually means going *back*—back to basics. And this means articulating the questions that *must* be asked before going on to plan any clinical trial:

What do I want to show in *this* trial?

Whom do I want to show it to?

In the next chapter I will deal with the first.

CHAPTER 3

Medical Product Attributes

CONTENTS

- Basic and applied science
- Endpoints
- Measurement: statistical and clinical roles
- Common attributes tested in trials:
  - efficacy
  - safety
  - performance
  - pharmacokinetics

INTRODUCTION

In 1923 a reporter asked George Mallory why he wanted to climb Mt. Everest. The famous reply "Because it's there"—whether actually Mallory's words or the reporter's—came to epitomize this characteristic of doing things for their own sake—and, in Mallory's case, of dying for them.

At one time or another most of us do things "because they're there," although Herculean mountain climbing, like good steak, tends to be rare. Success in these sorts of endeavors gives us satisfaction, proves some point or other, and begets admiration. As for practical use, that is not really the point.

Those doing basic science will tell you they seek to solve problems for their own sake. Much of their work goes unnoticed except perhaps by a handful of experts in some subspecialty or other. Yet, every so often their ideas *do* reach industry where necessity is the most common ancestor of invention. And because need is the fundamental driver of industry, it will unashamedly ask, "What is it good for?"

Now as far as questions go, this is a pretty good one. The answer will mark your target and, in our own particular language, define your product's intended use. It is certainly useful to mark your target if you hope to get there. It is also worthwhile repeating the "What is it good for?" question throughout the development process and even after. This is because targets can change, and, like children in math class, multiply. Aspirin, for example, was developed to treat pain and fever and is now also used for preventing heart attacks. Similarly, a drug for the treatment of colorectal cancer has been shown to be effective in treating a degenerative eye disease. And then there are drugs like Viagra.

So the question "What is it good for?" is basic, and it may be the most basic of all. At the same time it is often too general to be of practical use when planning a specific clinical trial. For example, suppose you have developed a device that is implanted in the body for monitoring blood flow from the heart to the lungs. This is important information for physicians treating patients with congestive heart failure (CHF). Specifically, this particular device is "good for" long-term monitoring of CHF patients. An appropriate test of it would see large numbers of patients implanted with the device for long periods of time and parameters like hospitalization rates and life expectancy measured. Yet, before exposing many patients to new technology over long periods, you had better conduct a more limited clinical trial. In this trial you would demonstrate in a small group that the device can be implanted safely and can function after implantation. Only after making your point in a relatively small study will you go on to conduct the larger trial meant to test the device's intended use directly.[1] Now this sort of early trial will provide a great deal of information on the product's functioning and very little about its clinical benefit. But it is necessary before embarking on a study designed to test "what it is good for."

Another example is the **dose-response** studies in pharmaceuticals where each group receives a different dose of the same drug (and a dose = 0 condition is usually included as well).[2] In this sort of study you aim to identify a drug's optimal dose rather than addressing the general "What is it good for?". Once the dose has been established, you can go on to test the product's intended use.

---

[1] Your initial study will likely have a short follow-up (say, two or three months), after which, if you succeed, you will go on to the larger trial with the longer follow-up (say, a year to two). At the same time, you will continue to monitor those patients from the first trial. You do not, however, want the initial trial to extend over a year or two, since this will greatly delay time-to-market. Just how long the initial "short and limited" trial ought to be is something to be discussed and decided upon with clinicians and regulators.

[2] There can, of course, be dose-response relationships of interest in devices as well. For example, when using a cardiac catheter for ablating (burning) by electrical current, there will be a relationship between the current's strength and the degree of ablation. You may then wish to conduct a study to determine the optimal "electrical dose" for a given application.

Thus, long before your reach the **pivotal trial** stage—*the* study or studies determining whether your product should be offered to the general public— you will need to address numerous preliminary issues.

Product development, by definition, takes place over time. In our particular industry much of the process is formalized with many conventions, including specific names for processes and stages. Thus, there are preclinical studies where your product is assessed in the laboratory and clinical trial Phases I, II, and III where your product is tested on humans. There are many variations on this broad scheme, and few development programs are staged exactly alike. Regardless, the "What is it good for?" question will only be answered definitively at the very end. Thus, when planning a specific study, you would do well to come up with *explicit questions tailored for the specific trial at the particular stage*. And the question most appropriate to begin with is "What do I want to show in *this* trial?"

Now this particular question has some very definite implications in the context of a given study. At the same time, you would do even better to subdivide it into the following two issues:

1. "What *attribute* of my product do I want to assess?"
2. "What *about* this attribute do I want to show?" That is, what do I aim to demonstrate with this attribute that I have chosen to assess?

In this chapter I cover the most common attributes tested in clinical trials. In the next I will enumerate goals you might set for these attributes—that is, what you would like to demonstrate about them. Finally, I will put the two together to create a sort of "matrix guide" to defining clinical trial objectives for clinical trials in general.

ATTRIBUTES

Efficacy

For a product to be "effective" it must do what it is meant to do. Simple. A blood test assessing a woman's risk for having a baby with Down syndrome should be accurate, and a pill for reducing pain should do just that.

Defining a product's efficacy is really another way of answering the question "What is it good for?". This then seems to bring us back to square one: when I said that "it is often much too general to be of practical use when planning a particular clinical trial." Well, I do not retract.

First, "often" is not "always." Second, as I showed in the preceding chapter, a product's ultimate use is not necessarily that assessed in a given stage of development. Finally, and perhaps most importantly, issues in clinical development will sometimes weave within and upon themselves, taking you back to places you have already been. Testing efficacy is only one of numerous attributes that a trial might assess. And it may or may not be a relevant question, depending on the phase of development you happen to be in at the moment.

A WORD ON ENDPOINTS

When setting up an efficacy trial, you need to define precisely what your product is expected to do and test it. Testing involves evaluation, which in turn requires *measuring* the product's effect. You will, for example, measure an anti-inflammatory medication's effect on inflammation and a drug-eluting stent's ability to remain clear of plaque. These effects will then be compared to some Reference, such as another treatment in the trial or perhaps historical data. So at some (early) point, you must ask, "What should I be measuring in this study to demonstrate efficacy?"

Measurement is a central topic in clinical trials and arises throughout. But it is most formally addressed when discussing a trial's *endpoints*—the particular parameters used for assessing product attributes such as efficacy. And there are of course endpoints measuring other attributes such as safety or pharmacokinetics.

On the face of it, measurement is a statistical issue. After all, endpoints are most commonly evaluated with numbers, which are the statistician's forte. Yet, at the more basic level they are a clinical issue. While the statistician can advise on the method of measurement and quality of the data it yields, the clinician must determine the substance—the clinical relevance of the measurement. Thus, it is the physician, not the statistician, who specifies whether pain should be measured in a particular trial. Once determined, the statistician can assist by exploring alternatives for measuring the parameter. Pain, for example, can be measured in a number of ways, including self-report questionnaires, the physician's impression, and counting the number of pain pills taken over a period of time. In the context of a specific trial, each of these measures has its advantages and disadvantages—some clinical, others statistical. To take another example, a clinician may wish to measure disease activity in a complex illness like lupus (SLE). Having difficulty in selecting the best measure (none are really good), the doctor will ask the statistician for an opinion on the strengths and weaknesses of each. Most likely the selection process will be done in collaboration among the statistician, the physician, and others.

As a general rule, then, clinicians choose the content of what needs to be measured, and statisticians assist in determining the form. And from experience I can say that once these discussions begin, neither clinicians nor statisticians limit themselves to their supposed areas of expertise. Nor should they be.

Depending on the product of interest, the choice of endpoints can be straightforward or not. Unfortunately, in some situations there are no agreed-upon choices at all—in which case you and the statistician will have quite a challenge coming up with them. Regardless, endpoints are a central issue in clinical trials and deserve their own chapter. I suspect they will get it.

Safety

If an effective product does what it *should do*, a safe product should *not do* what it is not supposed to do. For example, a drug for relieving migraine headaches should only relieve migraine headaches. It should not cause annoying side effects like fatigue or disorientation or any other bodily reaction apart from its intended effect.

To take a more complex example, some medications for autoimmune disorders, such as multiple sclerosis and rheumatoid arthritis, are designed to suppress one or another of the immune system's responses. More particularly, they aim to restrain that activity of the system that is most damaging in the disease—the specific immune reaction causing the system's misguided assault on the patient's own organs. But suppressing immune activity has its risks, not least of which is weakening the body's ability to defend itself from real threats. Thus, in the case of immunosuppressive agents, an important element in demonstrating safety is showing that while protecting the body from one kind of disease, it does not expose it to others.

ON THE CONSUMPTION OF CAKES

Now most pharmaceuticals and interventional device products are not *completely* safe, and you will rarely get efficacy without exposing the physiological system to some risk. As in life, having your cake and eating it too is a virtual impossibility. And while we are spouting clichés, I might also mention that there is no free lunch. Given these alas-too-true life principles, demonstrating safety often involves showing that a product's benefits *outweigh* its risks. In other words, rather than showing your product to be perfectly safe, your goal when assessing an attribute or combination of attributes is showing that the product is worthwhile "all things considered." This naturally leads to a risk-benefit analysis that is a section typically included in clinical trial reports.

Risk-benefit analysis need not limit itself to considerations of the safety-efficacy tradeoff alone. The section will often deal with issues external to the product, such as alternatives to it, cost, and the severity of the illness it treats. We would expect, for example, that physicians who are treating aggressive life-threatening illnesses will be more concerned with efficacy than safety relative to those who are treating minor ailments. Thus, the tradeoffs between any product's attributes must be considered in the wider context of the disease it treats, the intended use population, and other relevant factors.

Performance

In clinical trials, the term **performance** has been used to refer to different attributes. In this book I shall limit its use to refer to "manipulation"—that is, to operating the product successfully. To function properly some medical products require manipulation beyond relatively simple actions like swallowing a pill or injecting medication into a patient's arm. This issue is often encountered in interventional devices, such as surgical apparatuses or catheters meant for insertion into blood vessels.

For example, there have been a number of surgical techniques developed for eliminating uterine fibroids—benign growths in the uterus that can cause great discomfort, heavy menstrual bleeding, and infertility. A necessary but not sufficient condition for effective treatment is performing the specific surgical technique correctly. This can be assessed during the surgery itself or soon after. Evaluation of efficacy—assessing the ultimate goal of surgery of relieving the physical and psychological difficulties caused by fibroids—could take many months and even years to do properly.

To evaluate performance in uterine fibroid removal, you might measure the time it takes to conduct the procedure, its ability to remove the fibroid completely, and whether the procedure requires a particularly adroit surgical manipulation or can be done with average surgical skills only. Additionally, you may want to assess the degree to which the procedure can be done without affecting the tissue around the fibroid.

Note that none of the parameters mentioned in the preceding paragraph involve efficacy directly in the sense of evaluating the procedure's intended effect on the patient's ailment (e.g., its ability to reduce pain or menstrual bleeding). Performance is related to efficacy in that you must succeed with the former to achieve the latter. Yet the two are distinct in that acceptable performance is a necessary but not sufficient condition for efficacy. Not only should an operation succeed, but it is also recommended that the patient live. And because performance and efficacy do not completely overlap, they are often evaluated separately—in the same or different studies.

The term *performance* is also used to describe the physical aspects of the product itself. For example, many products are required to withstand a minimal force before breakage and/or be provided in sterile packaging. For these aspects of performance the manufacturer might be asked to test both the product's strength and the integrity of its packaging. Clearly, products of which the sterility may be compromised by faulty packaging and/or are likely to break when used should not be on the market. Such physical attributes of products are critical for both safety and efficacy, but they are usually not tested in clinical trials.[3] Physical performance of products is usually evaluated in **bench testing**, which typically involves assessing products in laboratory environments. Thus, for example, the strength of a guide-wire used in catheterization might be tested by stretching it to the breaking point while measuring the force applied. The force at which the guide-wire tears is then specified as that which it can withstand. You would then compare your results to acceptable standards for such products, determining whether your guide-wire's strength complies with that required.

Another use for the term *performance* relates to subject compliance with medical treatment. For example, a pill may be effective chemically, but it is useless if subjects are unwilling to take it for one reason or another (e.g., hard to swallow, must be taken too often, etc.). Here, too, performance—compliance—is a necessary but not sufficient condition for clinical efficacy. As noted at the beginning of this section, I will limit my use of the term *performance* to the assessment of the degree to which a medical product can be manipulated successfully.

---

[3] If, for example, breakage of the tested device occurs in a clinical trial, it will certainly be recorded. But it is unexpected, and the trial is not set up for this. Typically, a clinical study will be approved only after you have shown that the physical attributes of the product are acceptable.

Pharmacokinetics

Pharmacokinetics is the study of what a body does to a drug: the rate at which it is absorbed, the time it reaches its maximum concentration in the body, the time it takes to be eliminated from the body, and so on. For example, you may want to measure quantities of the active ingredient in the blood over time for an orally ingested drug and compare these quantities to the same drug administered intravenously. Other parameters of pharmacokinetic interest may be the drug's behavior when given in different **formulations** and doses, when administered before meals or after, and so on.

Like performance, a drug's pharmacokinetics profile is related to efficacy but distinct from it. Thus, a formulation will not be effective if it cannot be absorbed by the body and distributed properly. Yet, absorption does not guarantee efficacy. The latter has as much to do with the efficacy of the drug's active ingredient as with its kinetics.

Virtually all medications require some sort of pharmacokinetic analysis as part of the development process. At the same time, pharmacokinetics is especially central when dealing with **generic drugs**—medications that are copies of **brand name drugs** (sometimes erroneously termed **ethical drugs**) that are produced once the original patent of the latter has expired.[4] In most cases, approval of generic drugs involves demonstrating that their pharmacokinetic profile is equivalent to that of the original. In other words, generic drug producers are usually not required to conduct clinical trials for demonstrating efficacy. Such trials have already been conducted for the original drug, and what remains for generic producers to show is that theirs behave similarly in the body. The regulator reasonably assumes that if a generic drug is similar chemically to the original and behaves in the body similar to the original, it will also yield similar clinical outcomes to the original. Chemical similarity is shown through the production process itself, and behavior in the body is tested by comparing the pharmacokinetics of the generic and original drugs.

There are, however, exceptions. For example, topical drugs—those used on the skin or other external parts of the body—often do not enter the bloodstream, or they enter in quantities too minute to evaluate. As such, they are not assessed on pharmacokinetics (or assessed to ensure they do not enter the blood in detectable quantities). Here, a generic drug maker may have no choice but to conduct a clinical trial to demonstrate that the new drug's efficacy and safety are equivalent to the old.

---

[4] Ethical drugs refer in general to those that can only be given by prescription. In clinical trials the term commonly refers to a branded drug under patent protection.

SUMMARIZING AND SOME THOUGHTS

Before going ahead and planning your clinical trial you must be clear on the choice of attribute your study should evaluate. There are several to choose from. The most common are efficacy, safety, performance, and pharmacokinetics. These cover the majority of attributes you will encounter when assessing clinical products. Yet, there are others, and we shall make a note of them from time to time.

At the end of the day you will want to know what your product is good for, which is really another way of asking if it is effective. Thus, of the attributes enumerated, efficacy is typically most directly related to your ultimate goal. For example, patients suffering from rheumatoid arthritis (RA) will buy your product if it reduces pain and swelling and enables greater freedom of movement. At the same time, they will certainly expect your drug to be safe, so demonstrating adequate safety is critical to any medical product.

It would seem then that of all the attributes enumerated, efficacy is most directly related to the more general "What is it good for?". This is in fact the case. Yet, determining the attributes to be evaluated must be examined on a study-by-study basis. This is especially true in early development, where there is a great deal to be understood about a product in addition to its efficacy. For example, in some cases you might wish to launch your product as quickly as possible, even if this means marketing less than your final version for it. This in turn would imply a more limited trial—one that evaluates less than the ultimate "efficacy package." You might, for instance, have a diagnostic kit meant to measure breathing rate, heart rate, sleep apnea, and sleep stages. Now it is relatively easy to recruit subjects for testing, say, heart and breathing rates—all subjects have them. But recruiting subjects with sleep apnea will be more difficult and is likely to lengthen your trial and delay regulatory submission. As a result you might choose to conduct a clinical trial assessing your kit's ability to measure breathing and heart rates and leave the "apnea submission" for later. In this particular case you will have tested only a subset of "what the product is good for." Another reason for testing only a subset of a product's (planned, final) efficacy may be that your R&D people are ready to sign off on one of the product's attributes but feel the need for more time to perfect others.

So while the question "What do I want to show in *this* trial?" is typically related to "What is my product good for?," it often also differs from it in any particular study. And this difference—be it small or large—will have some very definite implications for what you expect your study to achieve. This in turn will influence many aspects of your trial, including its design.

It is therefore vital to emphasize that when planning trials you should *not*, at least initially, consider any one attribute more important than another. First, the regulator often views your attributes' importance differently than you do.

Second, the attributes enumerated are related to one another, so it may be artificial to rank their importance. For example, a surgical device with inferior performance characteristics is likely to be ineffective and unsafe as well. Similarly, few people will be willing to take a medication that frequently produces unpleasant side effects, even if it is approved. It will thus be ineffective in practice even if its active ingredient is, in principle, very effective.

To the statistician, safety and performance and pharmacokinetics sometimes *feel* like adjuncts to efficacy. Physicians, on the other hand, will typically raise the safety issue before all others. Since both safety and efficacy are important, as are pharmacokinetics and performance, personal preference in prioritization is somewhat beside the point. All must be tested before a product is to enter the market.

A FINE LINE CRISSCROSSED

Science has gotten us far. We now, for example, treat diseases like diabetes that once meant certain death. Additionally, we have developed fantastically complex and informative diagnostic techniques like computer tomography (CT) and magnetic resonance imaging (MRI). In developed countries life expectancy has increased dramatically in the last 100 years, and a large part of the credit resides with medicine. Moreover, at any given time scientists, clinicians, and entrepreneurs are continually working to provide us with newer and better products. We expect no less. And we want these products to be safe and effective, which they generally are. But not so fast—or, perhaps, even faster.

Let me explain: If you want to know the long-term effects of a drug, you will, alas, have to study it in the long term. Thus, you cannot *really* know whether an innovative drug is safe when taken over 10 years until you have tested it for this long. But if you wait 10 years before bringing it to market, you will have kept it from some very eager patients (not to mention the possibility of having gone bankrupt in the meantime). Similarly, when developing a vaccine you cannot really know how well it works without giving it to thousands of people and following up on them for months and even years. Yet, there are times when a vaccine is required on short notice, such as, for example, when a new strain of flu threatens to create an epidemic. So instead of testing the long-term effect of the product, you might test whether the vaccine produces the antibodies for the disease in question. Thus, many vaccines introduced to market have not had their intended use tested directly, nor will they have had their long-term safety assessed.

What are we to do? As a society we want innovation quickly, and we (and our lawyers) want these innovations to have positive effects only. Well, you cannot have both. And in the short history of biomedical development and regulatory approval there are numerous examples of drugs and devices approved that were later found harmful. This is a sad state of affairs. But there is really no way around it; while we might be able to improve the system of innovation and regulatory approval, the tradeoff between speed and safety has, in principle, no solution. The best you can do is design a process optimizing the two—creating a system of checks and balances that will yield innovation with "reasonable" speed while providing safety with "reasonable" assurance. You will then continually monitor the process and tweak it as necessary. And this tweaking will often come after discovering that a product reached market when it should not have.

Unfortunately, I have nothing original to propose here. I merely wish to point out that as long as people demand "new products *now*" and get them, they will also, from time to time, end up with products that are not as safe as they would like. So the next time you hear about an approved product turned sour, do not be quick to judge the regulator harshly. We—consumers, physicians, legislators—have placed agencies such as FDA and EMEA in a bind from which they cannot extract themselves to everyone's satisfaction. The line between speed and safety is a fine one, and "to approve or not to approve" is precisely the question. All decisions on approval come with their risks and rewards, costs and benefits. And, on occasion, the regulator will find itself on the wrong side of the line.

In sum, to get your product approved by regulatory authorities, prescribed by physicians, and purchased by customers, you will need to show that it possesses a reasonable combination of the attributes relevant for it. And to assess these attributes you will usually be required to conduct one or more clinical trials. To plan any trial correctly, you must know in advance what your product is good for in general and what you aim to show in the particular study. And while these issues overlap, they are not necessarily the same. This is sufficiently self-evident that it had better be put in writing.

CHAPTER 4

Setting Research Objectives

CONTENTS

- Judgement by trial: evidentiary requirements
- Development in antibiotics: an example
- Trial objectives:
  - superiority
  - non-inferiority
  - equivalence
- Single- and multiple-arm trials
- Superiority in oncology: some design challenges
- Equivalence in stroke drug pharmacokinetics
- Non-inferiority in a device for diabetes
- A "recipe" for designing clinical trials

INTRODUCTION

A clinical trial is, well, a trial. You conduct one by collecting evidence that you analyze and present before a judge and a jury that may consist of colleagues, managers, journal reviewers, investors, regulators, Aunt Augusta, and others. The verdict may be favorable or not, or, as sometimes happens in the industry, it may fall into the gray area between. And if the latter happens with some favorably leaning evidence as well, you will likely conduct a retrial.

Clinical studies are generally rigid affairs carried out according to guidelines, points to consider, and recommendations provided by organizations such as the **FDA, EMEA**, and **ICH**. A multitude of evidentiary rules and endless acronyms are used for both expediency and evidence of guild membership; cite the right ones and you will not only say a great deal with a few words, but you will also be identified as a bird of a feather. If you have not done so already, you may one day soon discuss IRB approvals for GCP studies handled by CROs collecting data with EDC in CDISC-ready format. And when you find yourself actually enjoying this kind of talk, you might make some friends in the process. And you likely lose others.

When rules are followed—when patients have been read their rights, the study is well designed, and its data analyzed correctly—you will likely have what you need for an informed decision. But study outcomes are not always as clear cut, and even meticulously planned trials, not to mention sloppy ones, may produce equivocal results. A hung jury is always a possibility.

I have been carried away with this courtroom analogy and will soon desist. But I will do so only after pointing out that like rulings in general, results of clinical trials are evaluated by *comparing*. In the courtroom you compare the data presented to a Reference called "reasonable doubt." If you are beyond it, you convict. In a clinical trial you compare your Treatment to a Reference like Placebo and conclude success or failure. Using statistics you will also associate a level of certainty with your conclusion; you might, for instance, be 90% sure the two groups differ or 95% or any other level of certainty but 100%. Absolute proof is for mathematics and vodka only.

In many clinical trials the comparator will be "built in," as when a trial includes two groups of subjects: the one being evaluated and a comparator. Alternatively, you might test the product by itself and compare the outcome to some predetermined level of performance. But whether the comparison of attributes is direct or indirect, internal or external, there will need to be one. Attributes, like Aunt Augusta, are relative.

Actual comparison of attributes can only take place after data have been collected. But the comparison's details must be prespecified. This is what I meant when I said that before a study begins, you must clearly state what you want to show—what the trial's main attributes are and what you aim to demonstrate with them. Translating this into practical terms, I provide the following examples of questions you might ask when planning your study.

- Does my drug reduce inflammation for longer periods than the standard of care?
- Is the accuracy of my assay for Kinitis above the minimum set by the regulator?
- Is the safety profile of my orally administered drug for portal hypertension at least as effective as that provided intravenously?
- Is my device easier to handle than the two already on the market?

Each of these questions implies both an attribute and a comparison. So when you undertake a trial, you must deal with each of the following at the outset:

- The *attribute* you wish to evaluate.
- The *objective* for the attribute—what you wish to show with it.

Together, these two elements provide the reason for your trial and must be determined before all else. Addressing them is about as good a place to begin as any.

Suppose you have developed an antibiotic and aim to compare its efficacy to that most commonly prescribed in the indication. You might, for example, want to show that the new drug reduces bacteria counts at least as well as the competitor. The implied comparison for this particular attribute—efficacy as measured by Bacteria Count—is that your drug is "at least as good as" the competitor. Formally this leads to the objective termed **non-inferiority**, which involves showing your drug is no worse than the comparator. Now showing that you are "not inferior" when you want to demonstrate "at least as good as" would seem a bit convoluted. And it is. But there is a good reason for it, which will be explained.

Moving on, you are also convinced that your product has some advantage over the competitor in that it is prescribed for three days as opposed to the other drug's seven days. As such, you believe yours to be more convenient, implying an analytic comparison between the two products meant to show **superiority**—that is, the new drug is more convenient than the other.

To this point you have made two comparative statements: "I am at least as good as" on one attribute (efficacy) and "I am better" on another (convenience). Having further considered your second statement, you feel that you can do even better. Specifically, you reason that a more convenient regimen will yield greater **compliance**—higher rates of patients taking the medication as prescribed. And better compliance will likely yield greater cure rates.

To summarize, you now have at least three possible attributes and objectives for the planned trial:

- *Non-inferiority on efficacy*: The new antibiotic is at least as good as the old in terms of eliminating bacteria.
- *Superiority on convenience*: The new antibiotic is, relative to the old, easier on the patient.
- *Superiority on efficacy*: The new product yields a better cure than the competitor.

Faced with three alternatives, you are now charged with setting up a trial to test one or more of them. And the choice is not obvious. The trials imply different designs, sample sizes, timelines, costs, and so forth. As always, you can do no better than conduct cost-benefit analysis based on relevant information.

It is generally easier to demonstrate non-inferiority than superiority, the former being a more modest **claim**. Thus, the chances for proving non-inferiority are higher, which translates into smaller required sample sizes than superiority for the same chance for success. Alternatively, given the same sample size, you have a higher likelihood for success with non-inferiority. In short, this particular objective has much going for it.

Yet, it is only natural that deciding on an inexpensive and less risky trial has its downside. Specifically, if your non-inferiority trial succeeds, you will only be able to claim your product is "no worse" than the competitor. And this is certainly a weaker statement than "it is better." So what do you do? As in most cases, your final decision will be based on a number of considerations, such as science, budget, timelines, and marketing. In this instance it may actually be marketing that provides the decisive argument. When faced with about equally effective products, your marketing people argue, physicians will choose the one that is more convenient for the patient. Thus, it would be nice to claim superior efficacy but unnecessary. Having listened to and learned, you feel you can have the best of both worlds: demonstrate non-inferiority in your trial and, once approved, point out to the market that taking a drug for three days is more convenient than taking it for seven. Physicians and consumers will then go on to do their own math.

In the preceding chapter I presented some of the more common attributes tested in clinical trials: efficacy, safety, performance, and pharmacokinetics. In the following sections I shall describe in greater detail "what about" these attributes you might wish to show—my objectives for them.

OBJECTIVES (OR COMPARISONS OR "WHAT ABOUTS")

When statistically comparing a product's attribute to another, your objective will be showing one of the following:

1. "My product is better": Superiority.
2. "My product is neither better nor worse": **Equivalence**.
3. "My product is not worse": Non-inferiority.

Let us take up each in turn.

Superiority

Superiority is basic. You run a trial, collect data, and use them to compare directly between products or your product and some **performance goal**. If the statistic obtained for your product (e.g., Percent Cure, Percent Complying, Accuracy) is sufficiently different in the favorable direction from the **comparator**, you will claim that your product is superior.

Statistical comparisons to a criterion, rather than to some Control group, are typically associated with **single-arm trials**—studies in which all subjects undergo the same procedure. For example, you have a noninvasive diagnostic device designed to detect a particular type of bacterium in the stomach. To test it you select individuals who are known to be either positive or negative for the bacterium by means of biopsy—the current gold standard test. You then assess each of your subjects using the new method for presence or absence of the microbe. Finally, you compute the proportion of correct diagnoses obtained with your product in comparison to the gold standard (which, for lack for a better option, we assume is always correct). This provides you with some proportions (e.g., 88% true positives, 84% true negatives), which you then compare to a prespecified criterion such as a performance goal or an **objective performance criterion** (OPC). If, for example, the performance goal = 0.80, you will claim success if you show that you are at 0.80 or above.

Alternatively, you will conduct a **multiple-arm trial** in which one group of subjects receives the treatment of interest, while other groups receive alternative treatments and/or Placebo. This sort of trial may include any number of groups, but to keep things simple I shall address the two-group case only. In each of my examples you will compare a **Test** product T to a **Reference** R. The principles of comparing two groups hold true for multiple groups as well, and what statistical differences exist need not concern us. So having conducted a superiority trial, your statistical analysis of its data will yield one of two conclusions: "T is superior to R," or "I cannot say T is superior to R."

ON PHILOSOPHY OF SCIENCE, APPLIED RESEARCH AND THEIR INTERACTION

The second conclusion—"I cannot say T is superior to R"—is somewhat tortuous, and it would certainly be simpler to say, "T is not superior to R" or "T is inferior to R." But according to statistical theory and prevailing philosophy of science, we are formally limited to "I cannot say T is superior to R."

Yet philosophy of science is usually not high on your list when stating conclusions about T and R after a trial comparing them. It is therefore reasonable to suppose that if your results were really bad, you would conclude that "T is not superior to R." You might, in fact, not hesitate to conclude that your product is "downright inferior." And this is fine. In product development we must make decisions one way or the other

and cannot be too concerned about splitting hairs. All the same, even when disappointed there is reason to be careful with your final judgment. Using the more cautious "I cannot say T is superior to R" as opposed to the more definite "T is inferior to R" may, in some cases, actually salvage a promising product. It leaves the door open for additional investigation, and we shall discuss this further when dealing with issues relating to sample size and **error of estimation**. For the moment I merely ask you keep in mind that despite its indecisiveness, the statement "I cannot say T is better than R" is not only scientifically and philosophically correct, but it can be useful as well.

Now the concept of "superiority" is indeed as straightforward as it seems. Yet, when you apply it in practice, it may not always be. An example: Most cancers have multiple treatments—in part because even effective treatments often slow the disease rather than cure it, and additional options are needed. Moreover, even an effective treatment will often become ineffectual after multiple administrations. When this happens the treating physician will seek an alternative. Unfortunately, there is no silver bullet for most forms of cancer, so researchers are continually developing new and hopefully better treatments for it.

Having developed a treatment for a particular cancer, you now wish to demonstrate its effectiveness. Specifically, you aim to show that it is superior to the current standard—the treatment that is recommended as **first line** by the American Society of Clinical Oncology. But your product is still at the development stage and will not normally be given an opportunity for direct comparison to a proven standard. After all, why would patients and physicians accept (and **ethics committees** approve) a study in which subjects receive an experimental treatment when a proven one is available?

So in this instance ethical considerations will likely prevent testing your new drug by itself on patients for whom a standard drug is indicated. What do you do? One solution might be to prescribe your drug in addition to the standard of care. Your eventual comparison would then be "accepted drug + new" versus "accepted drug only." But this is not always possible—for example, when subjects' physiological systems cannot tolerate two chemotherapy agents administered at the same time. And besides, it may not work. Another option might be to test the new drug on subjects for whom first-line treatment has failed. But as a rule you prefer to avoid this. First, patients who fail approved treatments are likely to have more advanced stages of a disease and so are more difficult to help; limiting your trial's subjects to especially difficult patients is likely to reduce your chances for showing efficacy. Second, even if you *do* succeed with these especially ill patients, you have not shown your drug superior to first-line treatment; you have only demonstrated efficacy for those who failed the first-line drug. Thus, the best you could hope for from this trial is that your drug will be approved for use only *after* standard treatment has failed, as a second line or third. This will narrow your potential market considerably.

Be that as it may, you will probably not be given the opportunity for head-to-head superiority testing versus standard-of-care. This may leave you with little choice but a single-arm trial—one in which only subjects failing standard treatment receive your drug. You would then determine success or failure by comparing results to some external standard or expectation—external, that is, to your trial. For example, from information in scientific publications you might estimate the survival time of individuals who failed first-line treatment and use this estimate as your Reference. But these criteria are often difficult to interpret because of the large variation of outcomes in the literature. An alternative might be to compare your drug's results to those of patients receiving no treatment after having failed all standard therapies. This is the preferred option and gets you back to a two-arm trial with a direct comparison. But recruitment of Control subjects may be difficult, since very ill subjects who are receiving no treatment have little incentive to participate in a clinical trial.

To summarize, you planned to test your drug for superiority and instead found yourself up against two difficulties: You are not permitted a head-to-head comparison versus current treatment, and there appears to be no agreed-upon benchmark to which you can compare results of a single-arm trial. How then will you determine whether or not your drug is superior to *anything*?

Well, we can go back and forth here, discussing different possible designs, hoping to identify the optimal approach. And mind you, there *must* be some such design. If there were not, we could not develop new drugs in this not uncommon situation. Well, I will let you puzzle this out for yourself. It is a good exercise. Here I only wish to point out while the concept of superiority is statistically basic, its application in practice can be tricky.

Equivalence

It is virtually impossible to show two products to be truly the same even if they are truly identical. Indeed, in statistics we assume that showing identity *is* impossible. For now I ask that you take my word for it; an explanation is forthcoming. And because you cannot show that two products are truly equal, we define equivalence using a *range* of values rather than a single number. Thus, you will declare one product equivalent to another if the performance of the former is within a predetermined range of the latter. For example, you might specify your product is equivalent to another if your obtained rate of cure is within ±5% of the comparator. Thus, to demonstrate equivalence you specify upper and lower **equivalence margins**. If your study shows product outcome is within these margins relative to the comparator, you will conclude that the products are equivalent.

STATISTICAL CONNECTIONS

In an earlier chapter I mentioned that the statistician's bag of tricks is limited. We have a case in point here where we approach one problem by framing it in terms of another. Specifically, equivalence is shown if your product's performance is between lower and upper margins. And how do you test this? Well, you aim to demonstrate that it is higher than the lower margin and lower than the upper. Now showing "lower" is the flip side of "higher" and entails the same statistical methodology. We have thus translated the concept of equivalence into two, superiority-like statements. So if you wish to add another acronym to your arsenal, try TOST—two one-sided t-tests, which combine two superiority-type tests for assessing equivalence.

So equivalence is defined by limiting your attribute at both ends. Using the preceding example, you wish to show that the cure rate is ±5% relative to the comparator, which implies the following:

$$-5\% \leq T - R \leq +5\%$$

While the principle should be clear, the logic seems less so; why would you ever want to limit performance at the upper end? Why reject a product for being better? Well, there can be at least two answers to this question, one of which has primarily to do with wording. To this point I have equated "higher" with superior and "lower" with inferior, and this is not always the case. As anyone who cooks, bakes, or carries out contracts for the Mafia knows, there is such a thing as "getting it just right."

Ischemic stroke involves a disturbance in brain function due to a lack of blood supply to it. This can, for example, occur when a clot (thrombosis) blocks the flow in vessels carrying blood to the brain cells. Patients with ischemic stroke are routinely given **anticoagulants** in an effort to prevent additional clots. One such anticoagulant is Warfarin, and there are many others of the same family.

In a severe ischemic stroke many brain cells will die due to lack of blood supply. And when this happens, cells in the vicinity of those that have died are at risk as well. This is the case even after the region's blood supply has been reestablished. Suppose your company has developed a neuroprotective agent—a drug that provides protection to brain cells at risk—for addressing this particular phenomenon. You believe the drug can be effective when given up to five hours after a stroke's onset. Having developed the drug and completed preclinical testing with it, you are now planning a superiority trial. Specifically, you aim to show via statistical analysis that stroke patients receiving your drug do better than those who do not—in short, a superiority trial.

Yet before testing your drug's efficacy, you will need to show that it is safe. There are many aspects to safety in a stroke, but I shall deal with only one: the possibility of your drug interacting with the anticoagulants. Recall that patients with ischemic stroke will often be given Warfarin-like drugs to prevent clotting. Well, if physicians are to use your drug, they must be sure that it will not interfere with existing treatments. In this particular example, you will need to demonstrate that administering your product will not affect Warfarin's behavior in the body. To show this you will likely set up an equivalence trial of which the goal is demonstrating that Warfarin "is neither better nor worse" when given with your treatment compared to when given by itself.[1]

---

[1] Warfarin is used here to model your new drug's interaction with the *class* of Warfarin-like agents rather than with this specific medication.

Here, as in similar situations, the equivalence trial will likely be done on healthy volunteers. This is a characteristic of Phase I clinical trials that typically aim to test safety only. The study itself will probably be conducted using a **crossover design** in which each subject is exposed to both treatments of interest as follows:

1. In stage one, half of the subjects will receive Warfarin alone, while the other half will receive Warfarin with your neuroprotective agent T. Pharmacokinetic measurements will be obtained from all subjects.
2. The second stage involves a **washout period**—an interval in which subjects receive neither of the drugs and is judged long enough for both agents to be eliminated from the body.
3. The trial's final stage will be the reverse of the first. In it, subjects who received Warfarin alone will now receive it with T, while those who received both drugs will receive Warfarin alone. Once again you will obtain pharmacokinetic measurements from all subjects.
4. You will then compare the behavior of Warfarin—its pharmacokinetics—between the Warfarin-alone and Warfarin-T groups.

To make this comparison, you might compute for each subject the following ratio:

$$\frac{R}{T} = \frac{\textit{Behavior of Warfarin in the blood when given alone}}{\textit{Behavior of Warfarin in the blood when given with new drug}}.^2$$

If there is no interaction between the drugs, Warfarin should be unaffected by T, and this ratio should be about 1.0—that is, the behavior of Warfarin in the blood will be about the same with or without adding your neuroprotective agent. You then compare the average of subject-ratios to 1.0. Showing that this average is neither too low nor too high relative to 1.0—that it is within an "equivalence range" of 1.0—will allow you to conclude equivalence. Here this means that Warfarin remains "just right" when taken with T.

Here you might state that a ratio no lower than 0.80 and no higher than 1.25 demonstrates equivalence. Determination of the range should be based on both clinical and statistical criteria. At the same time I should point out that equivalence testing in pharmacokinetics is usually simpler than non-inferiority with respect to the determination of clinically appropriate margins. While in most non-inferiority situations there are no acceptable criteria for "range of non-inferiority," in most cases of equivalence in pharmacokinetics there exists an acceptable range (typically, a ratio-range of 0.80 to 1.25). To learn

---

[2] In pharmacokinetics, "behavior" has several measures such as Tmax, which is the time it takes for the drug to reach maximal concentrations in the blood. Here then you would assess the T/R ratio for all relevant pharmacokinetic parameters.

more about **non-inferiority margins**, which I will discuss in the next section, I recommend that you take a look at EMEA's *Guideline on the Choice of Non-inferiority Margin* (2005).

Equivalence studies are most often conducted to assess generic drugs—new and chemically equivalent[3] versions of established drugs. When producing a generic drug, your statistical test aims to show its performance is equivalent to the established agent. This is generally done by demonstrating that the pharmacokinetic properties of the generic drug are similar to those of the comparator. We assume here that if the two active ingredients have similar pharmacokinetic profiles, they also have similar clinical effects. This is why trials for showing equivalence of generics usually involve pharmacokinetic comparisons rather than clinical efficacy. As a result, pharmacokinetic studies are generally much shorter than efficacy studies and require fewer subjects.

One last word on equivalence in generics: There are some cases where "higher" is indeed "better," and you will still be required to show equivalence. This is the second reason for using equivalence, despite the apparent advantage of the superiority approach.

Suppose you wish to show that your topical medication for eliminating some fungus can serve as a generic equivalent to some R. In this case, where the drug is topical and not meant to enter the bloodstream, a pharmacokinetic study is not an option. Instead, you will be asked to demonstrate that T's Fungus-Cure—a clinical efficacy parameter—is equivalent to that of R. Once done, you will conclude that T is equivalent to R and can be used as a generic substitute for it.

Now in this last example more (Cure) is indeed better. Thus, it may seem a bit foolish to use equivalence rather than non-inferiority. After all, if your generic drug turns out to be much better than the comparator, shouldn't everyone be happier? Well, yes and no. In fact, a drug that gets rid of fungus better than another *is* generally preferable. But if this is the case, T can no longer be considered equivalent to R. It is a different product and will need to be evaluated as such,[4] so it cannot be labeled "equivalent." When this happens—when your generic version turns out to be superior to the original—you will be required to go the longer route required for approving a new drug, since this is what you actually have.

---

[3] Generic drugs have the same quantity and structure of active ingredient, but they are not necessarily the same overall. The drugs' coatings, for example, may be different. Moreover, since they are produced in different plants by different companies, one cannot assume they are similar without some testing in humans.
[4] For example, different products cannot (like generics) be assumed equivalent on parameters relating to safety.

In summary, equivalence should be used in the following situations:

1. Demonstrating that a new drug does not affect the pharmacokinetics of another drug given with it—that is, showing that the established drug is equivalent when given by itself or with T.
2. Demonstrating that T is pharmacokinetically equivalent to R and, by implication, that it is clinically equivalent as well.
3. Demonstrating that T is clinically equivalent to R when it cannot be shown by pharmacokinetics.

I also noted that if in an equivalence trial T is actually shown to be superior to R, T will be considered a new product and will need to be tested in additional studies.

Non-inferiority

Demonstrating one product to be non-inferior entails showing it to be "no worse" than another. There are various designs for testing non-inferiority but the term as used typically implies at least a two-arm trial. Let us take the simple case of T versus R.

Having set up and undertaken a non-inferiority clinical trial, you are now ready to conduct statistical testing. As before, formal testing will yield only one of two conclusions: "Product T is non-inferior to R," or "I cannot say that product T is non-inferior to R." The second conclusion suggests that we are in the habit of making inconclusive statements. And we are. But these statements are both theoretically correct and, at times, useful. So we will stick with them.

The fact that there can be only one of two conclusions from a non-inferiority study has implications at both ends:

1. Highly unfavorable results will yield "I cannot say T is non-inferior to B" rather than "T is inferior to R."
2. Highly favorable results will yield only "T is non-inferior to R" rather than "T is superior to R."

The first scenario is not particularly interesting because you do not care whether an inferior product is simply that or "very inferior." The second scenario however, is at the very least annoying. This is because you cannot formally conclude superiority from a non-inferiority trial even if it is obvious. For example, suppose you have conducted a non-inferiority study comparing T to R with 100 subjects in each group and found T to produce a cure rate of 90%, while R yields a mere 40%. Even here—where if you had conducted a superiority trial, you would have shown it—you cannot formally conclude that T is superior to R.

Non-inferiority works similarly to equivalence except that its margin is at one end only. This number is referred to as a non-inferiority margin. For example, if you specified a non-inferiority margin on Cure Rate of 7%, your data will need to show that your product is "no worse than 7% worse than the comparator." This is the same as declaring that you are superior to the comparator's efficacy minus 7%. Technically then, showing non-inferiority requires demonstrating that you are no worse than the comparator minus some delta—a **non-inferiority delta**, which is an alternative term for non-inferiority margin.

The actual mechanics of conducting such comparisons requires some statistics. A simplistic account of these will be presented in the next chapter, and I refer you to standard texts if you wish to understand the analytical techniques as well.

In practice, regardless of the type of trial you conduct, if you observe a result greatly in your favor, you are likely to *believe* that your test product T is superior to R. This is reasonable, and there should be nothing to prevent you from thinking it. You might even consider shouting it from rooftops. But formally you are constrained to claim only that which was specified before the trial began. If your initial stated aim was non-inferiority, you will be permitted to claim no more than this. The principle underlying this is as straightforward as it is important: *Formal conclusions at the end of a trial must be perfectly consistent with the objectives set for the trial* (see Chapter 9). Much of the justification for concluding *anything* from clinical trials rests upon this principle.

The concept of non-inferiority gives rise to a number of issues, including the following:

- Why design a study to show "non-inferiority" if you believe you are "as good as"? Clearly, claiming "T is as good as R" is a more direct statement than "T is not inferior to R"—and stronger besides.
- Why would you ever want to demonstrate a product to be "no worse" in the first place? If your product is better, go ahead and show it. If not, there seems no practical use for it, since there is already one on the market meeting patients' needs.
- What *is* "non-inferior"? In other words, which criterion do you choose for establishing non-inferiority? For example, would you consider your product non-inferior if its true Cure Rate is 78% and the comparator's is 80%? And if yours is 79.5% and the comparator's is 80%, what then? In other words, which difference is sufficiently small to allow your claim that one product is non-inferior to another? This is crucial because when planning a trial you must determine in advance what constitutes *proof*—that is, you will need to specify in advance the outcome that will support your claim.

The first bullet suggests that it is better to show "as good as" than "non-inferior." And while this is certainly the case, it cannot technically be done. As noted, even identical products will rarely perform identically in different groups of individuals. Indeed, apply the same pharmaceutical or device to the same people twice, and you will not get identical results. Your options then become limited to (1) equivalence—showing your attribute within some range—or (2) non-inferiority—demonstrating your attribute better than some "comparator minus some delta."

A perhaps intuitive example can be found in election surveys, which are nearer to our everyday experiences. These surveys are rarely in precise agreement despite purporting to estimate the same parameters (e.g., percent who will vote for Peoria Joe). Keep in mind that at the end of the day candidate Joe will get exactly Y% of the vote. And yet different surveys aiming to predict this figure will come up with different numbers even when they have the same sample size and are taken from the same population at the same time. And while the methodology of clinical trials is typically different from that of surveys (with exceptions), the principle is the same. We "survey" two **samples** and expect that even if they were asked the same question—given the same treatment—the results will differ.

It is the nature of **sampling** that no matter how well planned, none of these groups will be *identical* to the population they purport to represent and, thus, to each other. Consequently, whatever it is you measure on the sample will virtually always yield results that differ from the truth in the population. We call this **sampling error**—the fact that samples typically err to some degree or another in representing the population from which they were taken. Now it is difficult to overstate the importance of accounting sampling error when conducting clinical trials. And to prove the point, I shall devote much of the next chapter to it.

So we require some statistical sleight of hand to deal with the impossibility of showing identity, and in the concepts of non-inferiority and equivalence we have it. Getting back to our initial questions, the answer to the first bullet is clear. You conduct non-inferiority because when you want to show "at least as good," you have no choice; even if you are identical, you will not, in a given trial, be able to show this.

This gets us to the two additional issues raised—namely, your motivation for showing "at least as good" to begin with and, having decided on it, determining a criterion for comparison. I will use a specific example to address both these issues and in the process suggest the relationship between them.

Diabetes is a disease that generally causes higher than normal sugar levels in the blood. This can lead to a wide variety of complications, many of which are sufficiently serious to endanger life and limb. For many diabetes patients the only treatment is injection of insulin, a hormone that in healthy people is produced by the pancreas and that reduces sugar levels. Diabetes patients who require insulin to control their disease are said to have *insulin-dependent diabetes.*

Treatment with insulin must be carefully managed. Injecting too little will insufficiently reduce blood sugar and may cause a *hyperglycemic episode* ("hyper" for short)—the occurrence of an abnormally high level of sugar in the blood. Conversely, injecting too much insulin will reduce the blood sugar level abnormally. A *hypoglycemic episode*, or "hypo," is the occurrence of an unusually low level of sugar in the blood. It is therefore imperative that in any given circumstance a diabetic patient must inject the right amount of insulin to prevent both hyper and hypo.

There is currently a standard formula for calculating the recommended amount of insulin to be injected in any particular circumstance. The formula is based on various parameters, including the person's current blood sugar level, the amount of carbohydrates the individual intends to eat, the individual's body's sensitivity to insulin, and others.

Suppose you have developed a new formula for determining the amount of insulin to be injected and a device to go with it. Using the device, patients enter the required information and are provided a suggested quantity of insulin to inject. Having conducted initial testing on your device, you believe it is about as good as that using the existing formula. In other words, you expect your new formula and device to be about as effective as the old. Thus, your product cannot be said to be superior to the one already on the market. Accordingly, you plan a non-inferiority trial comparing your device T to the existing standard R.

But why would you want to show non-inferiority to begin with? If there is already a device for precisely this purpose and yours is no better, why produce an alternative? Well, there may be any number of reasons. We shall choose *price:* Your device will cost much less than the competitor and as such will be easier on the wallet of those who would consider the alternative. Your product will also provide those who cannot afford the current device with an alternative. In sum, conducting a successful non-inferiority trial for your device will demonstrate that the device is "about as good" as that on the market. Coupled with its being less expensive, you will have shown it has a marketing edge over the product currently on the market. There can be many others. In fact, one of these was mentioned earlier when discussing drugs that have similar efficacy, with one being more convenient to take than the other. Whatever the reason, there are circumstances in which non-inferiority make sense.

Now that we have provided an answer to the second question, we come to the trickier issue of defining non-inferiority when comparing T to R. First, the formal definition:

> ...a non-inferiority trial aims to demonstrate [analytically] that the test product is not worse than the comparator by more than a prespecified, small amount. This amount is known as the non-inferiority margin, or delta (Δ).[5]

So in any particular trial aiming to demonstrate that T is non-inferior to R, you will need to do the following:

1. Quantify the concept of "non-inferiority" by attaching some number to it. For example, you might claim that as long as that amount of insulin your device recommends causes no more than 5% additional (and not serious) hyper and hypo episodes than the competitor, it will be considered non-inferior. Thus, you define a non-inferiority margin of 5% on efficacy as measured by incidence of hypo and hyper episodes.
2. Set up a trial of which the design will provide an acceptable test of whether or not your product meets the quantitative criterion specified at the higher and lower ends.

That there cannot be a one-size-fits-all criterion for non-inferiority should now be apparent. Thus, for example, you would expect a smaller allowable margin in life-threatening applications than in those that are not. Where the risk is great (e.g., life and limb), T will be allowed a non-inferiority margin that is smaller than when the risk is minor (e.g., stomach upset). Making use of the guidelines again:

> The choice of [non-inferiority] delta [or margin] must always be justified on both clinical and statistical grounds. It always needs to be tailored specifically to the particular clinical context, and no rule can be provided that covers all situations.[6]

Returning to our example, we noted that incorrect insulin recommendations can lead to either hypo or hyper episodes. As a general rule (with exceptions), hypo episodes are more hazardous to the patient than hyper episodes. Because of this, the regulator may require your non-inferiority trial to have two different margins: one for hyper episodes with a relatively large delta and another for hypo with a smaller delta. For example, you might be required to do the following:

1. Demonstrate that the number of *hyper episodes* when using T (new device) is no more than 8% higher than when using R (current device). More

---

[5] European Medicines Agency (EMEA). *Guideline on the Choice for Non-inferiority Margin*. 2005. London.
[6] European Medicines Agency (EMEA). *Guideline on the Choice of the Non-inferiority Margin*. 2005. London.

formally, demonstrate that the non-inferiority margin for showing efficacy with respect to hyper is −8%.

2. Show that the number of *hypo episodes* using T is no more than 3% higher than when using R. Formally then, the non-inferiority margin for demonstrating efficacy on hypo is −3%.

In this section I described circumstances where statistical considerations leave you no choice but to go the non-inferiority route. Underlying all this is the assumption that non-inferiority is a reasonable thing to show. Well, is it? At the more basic level there would seem to remain the following question: From the clinical standpoint, why would the regulator approve *any* product based on non-inferiority? Well, I noted a couple of reasons, and there are others. But having been with this topic for a while, I shall heed Chaucer's dictum that "it is nought good a slepyng hound to wake."

PUTTING IT TOGETHER

In the preceding chapter I dealt with attributes, while in this one I described some options for "what about" these attributes you might wish to show. Put these two together and you get what usually comes under the section headed "Study Objectives" in a clinical trial's protocol. Table 4.1 shows some of these combinations.

Following are some "Study Objective" statements taken (with appropriate modifications) from clinical trial protocols. You might try placing each in its respective table cell. If you cannot, then the objective does not contain all the information it should.

- "Show that T's safety is now worse than R when given twice daily in a population of recently diagnosed lupus."
- "Demonstrate that T is **substantially equivalent** to R in detecting severe heart arrhythmia."
- "Assess the safety and tolerability of T in patients with venous insufficiency."
- "Show that T is equivalent to R in the treatment of migraine."

Table 4.1 Clinical Trial Aims and Attributes

Objective (Analytic Aim)	Attribute of Interest			
	Efficacy	Safety	Performance	Pharmacokinetics
Superiority	A	B	C	D
Equivalence	E	F	G	H
Non-inferiority	I	J	K	L

You might have noticed that the third bullet did not include a "comparative statement" but simply stated that the study's objective is to assess safety and tolerability. This study's planners should have stated that they wish to assess these attributes "relative to. ..." They could have chosen a comparator within the trial, external to the trial, or some acceptable reference if there is one. Since they did not, the objective cannot be identified with a cell in the table and is lacking.

In this chapter I dealt with planning a clinical trial by focusing on its objectives. These in turn imply testing product attributes with a specific goal in mind. In the chapter that follows I shall begin dealing with actual statistics—those associated with describing results obtained from trials and more complex issues relating to statistical comparisons.

CHAPTER 5

Statistical Thinking

CONTENTS

- Classification, science, and statistics
- Descriptive statistics in a hearing implant
- Statistical versus clinical thinking
- Classification, grouping, and descriptive statistics
- Intended use populations and statistical populations
- Intended use and accuracy: an example from oncology
- Samples and populations
- Phase I and Phase II trial population differences

INTRODUCTION: A MENTAL ACTIVITY

- Cats and dogs are biologically different.
- Cats and dogs are domesticated.
- It's raining cats and dogs.

The first two statements are very simple—banal even. But they are also examples of a central cognitive process of ours: *classification*.

When I say that cats and dogs are different, I call attention to their dissimilarity and place each in a separate group. And when focusing on their similarity, I put them in the same class of domesticated animals. This mental activity is very basic and sufficiently important for there to be many words in English for it: traits, groups, classes, characteristics, types, categories, and taxonomies. The third statement, when I think about it, makes little sense.

Strategy and Statistics in Clinical Trials

Alexis de Tocqueville (1805–1859) contrasted this cognitive process with that of the Devine:

> The Deity does not regard the human race collectively. He surveys at one glance and severally all the beings ... and he discerns in each man the resemblances which assimilate him to all his fellows, and the differences which distinguish him from them. God, therefore, stands in no need of general ideas; that is to say, He is never sensible of the necessity of collecting a considerable number of analogous objects under the same form for greater convenience in thinking. Such is, however, not the case with man. If the human mind were to attempt to examine and pass a judgment on all the individual cases before it, the immensity of detail would soon lead it astray and bewilder its discernment: in this strait, man has recourse to an imperfect but necessary expedient. ... Having superficially considered a certain number of objects, and remarked their resemblance, he assigns to them a common name, sets them apart, and proceeds onwards.[1]

So no two dogs are identical, and even two door handles coming off the same production line differ. But some objects are sufficiently similar that we lump them together.

Jean Piaget (1896–1980), whose theory of child development is one of the few constants in psychology, observed that the ability to classify starts early and refines as we go along. The young child being no deity (despite some parental behavior to the contrary), she will learn early to distinguish between toys and knives, and upon seeing one or the other will, to use Piaget's and de Tocqueville's term, *assimilate* it into its category—that is, she will place it in the appropriate "pigeonhole" in the brain. Once assimilated, the object is *understood* and can be treated accordingly. For example, a wooden train set and Lego blocks will be distinguished from a Swiss Army knife and bread knife, with the pairs assimilated into the respective categories formed.

Time goes by and the child's universe expands. Her experience grows and her brain matures. Her distinctions become finer. She will learn to differentiate sharp knives from dull ones and between toys needing electricity and those that do not. She will know that "batteries not included" means a gadget will not work when she gets home, and that inside the home or out, some knives should be handled with greater care than others.

Every so often the child will see an object for which she has no ready-made category. She might, for instance, observe a zebra and instinctively place it in

---

[1] de Tocqueville, A. (1840). *Democracy in America*. Project Gutenberg EBook.

her "horse" pigeonhole. Then focusing on the difference in coloring and the fact that she is at the zoo and not a racetrack, she will have second thoughts. Confused, she is motivated to update her classification system—to create a new category. If her brain has sufficiently matured, she will. If not, this will have to wait. Piaget calls this constructing of new mental classes *accommodation*. For the young child it involves creating a "zebra pigeonhole" separate from the "horse pigeonhole" she already has. Once done, she can assimilate the two animals into more suitable categories. As the child's distinctions multiply, she is better able to make sense of the world around her. Without this shared understanding, she could not communicate with the rest of us, and we could not communicate with her. Life itself depends on it. Thus, it would be impossible to keep out of harm's way if we could not distinguish between cats and cars, bipeds and mopeds.

Classification is a central activity of science as well. Geologists will group rocks, physiologists type tissues, and zoologists categorize animals into taxonomies. Some of these systems are theoretical and have little immediate application, although one day they might. Thus, you might classify planets outside the Milky Way by density and orbit, using this information to estimate when and where they were created. This is interesting—even fascinating—but of no immediate use on *terra cognita*. On the other hand, classify human tissue properly, and you might know how to treat it and, perhaps, even find a replacement for it; correctly identify geological strata, and you might know the chance for a landslide or something about resources underneath.

Statistics provides methods for classifying objects into groups. With the aid of **statistical testing**, also called **hypothesis testing**, we can, to use Piaget's terms, both assimilate and accommodate. In this sense statistical techniques are formalizations of one of our central thought processes. But first things first.

DESCRIPTION

The discipline of statistics is typically divided into two parts and taught that way. The first of these is **descriptive statistics**, which provides methods for summarizing and organizing data. When I obtain data, the first thing I do is describe the data using the methods available to me. This helps me get a feel for the numbers, which is important. But in doing this I am more an observer than a participant. It is only at a later stage of data analysis that I will be concerned with arriving at specific conclusions from the data. It is when doing the latter that I am more directly affecting product development.

Now looking at data—even to merely get a "feel" for them—is no trivial pursuit. A multitude of numbers are usually involved, and simply looking at them will not get me very far. On the other hand, reducing all data into one or two summary statistics—say, the mean and standard deviation—will likely mask a great deal of essential information. So my first task is to summarize the data sufficiently to make them comprehensible—that is, to reduce the jumble of numbers into a few meaningful statistics. Now there can be no summarizing of data without a loss of information. As we well know, the whole of the information is present in the individual objects only—in *all* the measurements taken. Thus, the challenge is to summarize while retaining the essential storyline of the data.

Let us suppose that a company wishes to test the efficacy of an implantable hearing aid and conducts a trial with 248 subjects. All subjects are implanted the same device, and their hearing is evaluated both before and after the implantation. The trial done, my first task is to describe the data in a manner that best tells their story. To do this I will use techniques that come under the heading of Descriptive Statistics, which provide numerical and graphical methods for summarizing and simplifying the numbers. If I do my job well, I will have transformed the data into *information*.

I will not provide here an overview of Descriptive Statistics. Many good books on the subject are available. In this section I shall merely present an example intended to give a taste of the challenges associated with "simply presenting data." Yet, before going on, I should say a word about how the data in this example were generated.

The Audiometer Hearing Test (AHT) evaluates individuals' sensitivity to tone as a function of Frequency and Loudness; Frequency is measured in Hertz (Hz) and Loudness in decibels (dB). In this hypothetical study each subject was exposed to frequencies of 500 Hz, 1,000 Hz, and 2,000 Hz. At each of these, the audiologist varied Loudness in decibels (dB), aiming to identify the minimal dB level at which a subject perceives a specific tone. The greater the Loudness required for perceiving a tone, the poorer the hearing.

Testing was done before and after implantation of the device,[2] so each subject has a "hearing profile" at two time points. For example, a profile of 30 dB, 45 dB, and 38 dB indicates that these are levels of Loudness needed for a subject to perceive tones of 500 Hz, 1,000 Hz, and 2,000 Hz, respectively. Figure 5.1 presents pre- and postimplantation profiles for one of the subjects in the study.

In Figure 5.1, we have what audiologists call an *audiogram* and what statisticians call *graphical descriptive statistics*. Using this simple tool—a plot of Loudness against Frequency for two time points—we have a presentation that is much more informative than a mere list of six numbers. You can now conveniently see the subject's profiles before and after implantation without

---

[2] Testing before implantation was done using the best available (external) hearing aid for the subject.

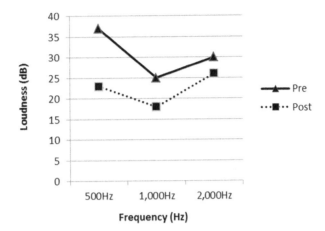

FIGURE 5.1
Pure Tone Audiogram for Patient 054

delving too deeply into the numbers. And you can go on to make statements like the following:

- Implantation seems to have led to hearing gain at every Frequency.
- The greatest gain was at 500 Hz and the smallest at 2,000 Hz.
- There may be a relationship between efficacy and Frequency such that the higher the Frequency, the lower the device's efficacy. (This is based on the observation that improvement seemed to decrease as Frequency increased. Keep in mind, however, that these data are for 1 of 248 subjects only—a subject that may or may not be representative of the others. As will often happen when doing Descriptive Statistics, you will notice patterns in the data that will be "filed away for future testing.")

While these statements may seem simple (and they are), they are also a fine example of how selecting an appropriate method for presenting data can make the data's meaning accessible. Also note that in my statements I have gone beyond mere description and hinted at inferences—for example, "Implantation seems to have led to hearing gain. …" It appears, then, that my separating of processes—in this case, separating between mere description of data and reaching conclusions from them—is somewhat artificial, and once again we find that "everything is connected."

Getting back to my description and resultant statements, they seem useful. Still, they are based on one subject only. As a matter of fact, we have 248 subjects, each assessed at three frequencies at two different time points. So in all we have 1,488 data points, and presenting 248 separate audiograms will not do. While each is informative by itself, there are simply too many to make examining each and every one feasible.

ON STATISTICIANS AND CLINICIANS

Working with physicians, I often present statistics in numerical or graphical form. Almost inevitably some physician will place her finger on a data point or specific chart and say something like "This makes perfect sense. You can see from here how the treatment works. ..." This might have occurred, for example, when presenting Figure 5.1, which is only 1 of 248 and should not be interpreted in isolation. In my infinite statistical wisdom I smile inwardly and point out that our aim is to look at the pattern in the data rather than at the individual patient. And in this particular instance I am probably right, since research is designed to evaluate what happens "on average" (though, admittedly, my smile is likely smugger than it should be).

Still, it is not as simple as all that. Physicians work with real people, not numbers. And while averages may guide medical practice in general, the doctor deals daily with "individual data points." And each point is distinctive, being a patient with a particular Age, Gender, Medical History, Level of Family and Financial Support, Ability to Withstand Pain, Severity of Disease, and many other characteristics relevant to treatment. Consciously or not, these individuals' data and others will be taken into account by the physician deciding on treatment. And these very characteristics are lost on statisticians computing summary statistics.

Over the years I have found these natural tendencies of the two disciplines to be a barrier in communicating between them. Simply put, I have often been frustrated when talking with physicians, and I am sure they are no less frustrated with me. Different professions being what they are, there is no ideal solution for this. At the same time, both disciplines must be aware of the others' natural tendencies and use them to the best advantage. Thus, for example, observing overall patterns is the essence of statistical investigation. At the same time, understanding the individual case can go a long way to gaining a deeper understanding of the clinical, physiological, and psychological processes involved. And this in turn can provide the statistician with an understanding that will guide him to more insightful analyses. Analyzing data without at least some understanding of the medicine involved is as an egregious an error as focusing exclusively on the individual when doing statistics.

A statistician given these numbers has many options for organizing (read "reducing") the data both numerically and graphically. Following are a few possibilities:

1. Plot the Average *Change* Profile for all subjects by:
   a. For each subject, compute pre-post difference at each Frequency.
   b. Compute the average pre-post difference for all subjects at each Frequency.
   c. Graph this average in a manner similar to that shown in Figure 5.1. You now have a similar graph but with a single profile representing Average Change over all subjects.
2. Repeat (a) and add an interval around each point in the graph representing the smallest and greatest change encountered over all subjects. That is, at each point show a line parallel to the *y*-axis representing the range of change achieved; the upper limit and lower limits of this line represent the range of measurements observed across all subjects.
3. Compute pre-post differences at each Frequency and present the average along with an interval describing the **standard deviation** at each point. You now have a single "difference line" rather than lines representing "before" and "after" measurements.

4. For each subject, compute Percent Change by dividing the pre-post change in dB by the preimplantation dB value and multiplying by 100. These new plots describe Percent Change rather than Absolute Change.
5. Compute Average Percent Change over all subjects and present a single number representing Percent Change from preimplantation to postimplantation.
6. Define "Success/Failure" for each subject as follows:
   Success: A hearing improvement of at least 20% at each Frequency.
   Failure: At least one Frequency in which Percent Change is less than 20%.

Once Change is transformed in this way, compute the rate of Success over all subjects—that is, the proportion of subjects for whom the procedure was successful given the criterion of "at least 20% improvement at each Frequency."

As an exercise, you might try coming up with additional possibilities. There are many more, and, as a rule, one cannot be said to be more correct than another. Rather, each description tells its own story, addressing a different aspect of the data. Depending on the question of interest, some of the descriptions will usually be more informative than others; change the question and you will likely change the appropriate analysis. Thus, it is your challenge to select the one most suitable description for the specific circumstance. All the while you must keep in mind that while the techniques can be simple or complex, the goal is always the same: Present the data in an accessible and meaningful fashion.

Now there is another important issue here that relates to the grouping mentioned in the preceding section. For example, had the subjects in this trial come from two groups—for example, each implanted with a different device—would you have combined their data and presented their statistics as a single group? This is not such an innocent question, and we shall deal with it at length. But for now I will give the simple answer: "No." When a trial includes two or more groups, the data should be presented separately for each. (The exception is if you conclude that the groups do not differ and are, despite being treated differently, a single group in terms of outcome. Here, then, is a hint of things to come—of issues connecting between description and statistical testing.)

You see, descriptive statistics make most sense when they are done within a specific category. Thus, we will compute the average weight of apples from Annie's Orchard separately from that of oranges from Shady's Grove. Statisticians, like the rest of us, should not confuse the two.

I shall thus formally define *descriptive statistics* as providing procedures to summarize, organize, and simplify data collected from a *specific group*, a *population*. The latter part of this statement is not typically articulated when defining descriptive statistics. But it is correct, it suits my purpose, and I shall keep it.

I should also point out that our usual conception of categories typically includes descriptive statistics, although we may not call them that. A child, for instance, will see an animal that walks like a duck and quacks like a duck and decide it is a duck because it fits the descriptive statistics she has accumulated for the category. Over time she has collected data on ducks and knows their distribution of sizes, colors, and behaviors. Upon seeing an animal that might be a duck, she matches its individual characteristics to the group-descriptive statistics she has constructed. Similarly, she has amassed data and organized them for numerous categories such as houses and trees and trolls. Thus, viewing the process, the methods encompassed by descriptive statistics are in fact a formalization of the thought processes we engage in continuously.

In the first section of this chapter I considered the mental activity of categorization, and in the second I discussed the area of statistics meant to organize and simplify data collected from a category. In the section that follows I discuss how statistics approaches the *idea* of category and how it resembles its application in everyday life.

POPULATION

In an earlier chapter I mentioned the term *population* for the first time and have been using the term quite a bit. In both statistics and everyday life, it is defined as a group of objects—persons, places, or things—that have an attribute in common. Thus, Swedes are individuals who have Sweden in common, and the population of individuals suffering from migraines share a similar disease. Now the child—or adult for that matter—may not formally define her mental bins as populations, but this is precisely what they are. And when she assimilates an object to one of these bins, she has, in our language, assigned it to a population.

Everyday communication requires that we understand one another more or less, which is usually enough. You do not need to properly define "cars" to drive them nor "dogs" to pet them. But this is not the case in the science of clinical trials. If, for instance, you claim that a product straightens teeth, you must specify the relevant population for it. Do you mean for young or old people? Are you talking about very crooked teeth or only slightly askew? And are you referring to the population of individuals who must align a single tooth, or must there be at least two teeth involved?

For each clinical trial you specify inclusion and exclusion criteria, which define the population of interest precisely. And if your product is found safe and effective in the trial, you will claim that it works for the population of subjects represented by those participating in the study—for them and not for others.

There are many possible definitions for the term *population*, and I shall use one that suits my purpose: A population is a group of elements[3] that have a characteristic of interest in common that those in other populations do not have. For example, if your trial includes subjects that have experienced a myocardial infarction (MI), this is the characteristic common to your group (and that excludes those who have not had an MI).

So it is *you* who decides on the population of study in a manner that suits *your* purposes. And here is a difference of sorts from the term's use in everyday life, which typically refers to self-evident groupings, such as cats, cucumbers, and communists. For example, when studying immune disorders you will lump AIDS and minor allergies in the same population. And when studying people who experienced life-threatening ailments, MI, AIDS, and car crash victims will find themselves in the same group.

So you create populations by *defining* them; they are figments of your application and are specified for a purpose. Statistics is a tool for describing and demarking populations, and as such can no more dictate the population of interest than a hammer suggesting where to place your blows. The choice is yours, and you must be careful with it. Once made, statistics will provide you with the tools for extracting information from the population and determining who or what belongs to it.

Belaboring the point, one characteristic of populations is that they can be as shifty as the Sahara's sands. But unlike those particular particles, it is you who determine the rules of motion. Thus, your population can include anyone who is currently suffering a cold, in which case individuals will move in and out of your group as their condition changes. Alternatively, you can define a population as anyone who has ever experienced a cold, in which case your group is much more inclusive. A third option might consist of all who *will* experience a cold in the future, in which case the population of interest is not readily available for study. While available in theory, it is only after a particular individual experiences a cold that you will know he actually belonged to this population.

Now the "cold-groupings" enumerated are neither right nor wrong in any absolute sense. Rather, each is appropriate in a particular context. If you want to know "what it feels like to have a cold," you will interview those who have experienced one. But if you wish to examine the effect of your medication on alleviating cold symptoms, you had better give your drug only to those who are currently ill. And if your goal is to estimate market potential for a new medication, people who will have the illness in the future are of greatest interest.

---

[3] People, places, things, concepts, and so on—anything of interest.

A CATCH (FOR EXAMPLE)

Regulators require that you define an intended use population for your product—people with particular characteristics (that others do not share) for whom your product is meant. Frequently, defining and studying a population can be straightforward. But this is not always the case.

Suppose you have developed a blood test for diagnosing a rare cancer—one that currently can be positively diagnosed by biopsy only. Your first step might be a simple feasibility trial in which subjects sent to biopsy undergo your test as well. Once the results from both tests are in, you compare your diagnosis with that obtained from histology and determine your test's accuracy. Let us assume that you have already done this and found your accuracy encouraging but not perfect. This is fine. After all, you do not expect a blood test to be as accurate as an invasive procedure. Instead, your blood test is intended to aid diagnosis rather than as a gold standard for definitive determination of whether or not the disease is present.

Having completed the feasibility trial and obtained satisfactory results, you now plan a pivotal trial—a study aimed to prove to both regulators and consumers that your test is useful. When developing the trial's protocol, you will need to provide complete information on the planned trial, including (1) the intended use population for your product and (2) where and how you will obtain subjects for it.

Considering the first issue, you would like your test to be used for screening in general—for everyone. But this is impractical; you cannot expect physicians to routinely screen all their patients for a rare disorder, nor can you expect health care providers to pay for it. So you decide to be less ambitious and define a limited intended use population. For example, you might state that your test is meant for "all those who underwent biopsy for the specific cancer." Upon further consideration you realize that this too makes little sense. If patients have already done the gold standard test, why trouble them with one that is less accurate? In other words, your intended use population should not be those who have already undergone the test.

So you decide to take one step back in the diagnostic process and define your target group as those "at risk for the cancer or suspected of it." These are patients who the physician may or may not ultimately send for biopsy. The physician's final decision regarding biopsy will be based on the best available information on the patient—data obtained from physical examination, family history, routine lab tests, and other information. The goal, you decide, is to have your blood test included among this collection of assessments that comes under the heading "best available information" (excluding biopsy, which may or may not follow the initial assessments). This is reasonable, since a biopsy is a serious procedure, and one should use noninvasive tests before deciding on it.

More formally, you specify that your blood test is intended as "a *diagnostic aid* for individuals at risk for the cancer." The test, you claim, is "an aid" and not meant to be definitive by itself.

Now that you have defined your intended use population, you begin recruiting subjects from this population for the trial. This, then, is one, basic function of a well-defined target population: It determines the group of people from among whom you will select for study.

Since your product has yet to be approved, the information it provides will not be used in the trial. Participating physicians will be asked to decide on referral to biopsy in the usual manner.[4] Your aim in this trial is to demonstrate your diagnostic efficacy—your test's accuracy—by comparing its results with those obtained from the gold standard biopsy. Once demonstrated, it can actually be applied in the diagnostic process, but not before.

The trial has begun, and the physicians proceed as usual. Subjects in the trial undergo your test, and a good portion of them—let us say, about 40%—are sent on to biopsy. Some of these turn out positive for the cancer and others negative. You conduct statistical analyses comparing your test's outcomes to those of biopsy, find the blood test's accuracy reasonable, and present your data to the regulator for approval.

All seems to be going smoothly until the regulator's statistician asks, "What about the 60% of patients who were not sent for a biopsy? Do you know how accurate your blood test is in *that* group?" Some of them were diagnosed negative by your test and others positive. And having no gold standard reference diagnosis for them, you cannot evaluate your test's accuracy for them. Now this would seem

---

[4] Indeed, it would be best if in this trial the physician would not be made aware of your blood test's results. Until the time that your test is approved for marketing, it should not be used for treatment decisions.

A CATCH (FOR EXAMPLE)—CONT'D

an impossible question to answer, since there is no definitive diagnosis for these patients. All you know about them is that the physician was convinced they do not have the cancer and so did not send them for invasive testing. But a physician's decision, unlike a biopsy, is not a gold standard diagnosis. Technically, then, you cannot evaluate your test's accuracy in this group.

You think about it for a few moments and give what seems to you an obvious answer: "There is no reason," you say, "to assume that my test performs any differently in this group than in those referred to biopsy. I would therefore like your decision to be based only on those 40% of patients who underwent both diagnostic tests." In other words, you assume that the accuracy obtained when comparing your test to the gold standard is similar in those not referred to a biopsy.

Your reply seems to have no effect on the regulator's statistician, who replies, "Those not referred to a biopsy are different in that the physician did not suspect them of having cancer. Your blood test's accuracy may or may not be the same in that group as in the other, but we do not know. In fact, there is reason to believe that your test is less accurate in the nonbiopsy group. After all, those who were not sent to invasive testing have milder symptoms than the others, and it may be more difficult to separate the positives from the negatives in this milder-symptom group. Regardless, you cannot assume that the results obtained in one group apply to the other as well."

Your face darkens. Then you consider suggesting that all those not sent for invasive testing should be assumed negative; while they have not been diagnosed by a biopsy, the physician decided that they are negative, and you will use this diagnosis to test your accuracy in this group. Now you must consider the following:

1. You do not know whether the regulator will accept this answer. After all, it is a biopsy, rather than a physician's decision, that is considered the gold standard.
2. Even if the regulator accepts your argument, you have no idea how many of the nonbiopsy patients were diagnosed negative by your blood test. This is one analysis that you have not done. In other words, you have no idea how accurate you are versus the physician's "negative" diagnosis.

So before making this second suggestion, you plan on reanalyzing your data to assess their agreement with the physicians' negative diagnosis. And even if your results turn out to be favorable, you still do not know whether the regulator's decision will be favorable as well.

It seems, then, that intended use populations are not always easily defined. And once defined, they can be difficult to study comprehensively. How would *you* suggest solving this problem? For those of you particularly interested in this sort of scenario, I should mention that this issue is called **referral bias** (or **verification bias**), the statistical treatment of which is beyond the scope of this book.

SAMPLES

Another characteristic of populations is that they are virtually always very large. Indeed, they are so large that in almost all cases our attempt to learn something about them must be from a **sample**; we do not, and usually *cannot*, study the whole population. I shall define a sample as *a subset of a population that is obtained by sampling from the population*. Simple.

There are many sampling methods in clinical trials, and I shall discuss a few of them in future chapters. Here, I wish only to point out that samples are designed to represent the populations from which they are obtained. Putting this together with the preceding chapters, we get the following standard procedure for a clinical trial and for research in general:

1. Define the product attributes of interest for the specific study, including efficacy, safety, compliance, and so forth.
2. Specify the intended use population for the product.
3. Identify subjects from the intended use population and select a sample of them.
4. Measure the relevant endpoints—those relating to the attributes of interest specified—on each member of this sample. For example, if your study assesses efficacy, you might measure Cure for each subject scored as 0 ("not cured") or 1 ("cured").
5. Use your results to estimate the parameter of interest in the population. For example, compute % Cure in your sample, which becomes your best estimate for % Cure in the population; in other words, your trial's outcome is meant to estimate what the outcome would have been had you studied the whole population (which you cannot).
6. Report the results obtained with the suggestion that they represent the true values in the population more or less.

Suppose you are testing a new product for migraine headaches and are at the very beginning of trials in humans. Your natural first step is a Phase I study in a sample of healthy individuals—people who do not suffer from migraines. Once you show your drug is safe in Phase I, you will move on to testing feasibility in Phase II on those experiencing the disorder. Phase III is far into the future, and you are not thinking about it at the moment.

Earlier I noted that it is you who determines the population, which is based on your particular interest. Well, you already seem to have a problem here in that the healthy volunteers of Phase I do not really interest you. Still, they have now become your population of interest. Why is this so? Truth be told, you have no choice in the matter. Your drug has yet to be tested in humans, and before testing it in those who are ill, both regulator and ethics committees require that it be tested on the subjects who are most resilient—on those who do not have the problem. At this early stage the medical community is most concerned that your product does no harm, that it is *safe*. Once that is established, you will be allowed to test efficacy in the diseased population.

So for the moment, healthy volunteers *are* your population of interest, and this is because (1) they are hardier than your ultimate intended use group and so most appropriate for testing safety early on, and (2) their biological system is sufficiently similar to those with the ailment so that what you learn about the drug from the healthy group can, with respect to safety, apply to the other. In other words, we expect results in healthy humans to **generalize** to those with the illness. This, of course, should not be a new idea. After all, your research began in test tubes of which the results you generalized to mice and continued with generalizing results from mice to humans. Clearly, neither test tubes nor mice were your intended use population.

Moving on, you have collected data from a sample of 20 healthy volunteers and found two safety problems of note. Specifically, two of the subjects experienced a mild bout of sweating after taking the first pill. The trial's principal investigator believes that these **adverse events** (AEs) are related to the drug but judged them mild enough to allow both subjects to complete the trial. Based on the results obtained in Phase I, you conclude that the drug is safe enough to be tested in those who have migraines. Have you made the right decision? Assuming that Phase I was conducted properly, the short answer is "yes." At the same time, we should take a more careful look at what exactly was done here.

You sampled 20 people from a very large population and obtained (mostly) favorable results. You then concluded that this sample of 20 provides enough information to conclude that the drug is safe in general. Now you may recall my emphasizing that scientific enquiry requires precisely defined terms. And here I described a population as "very large," which does not seem particularly precise. So at this stage I will formally state that populations are sufficiently large that, in statistics, they are considered *infinite* in size. Now while this may not be the case every time, for all practical purposes this is so. You see, you could have selected 200 or 2,000 and would still have obtained only the tiniest of fractions from the population of healthy individuals. And when you go on to conduct a trial in subjects with migraines, whatever numbers you choose will still constitute a very small portion of all those with the illness. Thus, in virtually all clinical trials the number of subjects participating is a minuscule proportion of the population they aim to represent.

The fact is that when sampling you will never know *exactly* how safe your pill is in any population. To know this, you will have to measure each and every member of the population. And since this cannot be done—since you are forever constrained to learning about the whole from subsets of it—populations are, for all practical purposes, so "very large" that they are infinite. Now if I really want to get technical here, I would provide examples of finite populations that can be measured in their entirety. Instead, I shall compromise and provide additional details in a footnote.[5]

---

[5] For example, we might define all girls in a specific fifth-grade class at a specific school as our population and go on to measure all of them on a parameter of interest. Similarly, there might be a very rare disease where it is realistically possible to measure all individuals known to suffer from it. But we must consider that (1) these cases are sufficiently rare and are not particularly relevant to this book, and (2) even in cases such as these, one is, in fact, often sampling. Let us take the rare disease where the researcher's goal is typically to learn something about this disease in general and thus about those who will contract it in the future as well. In this sense, even measuring all who currently have the disease is sampling from a population. It is just that some in this population are not at this time available.

Getting back to the initial question, why could you conclude that your drug is safe based on a sample of 20 subjects? Indeed, why not 200 or 2,000? Well, in Phase I there is usually no formal statistical justification for this. It is just that over time certain conventions have developed, and one of these is that relatively small numbers of subjects are enough for testing safety early on.[6] There is some statistical logic to this in that the size of Phase I trials is based on experience, which is another way of saying "empirical data." But while there is statistical logic here, there is usually no hard and fast statistical justification for the specific sample size of the kind you find in later stages. And, as all my general rules, this one has exceptions as well.

In summary, samples are subsets of populations, and the results obtained from them are designed to generalize to the population. Whether or not this is actually what happens is a crucial question that we shall address in the following chapter.

---

[6] Keep in mind that Phase I is only done after extensive preclinical testing, much of which is designed to demonstrate a drug's safety in biological systems similar to humans. Moreover, Phase I testing is usually very thorough, with subjects kept in the hospital throughout and tests—vital signs, blood chemistry—taken continuously.

Estimation

CONTENTS

- Clinical trial data: sampling, estimating, and knowing
- Sample statistics and population parameters
- Using point estimates in a drug trial
- Quantifying intuition in the treatment of migraine
- Sampling error
- Confidence intervals

INTRODUCTION: FACT AND FICTION

Imagine that you run a two-arm trial testing a drug for reducing fever, with the goal being to demonstrate safety and efficacy. There are 22 subjects in Treatment, 26 in Control, and you take their Temperature at baseline and at three-hour time points. The protocol specifies that baseline Temperature should be measured no more than 10 minutes before taking the drug and not after; final assessment should be within 10 minutes of the three-hour time point.

Assessing one of the subjects at baseline, you find his temperature to be 38.5 °C. The subject's temperature was measured about two minutes before he took the pill. At three hours and four minutes, his temperature was 37.2 °C, a 1.3 °C reduction. Depending on his group, the result may be favorable, unfavorable, or somewhere in between. Be that as it may, I will focus on the more basic question, "Can you believe what you see?," and in way of an answer, I shall ask a few more questions:

- If you had taken the subject's temperature seven minutes before he took the pill instead of two minutes, would his temperature have been 38.5 °C exactly?

- If you had assessed the subject at three hours minus six minutes instead of three hours and four minutes, would you have gotten an identical 1.3°C reduction from the baseline?
- If another individual were randomly selected to participate in the trial instead of this one, would she have shown a 1.3°C reduction as well?
- Having completed the trial, you find that the average reduction was 1.8°C in Treatment and 1.0°C in Control, a difference of 0.8°C in favor of Treatment. If each group had consisted of 31 subjects (instead of 22 and 26 in Treatment and Control, respectively), would you have gotten the same result?

I will give you a hint: The answer to all of these questions is "Not much of a chance." In other words, "No."

Now the implication of all this is that *you cannot trust what you see*, which is something you likely learned long ago along with "Don't talk to strangers." This particular issue has also been central for some great personages like Kant, Schopenhauer, Berkeley, Locke, Holmes, and Houdini. So when you see a 0.8°C difference in reduction between two drugs, you cannot really believe it. Nor could you have trusted another number had it emerged. And if this is the case, how can you conclude *anything* from clinical studies? In fact, if empirical data cannot be trusted, what is the use of science? Well, let us not go overboard.

SOME TERMINOLOGY

In the preceding chapter I described a Phase I study in which you obtained a sample of 20 healthy volunteers to test the safety of a drug for migraine headaches. Having found only two subjects experiencing mild AEs, you concluded that the drug was sufficiently safe to advance to the next stage of testing.

Claiming that your product is "sufficiently safe" is a good start, but you need to be more precise. Specifically, you must *quantify* the statement, which you do by stating that about 10% (2 out of 20) individuals who take the medication may experience mild bouts of sweating. You also add that to the best of your knowledge there are no other AEs associated with the drug—and certainly no **serious adverse events** (SAEs).

Notwithstanding what I just wrote, these statements are based on data, so they seem to be sound. They very well might be. Still, as noted in the preceding section, you cannot take the process generating these data for granted. You have, in statistical terminology, engaged in **estimation**—approximated a population value from a sample. Specifically, you obtained a sample of 20 individuals, measured some endpoint on them (occurrence of AE), and computed a statistic (10%). In statistical terms you have obtained a **sample statistic**. Here this is the proportion of subjects experiencing AEs in the sample, which is your best estimate of the **population parameter**—the value of interest in the population and, as such, *the truth.*

Keep in mind that I have done no more than attach some terminology to the familiar activity of making statements about populations from samples. We engage in this activity continually. Thus when meeting Sheldon for the first time, you form an opinion of him; you use a single encounter (a sample of behaviors) to conclude something about Sheldon in general (his population of behaviors). And when a teacher makes up an arithmetic exam consisting of 10 questions, she expects her sample to represent all arithmetic problems of this type. She aims that the grade obtained by a pupil on *this* test with its *specific* problems will be a good estimate of the pupil's ability *in general.* The teacher has little interest in how well a pupil can solve arithmetic on a specific test. She wants to assess arithmetic ability in general, so she uses samples from the infinite population of arithmetic problems. The grade obtained is a sample statistic estimating the population parameter "true ability in arithmetic."

You may have noticed that I inserted the word "truth" here, which can mean anything from the trivial to the transcendent. In statistics its meaning is straightforward: Truth is the value in the population—the population parameter.

ESTIMATION AND CERTAINTY

You are about to start a Phase II trial testing a prophylactic drug for migraines, and I will not detain you. After extensive planning and consultation, you settle on a simple two-arm, one-month trial of 80 migraine sufferers. Half of your subjects will be randomly assigned to receive the investigational drug (Treatment) and half a placebo (Control).

The trial is done, the data have been collected, and you find that 20 subjects in Control had at least one migraine during the trial. The number experiencing migraines among those in Treatment was 10. Based on these results, you conclude the following:

1. My best estimate for the One-Month Rate of At Least One Migraine *in the population of those receiving placebo* is 20/40 = 50%.
2. My best estimate for the One-Month Rate of At Least One Migraine *in the population of drug takers* is 10/40 = 25%.
3. My drug is superior to the placebo in this trial (25% vs. 50%).
4. My drug is superior to the placebo in the population.

These are reasonable statements but this is a clinical trial and you will have to do better. You need to be *right*. Well, are you? The short answer is that you will never know. Populations are infinite in size and one cannot know the exact truth about them. As you might imagine, this is not a satisfactory answer. Both consumers and physicians expect to know how safe and effective your medication is, and here you are suggesting that it is impossible to know. That is just not good enough.

Clearly, we need some compromise, and it is this: Instead of providing definitive statements about your product, you will provide information you believe is true with "a great degree of certainty." It is the best you can do. So instead of making statements like, "I'm certain my drug causes mild AEs in 10% of subjects," consumers will have to settle for statements like "I'm pretty sure that. ..." In other words, having given up on *certainty*, you will report numbers that have a *high probability* of being true, and report the probability as well.

A WORD ON CERTAINTY

The solution suggested—foregoing definitive statements in favor of those with high probability—is not perfect. But it is the rule in life as it is in statistics. Thus when you buy a toy for your child, you assume with some degree of probability that it will function properly. It usually does, but sometimes it doesn't. Similarly, when you drive your car or fly to a distant city, you are "pretty sure" you will arrive safely. But accidents happen. Over time you have learned to live with uncertainty and minimize it to the degree you can. You buy products and make travel plans (and do much else) based on probabilistic assumptions. And while you do not formally compute these probabilities, let alone articulate them, you make intuitive use of them. In science, with the aid of statistics, we transform intuition into numbers.

Now many scholarly works are available that describe how we humans go about computing probabilities intuitively. Many of these show that we do it often—and badly. Yet we muddle along regardless, building roads and cities, bearing children and raising them, and engaging in a variety of other activities with a fair degree of competency. Still, in both science and life we must live with uncertainty.

At the same time, it should be obvious that our "probability requirements" differ between situations. For example, when you decide to take an umbrella to work, you would like to have made the right decision, but if you did not, it is not a disaster. At worse, you are inconvenienced by an unnecessary umbrella when it does not rain or, having decided to forgo the umbrella when it does rain, you get a little wet. This is not the case in medical products, where incorrect decisions typically have more serious consequences.

So let us agree that while we are generally reconciled to uncertainty, its acceptable level varies from one situation to another. Specifically, where life and limb are concerned, we aim to keep uncertainty at a minimum. And what this "minimum" should be, and how we go about obtaining it, is something statisticians are particularly concerned with.

Getting back to the issue at hand, we agree that empirical studies cannot yield the perfect truth. Still, some studies will provide better information than others and when planning a trial you try to make yours one of the good ones.

Now there are many factors that determine the accuracy of a particular study's information, including:

- The degree to which measures can provide consistent results—that is, the extent to which they are **repeatable** and **reproducible**.

- The degree to which measures are relevant to the issue under investigation—in other words, **valid**. For example, you can measure shoe size with both accuracy and repeatability, but doing so will usually not be terribly relevant for most clinical indications.
- The degree to which subjects are similar to those in the intended use population—that is, the degree to which your sample is representative of the population.
- The number of subjects in your trial—that is, your study's sample size.

There are many other factors, and I shall cover the most important ones when discussing clinical trial design. For the moment I will focus on the issue of sample size only.

While we agree that you can never know the truth in the population, we can also agree that the larger your sample size, the nearer the truth you can expect to be.[1] For example, you put greater trust in the results of a poll of 500 people than you do in one of 50. Similarly, you are more comfortable labeling someone a "good student" if you know that she achieved good grades on several tests as opposed to one. Examples like these abound and have found their way into our language as well. For instance, you "take a second look" when you are unsure of something, which in statistical terms means that you have enlarged your sample from one to two in an effort to get nearer to the truth.

Summarizing thus far:

1. Knowing the truth in the population with absolute certainty is virtually impossible in both everyday and clinical trials.
2. We are thus forever constrained to probability-like statements.
3. The degree of certainty associated with any statement is in great measure determined by the sample size it is based on; the larger the sample, the greater the level of certainty.

Now long before reading this book you knew that more observations lead to greater certainty. At the same time, there is something you may not know that is essential: the *functional* relationship between sample size and certainty. This is the actual amount with which certainty changes as sample size changes. Consequently, you cannot *quantify* just how sure you are of a particular result given a specific sample size. And in clinical trials you will need to know this.

So we agree that a poll of 500 provides more confidence in results than one of 50. But without some mathematics, we will not be able to say just how much greater our confidence is. And if team A beats team B twice in a row, you are more confident of A's superiority than if it had won once only. Yet here too you do not know how to *quantify* by how much your certainty has increased in the second instance relative to the first.

---

[1] Assuming, of course, that the other factors affecting your data's accuracy are, more or less, taken care of.

Let us agree that using phrases like "fairly certain" or "pretty sure" is fine in our everyday lives but not sufficient in clinical trials. To get your product to market, you will need to make some very specific *quantitative* statements about its attributes. These consist of two types:

1. The first type of statement relates to the attributes of the product itself—attributes such as safety and efficacy. For example, you might claim that the drug (a) causes mild AEs in about 10% of those who take it and (b) reduces the incidence of migraines by 50%.
2. The second type of statement relates to the degree of confidence you have in the estimates provided. You might, for example, wish to say that you are 99% confident of the numbers reported. Unfortunately, you cannot.

Now the first statement is straightforward and simply involves computing sample statistics from study data. You then cite these sample statistics as your best estimates of population parameters—of how the drug will perform when used by a large number of people. The second statement is more involved, in part because it is also dependent on the relationship between sample size and accuracy.

POINTS ESTIMATES AND INTERVAL ESTIMATES

At this stage I have already defined sample statistics, presented examples of them, and noted that quantities like Rate of Migraine obtained in a trial provide your best estimates of the truth. And they do. But they are also *wrong*. This should come as no surprise, since I have emphasized all along the limitations of samples in representing populations. Because populations are infinite and you cannot measure all of the elements in them, you also cannot know the absolute truth about them. In other words, you have *zero* certainty about any estimate of a population parameter.

Oddly, this logic makes no distinction between small samples or large; with both you are equally certain that your specific estimate is wrong. Yet, this is the way it is: For large samples or small, you can pretty well take for granted that your **point estimate** of the population parameter is incorrect. But if this is the case, how can we express the apparent "accuracy advantage" of larger samples over small ones?[2] It seems, then, that we require a somewhat different approach.

---

[2] I write "apparent" because on occasion a smaller sample might, by chance, yield a better estimate than a larger one. But this hedging my bets with "apparent" is cumbersome, and I shall omit it in the future. Be that as it may, you should keep in mind that on occasion, smaller samples yield more accurate estimates than larger ones by chance.

While all samples provide wrong estimates, we expect larger samples to yield values *nearer* to the truth. Thus when discussing an estimate's accuracy, you should not be asking whether or not you have hit the nail on the head (you *know* the answer to that one). You should rather be asking how close to the nail you pounded the hammer. In estimates, as in hand grenades, close counts. So from here on I shall be dealing with *distance* of point estimates from the truth rather than assessing whether a specific value is right or wrong.

Recall that in the preceding section I mentioned that there is a functional relationship between sample size and level of certainty—a mathematical formula relating the size of samples to the accuracy of the estimate yielded by them. Using the rationale presented, we can expect this relationship to relate to distance. Specifically, the functional relationship describes how increases in sample size yield values that are nearer to the truth in the population.

Now all of this appears to be reasonable, but it seems to have a basic flaw—in fact, a seemingly fatal one. Recall that we wish to know the truth in the population and have reconciled to never knowing it. So instead, I suggest an alternative that involves determining just how near the truth an estimate might be given the sample size derived from it. *But if I cannot know the truth, how am I ever to know my distance from it?*

Well this is indeed a problem, which I will summarily dismiss by noting that mathematicians have already taken care of it. And this elegant theory formulated hundreds of years ago has been tested with the brawn of modern computing and found to work. In short, it can be trusted.

Having set the backdrop, I will now move forward on the issue of distance using the concept of **interval estimate**—estimation that takes into account an interval-distance from the truth, as opposed to the point estimation. To do this, I will appeal once more to your Phase II clinical trial of a drug for migraines and make the following statements (with absolute certainty):

1. Before conducting the trial, you have no empirical information on the efficacy of your drug. So all you can say with complete certainty is that among those taking the medication, between 0% and 100% will experience at least one migraine a month.
2. Having conducted the trial and found that 25% experienced migraines, you can now say for certain that the true rate in the population is neither 0% nor 100% exactly.

Now let me introduce into this mix the more intriguing, if more distressing, uncertainty.

Whatever the truth about your drug, you can, after having conducted the trial, state the following:

1. The population parameter—the true Migraine per Month Rate for those taking your drug—is over 0% and less than 100%; it cannot be 0% because some subjects experienced migraines, and it cannot be 100% because some did not. Where exactly between 0% and 100% you do not know, but you *can* say the following:
   (a) The true value is very likely between 1% and 99%.
   (b) It is less likely to reside between 15% and 35%.
   (c) It is even less likely to reside between 24% and 26%.
   (d) It is not 25%.

Statements (a) to (d) can be summarized by saying that the narrower the interval, the less confident you are that the true population value is in it. Unfortunately, the more informative the interval—the narrower it is—the less certain you are of it. Thus, you are absolutely sure the true rate is between 0% and 100%, which is useless information. And you are absolutely sure that the 25% obtained is wrong, a specific value that (had it been right) would have been most informative of all. In short, the narrower the interval I specify around my point estimate, the less likely the true population parameter is to be in it.

Now all these statements are associated with the idea of **sampling error**, which is the statistical term for saying that samples do not perfectly represent populations. Sampling error can be small or large; it may yield an estimate of 25% when the truth happens to be 25.76%, or 33.0%, or any other rate between 0 and 100. The particular inaccuracy of a given estimate is subject to sampling error and cannot be known because the true population parameter is unknowable. Yet, what you do know is this: *Larger samples yield, on average, smaller sampling error.* And what you know intuitively, in statistics translates into probabilities. Specifically, it enables you to state the probability with which the true population value falls within a specified interval and thus:

- The larger the sample, the smaller the sampling error.[3]
- And the smaller the sampling error, the narrower the interval I can specify with a given probability that the true value is in it. For example, if I obtained 25% from a sample of 20, I am less certain that the true population value is between 20% and 30% than if I obtained 25% from a sample of 100. I recommend that you read the preceding sentence a few times until it makes completes sense to you.

---

[3] I just want to remind you again that this is true "on average," since small samples may, by blind luck, yield better estimates than large ones.

So for any given sample size, statistics provides us tools to construct intervals of a given width with a specified probability that the true value is in the interval. And, once again, we have a sentence that you should probably read a few times before moving on.

In statistics we translate this reasoning into numbers using the concept of **confidence interval** (CI). For example, stating that the 95% CI is between 20% and 30% is saying that I am 95% confident that the true population value lies between these two values.[4]

The mathematical formulation relating the width of a CI to the sample size can, in most cases, be provided by the **central limit theorem**. The theorem came into its final form early in the twentieth century, though elements of it have been with us for almost 300 years. Applying the theorem, I can construct an interval around the sample mean—an interval within which the true population mean is likely to be. I construct this interval using the sample size and other parameters. For the moment, I remain with sample size.

SUMMARIZING AND A BIT MORE

In statistics we deal with two types of estimates: point and interval. A point estimate is my best guess of the truth but is wrong, and an interval estimate provides a range within which I believe it likely that the truth resides. The probability that the population parameter is indeed within a given interval is in great measure a function of sample size. Thus, constructing a 95% CI will yield a wide interval when the sample is small and a narrow interval when the sample is large. At the extreme, when my sample is infinite—when it is actually *the* population—the width of the interval is 0; the value obtained is exactly the value in the population. In other words, it is no longer an estimate, and I no longer have an interval.

I use the 95% CI example because, for reasons unknown, it is the most frequently used in clinical trials; it is the standard. Yet applying the same type of computations, I can construct intervals of varying confidence as well. As you might expect, a 90% CI is narrower than a 95% CI, and an 80% CI is narrower still. If this is not apparent to you, give it some thought. Understand why this is so, and you will understand the concept of CI.

---

[4] The formal (technical) definition in statistics of a CI is different. It is actually "I am certain with some P% that repeated samples of this size will yield statistics within a particular interval." In practice, however, it is used as described here: the interval within which the truth—the population parameter—resides with a given probability. For the sake of completeness (and correctness), the formal definition of a confidence interval is the interval within which a specified percent of results will fall when your study is conducted repeatedly. From this point on, however, I shall use the more practical definition.

Being able to compute CIs opens a whole new world for us—one in which we can make decisions and attach specific probabilities to them. It allows us to make informed decisions quantified in probability terms. As such, *CIs enable us to know just how informed our decisions really are*. And this is very different from everyday statements such as "I think that…"

In chapters that follow, I will relate CIs to statistical testing, which is central in clinical trials. At this stage I would like to present a practical example of decision making aided by the CI, which is presented in the box below.

HOW CONFIDENT IS CONFIDENT ENOUGH?

You are running for public office, and you commission a poll among independent voters. Before conducting your poll, you determine that as long as at least 20% of these voters support you, there is no need to invest more resources in them; 20% is all you will need from this population to win the election. This is important information because your resources are limited and you must optimize their use.

At this stage of the campaign you believe that you are at least there—that your support among independent voters is at 20% or higher. But while you "believe" this is the case, you are sufficiently unsure to be worried about it. And now you must decide just how many resources to invest in the poll itself. The larger the sample you commission, the nearer to the truth your outcome will be. But larger samples are more costly, and you have other activities to fund as well. Consulting with a statistician, you learn that if you sample 100 people, the 90% CI will be about 14% wide. For example, if the result is 22%, you will know with 90% confidence that the true proportion of supporters among the undecided is between about 16% and 30%. Is this good enough? Probably not. But this is for you to decide, not for the statistician. If, on the other hand, you believe yourself nearer to 30%, a poll of 100 will do, since the confidence interval around 30% (or a similar value) is between 23% and 38%. In other words, if your result is near 30% and the size of your poll is 100, you will be 90% sure that you have exceeded the 20% minimum set for yourself.

As noted some time ago, one's "confidence requirements" depend on the circumstances. It will be you (and regulators and others) who will decide just how confident you must be of any particular estimate. The statistician cannot help you a great deal with this, since these requirements usually relate to considerations other than mathematics.[5] Once you decide how confident of your estimate you need to be, the statistician will tell you how many subjects will get you there. And even after the study is done, you will not have perfectly precise information. Yet you will have enough data to make informed decisions. And this is not bad at all.

---

[5] I am being a bit harsh on the statistician here. It is true that his forte is computing numbers, and it is generally up to you—the drug developer—to interpret these numbers in the most appropriate manner. At the same time, your run-of-the-mill statistician has been exposed to numerous medical product development projects. As a result, he can likely provide useful tips on what is and what is not acceptable when estimating true population values in varying circumstances.

CHAPTER 7

From Description to Testing: A Beginning

"God, therefore, stands in no need of general ideas; that is to say, he is never sensible of the necessity of collecting a considerable number of analogous objects under the same form for greater convenience in thinking. ...

General ideas are no proof of the strength, but rather of the insufficiency of the human intellect; for there are in nature no beings exactly alike, no things precisely identical, nor any rules indiscriminately and alike applicable to several objects at once. The chief merit of general ideas is that they enable the human mind to pass a rapid judgment on a great many objects at once; but, on the other hand, the notions they convey are never otherwise than incomplete, and they always cause the mind to lose as much in accuracy as it gains in comprehensiveness."

—Alexis de Tocqueville[1]

CONTENTS

- Statistics, "an imperfect but necessary expedient"
- Our psychology and descriptive statistics
- ANOVA: analyzing variation to compare means
- Statistical and clinical thinking
- Significance: a hint of things to come using a diagnostic device
- Sensitivity
- Specificity
- Type I Error and Type II Error in diagnostic accuracy

---

[1] de Toqueville, A. Democracy in America (Volume 2, Chapter 2). 1840. Project Gutenberg, 2006. netLibrary. http://www.gutenberg.org/files/816/816-h/816-h.htm.

INTRODUCTION

What the deity is or is not credited with has been a matter of faith and speculation for some millennia. I will attempt no contribution to the issue. But I *will* discuss statistics, readily admitting its ungodly nature as an "imperfect but necessary expedient" in the sense that de Tocqueville meant. Viewed thus, science itself represents intellectual insufficiency being a symptom of this need for "general ideas." But for weakness or strength, statistics does its best to support the research process. And I shall attempt here to show how.

In Chapter 5 I observed that both child and statistician look for commonality in objects so as to lump them together. Like the rest of us, they collect "a considerable number of analogous objects under the same form for the greater convenience in thinking." In statistics we call this collection of analog objects a *population*. I then described the process of selecting samples from these large collections to learn about the many from the few.

Sample data in hand, the statistician's natural inclination is to *describe* them. He does this by computing sample statistics like proportions, means, **medians**, **ranges**, and standard deviations. This activity constitutes a large part of statisticians' efforts and comes under the heading of descriptive statistics.

Many descriptive techniques are straightforward and easily done with Excel or any of the many available statistical software packages. We thus compute "mean Income," "median House Price," "proportion of Waking Hours Spent in Front of the TV," and so on. There are also graphical descriptions such as **histograms**, **scatterplots**, and others. Yet, be they numeric or graphical, simple or complex, descriptive statistics must be applied wisely because they "always cause the mind to lose as much in accuracy as it gains in comprehensiveness." You see, when doing descriptive statistics, I make the inevitable compromise of presenting a few numbers in lieu of all the data collected. And while the former are simpler to understand than the latter, they are also incomplete. I thus forgo the whole of the information in favor of comprehension—a necessary expedient.

A less complementary word for descriptive statistics is *stereotyping*, which the *Oxford Dictionary* defines as a "simplified idea of the characteristics which typify a person or thing." Substitute "population" for "person or thing" and you have described sample statistics like the mean and median.

Now the activity of stereotyping has gotten a bad name, and there is some justification for that. But, as de Tocqueville pointed out, we have no choice in the matter. Our mind is simply not built for handling each and every peculiarity of each and every member of a population. So, for example, when I say that the average height of women in New Zealand is 163 centimeters, I well know that most of them are taller or shorter. Indeed, there are probably very few at the mean exactly; in presenting 163 centimeters for the mean, I sacrifice accuracy "to gain comprehension."

Simplification is a central goal of descriptive statistics, but there can be such a thing as too much of it—of summarizing the original data to a point where the result is more misleading than informative. The statistician's challenge is to present summary statistics that tell the data's story as accurately as possible, which is often harder than it seems. Consequently, we should keep in mind that any particular sample statistic may be a good descriptor of the data or less than that. And by way of an example, I will present the following four hypothetical **distributions** of numbers:

> A. 8, 8, 8, 8, 8, 8, 8, 8
> B. 6, 7, 7, 7.5, 8.5, 9, 9, 10
> C. 4, 4, 4, 4, 12, 12, 12, 12
> D. 0, 0, 0, 0, 0, 0, 64

In all four sets the mean is 8, and in three of the four none of the individual numbers are at the mean exactly. From this standpoint alone, 8 is an imperfect simplification of all but the Distribution A, which it represents perfectly. At the same time, further examination of the numbers suggests that the number 8 varies in the degree to which it appropriately represents the other three distributions. Clearly it is a better descriptor of B than of C and D; in B all of the numbers are distributed uniformly around 8, even though an actual "8" does not appear in it. This is not the case in C and D, where the numbers are generally further from the mean. At the same time, in C the numbers are symmetrically distributed around 8 (all are equally far from it), which makes the number a better descriptor than in D, which is "lopsided" distribution.

I have little doubt that you can find additional reasons for one distribution being more appropriately described by the mean than another. You might also come up with alternative summaries that may be more informative, such as the following:

1. When describing D, one should exclude the large number (64) for being an **outlier** and only then go on to compute descriptive statistics.
2. No summary statistic is appropriate for C as a single unit, since its numbers appear to have been sampled from different populations.

Indeed, C is particularly interesting in that one might claim that the numbers in it originated from two populations: one with a mean of 4 and the other of 12. And if this were the case, it is inappropriate to compute an overall mean for C, since, as noted, descriptive statistics should be done separately for each population. Two or more groups should not be combined when computing sample statistics like means and standard deviations because they provide misleading information.

FROM DESCRIPTION TO TESTING

I have been talking about descriptive statistics and will soon discuss hypothesis testing, which is at the heart of the **scientific method**. In both I avoid formal technique to the degree possible. At the same time, it is difficult to resist something as elegant and intuitive as **analysis of variance** (ANOVA) when it rears its attractive head.

Look at C, and you will find that even though all of the numbers are presented in a single list, it consists of two groups: one with a mean of 4 and one with a mean of 12. If I told you that the first four numbers came from the Control group and the remainder came from the Treatment group, you would likely conclude that there is a (significant) difference between them. "Treatment," you would say, "seems to differ from Control." Formalizing, I can do the following:

1. Compute the standard deviation—a description of spread—for all the numbers combined and obtain 4.3.
2. Compute the standard deviation for the two groups separately and come up with 0 for each.

The difference between the standard deviations obtained suggests that the "variation within each group" is much smaller than the "variation overall." In other words, comparing these variations, I get an indication of whether they ought to be combined or separated. Thus ANOVA, like all methods of hypothesis testing, provides us with a quantitative index of whether data should be separated or combined. In the current context, its logic is as follows:

1. Computing the mean for all the numbers in Distribution C, I obtain 8.
2. 8 is a pretty bad descriptor of this list of numbers because:
   a. There is not a single number 8 on the list.
   b. The numbers are stacked in two groups—one at 4 and the other at 12, and there are no numbers in between.
   c. Each of these stacks is uniform and pretty far from the mean of 8.

I will thus conclude that while 8 is in fact the true mean of Distribution C, it is a bad descriptor of it. A better option might be to provide the mean for each group separately—4

for the first and 12 for the second. And by doing this, I indicate my belief that these numbers represent two populations.

It is important to note that all this makes sense only if you also have some additional information suggesting that there are two populations here—for example, when the first group includes only subjects receiving Treatment and the second Control (or, for instance, when one group includes females and the other males). Simply taking a distribution and arranging its numbers by size and calling the different sizes "groups" is usually not very useful.[2]

Now this should be very familiar to you, since it is very much how you identify populations. For example, you might observe a group of people in which there are both adults and children. Unconsciously you might note that on the variable Size there is little variation within each group separately. But when combining the groups, the variation of Size is great. Thus, you would conclude that there are two populations here. It is the same when looking at trees and cars. While trees differ greatly from one another, as do cars, the variation within each group separately is much smaller than that of the groups combined. Thus, comparing the variation within a group to that overall provides an efficient method for identifying populations.

While the formulas associated with ANOVA are somewhat more complex than presented, the principle is the same: Examine the relative size of variation computed in different ways on the same numbers. Hence you are analyzing variance.

As it turns out, both the logic and mathematics of ANOVA are the workhorses of a large number of statistical techniques grouped under the heading of the **General Linear Model** (GLM). These include often-used procedures like ANOVA itself, correlation, regression, and t-test. And they are fine illustrations of how descriptive statistics are closely tied to hypothesis testing even though they are typically presented as separate topics.

---

[2] I write "usually" because there are techniques such as **cluster analysis** that do this, which in some circumstances can be informative. But such techniques are seldom applied to clinical trial data.

Getting back to the issue at hand, statisticians recognize that some descriptive statistics are better than others in particular situations. Consequently, in any particular application, they usually present several of them, thus providing a more complete picture of the data. In the case of Distributions A and B, I might also want to present the standard deviation, which indicates the **dispersion** of numbers around the mean. I may also add some indication of *shape* using **kurtosis** and **skewness**. Depending on the numbers' characteristics, one should select those descriptors that best tell their story—that present as complete a picture as possible despite the information lost when computing summary statistics.

I should emphasize that this is not a trivial message. Presenting your data well—in an elegant and understandable fashion—will go a long way to getting your project to succeed. When trying to understand your data, as well as help others understand it, it is well worth the effort to select the most informative descriptives for it.

As we all know, numbers can be very elastic in the hands of statisticians (and politicians, journalists, Ponzi scam artists, lawyers, etc.). Indeed, much has been written about how to present the same data in different ways depending on the story one wishes to tell. There are also jokes about this and even a well-known expletive attributed to a nineteenth-century politician. I thus feel the need to emphasize that I am *not* writing in cynical mode here. I take for granted that you who conduct clinical trials and I who analyze them wish to get at the truth. And this means that we both aim to present sample statistics in a way that will represent the data as precisely as possible. And just to make sure that both you and I keep to our resolve, regulators have put in place various procedures to keep us honest. I will deal with some of these in chapters to come.

So let us agree that summarizing data is both necessary and problematic and that de Tocqueville had a point. Yet he himself generalized and so simplified. In particular, we know that our tendency to stereotype is not equally applied—that it depends in great measure on the situation we happen to be in. Thus, to know how financial markets fared in general, I might look up one of their many summary indexes like the Dow or FTSE or DAX. Such indexes lump many stock prices into a single number, which is enough information for some purposes. But if I were interested in the performance of a specific stock, I would seek out *its* value rather than that of any index it might belong to. In other words, some situations call for generalization, while others require more precise and limited information.

I should also note that statisticians sometimes deal with individual points in their data as well. But this is most often done to identify and understand outliers—values that do not fit the general pattern of the data. As a rule, individual points do not interest the statistician, and in this we differ from clinicians, whose primary preoccupation is the individual patient.

ON STATISTICAL AND CLINICAL THINKING

An editorial in the *British Journal of Medicine*[3] explains that **evidence-based medicine** refers to "integrating individual clinical expertise and the best external evidence." The writers go on to explain that by "best available external clinical evidence we mean clinically relevant research, often from the basic sciences of medicine, but especially from patient centered clinical research." The term *evidence-based medicine* has been around for some years now and is generally accepted as good medical practice. Its application requires physicians to base treatment on both personal experience and sound clinical research.

Now this seems sufficiently obvious that one may wonder why it needs to be said at all. Well, it turns out that evidence-based medicine is often counter to everyday medical practice in which physicians tend to "think clinically" rather than statistically. You see, each patient's profile is unique, differing from all others on parameters such as Medical History, Laboratory Test Results, Age, Sex, Social Support, and Tolerance for Pain. By nature, physicians focus on the individual, and this often obscures the fact that patients are exemplars of larger groups and should be treated as such. As a result, physicians will sometimes ignore empirical research and base their decisions on their own (at times limited and erroneous) experience and intuition. This is considered sufficiently problematic to have made the issue of evidence-based medicine prominent in medical journals, as well as in formal and informal discussions between practitioners. After all, if each patient were to be viewed uniquely, there could be no general treatment guidelines, and much of medical research would be superfluous.

In this book I am most concerned with statistics in clinical trials. Thus I am more interested in statistical thinking than in clinical thinking. When planning a clinical trial, the general approach is naturally statistical; we wish to show that "in general" our product works when used by a relatively large number of individuals. And when interpreting the results of clinical trials, we typically look at summary descriptive statistics, such as the mean, rather than at individual patients. Thus, when planning clinical trials, clinical thinking can be a handicap. Yet, clinical trials are also about treating individual patients, each of whom is unique. So when considering clinical research, both statistical and clinical approaches are necessary.

The difference in approaches described often makes it difficult for physicians and statisticians to communicate with one another. Indeed, I have frequently encountered this difference in approaches to be a source of misunderstanding and even frustration (on both sides). Thus, for example, when presenting data to physicians I have found them interpreting individual data points while I obstinately maintain that they should be looking at summary statistics instead.

This difference between statistical and clinical thinking is often difficult to bridge. Yet it must be bridged. And there is no question of right or wrong here because both are required. The *British Journal of Medicine* suggests that, in the clinic, physicians should be "integrating individual clinical expertise and the best external evidence." This certainly is good advice for those conducting in clinical trials as well.

[3] Sackett DL, Rosenberg WM, Gray JA, Haynes RB, Richardson WS. "Evidence-based medicine: What it is and what it isn't." 1996, BMJ 312(7023): 71–72.

To this point I noted the fact that statisticians compute sample statistics and focus on them. By doing this they primarily emphasize the similarity of subjects in a group rather than differences between them. This, however, is only half the story.

DIFFERENCES

Say you have developed a device for detecting **sleep apnea**, a disorder characterized by pauses in breathing during sleep. A gold-standard reference (R) for diagnosing the disorder already exists, but it involves using a large and cumbersome device that requires patients hooking up to it with several wires during the night. Thus, assessment with R usually involves patients spending nights at a sleep lab, with diagnosis obtained via multichannel recording.

Your new test product (T) is simpler to use and requires only a single contact point with the body. Additionally, it is compact and can be used at home. The device includes software that records and interprets single-channel data, which can later be downloaded at the doctor's office.

You have completed the prototype and are now ready to conduct a pivotal trial for marketing approval. Many aspects of your product must be tested to obtain approval. These include procedural and material safety, efficacy, software validation, and others. In this section I will deal with efficacy, which in diagnostic devices translates into *accuracy*—that is, demonstrating that your device actually measures what it purports to measure, and does this reasonably well.

You have decided to assess T's efficacy by comparing it directly with R.[4] The trial will include 250 subjects and will take place in a sleep lab. Each subject will be connected to T and R, both of which yield a large quantity of continuously recorded data. Your primary aim in this trial is to demonstrate T's accuracy in providing a **dichotomous** diagnosis of "positive" or "negative" (respectively, sick or healthy), which is done as follows:

- For each subject, both T and R provide a count of sleep apnea episodes during the night.
- If a subject's count is below 20 (for the night), he or she is diagnosed "negative" (healthy). If the number of episodes is 20 or above, the subject is scored "positive" (sick). Thus, each individual in the trial is scored as follows:
  - 0—Negative (# of episodes < 20)
  - 1—Positive (# of episodes ≥ 20)

Here, as in many diagnostic devices, you dichotomize a continuous score by transforming it into positive or negative. The continuous score is the apnea count that can vary from 0 to infinity, while the dichotomous diagnosis is determined by assessing whether a subject's score is above or below the cutoff of 20. This is useful for physicians who find it convenient to think of patients in terms of positive or negative. Yet, in many cases—and ours is one of them—the continuous score itself is also meaningful. For example, you would expect

---

[4] Depending on the regulator and the device, there may be other options as well. For example, you may compare your device to a **predicate** (P)—an approved device, though not itself a gold standard. Your own device, if approved, may serve as P for future devices in their approval process. You might also conduct a trial in which each subject undergoes measurements with T, P, and R, aiming to show that T agrees with R more than P does. Doing the latter will allow you to claim that you are more accurate than a competitor, P. There are other options as well, with the one presented in this section among the simplest.

a subject having 7 episodes during the night to have less of a sleep apnea problem than one who has 19. Yet, transforming the number of episodes to positive or negative yields the same diagnosis for both, which in turn results in loss of information. Dealing with continuous scores in diagnostic devices is an important issue and often difficult to deal with. Here I shall remain with the relatively straightforward case of comparing T to R, each providing a dichotomous score.

Table 7.1 presents your trial's results. Specifically, it shows the dichotomous diagnosis of positive or negative by both T and R for the 250 subjects participating in the trial. Let us first understand how to read the table and then examine how to interpret the numbers in it.

- The columns represent the gold standard (R) diagnosis. Looking at the bottom row (margin), you can see that R diagnosed 100 subjects "negative" and 150 "positive."
- The rows represent the diagnoses yielded by your device, T. Looking at the leftmost column (margin), you see the sum of each row for T. Overall, T diagnosed 109 of the subjects "negative" and 141 "positive."

In other words, T and R yielded very similar results overall, with the former diagnosing 60% of the sample positive and the latter diagnosing 56% positive. However, figures relating to overall agreement of group proportions are not particularly relevant to the devices' intended use. Keep in mind that doctors wish to diagnose individual patients, not groups. Thus, you and the regulator are primarily interested in the degree to which T's and R's diagnoses agree on each subject's diagnostic status. To explore this issue, you must examine the cells inside the table rather than the **marginals** that we discussed before.

Before going on I should emphasize that the gold standard R is, by definition, correct; in the context of this particular study, it provides a subject's *true* diagnosis. Now there is no perfect measurement, and even gold standards err every so often.[5] But because they are the best we have, we treat their diagnosis as true

Table 7.1 Outcome of Test Diagnosis by Reference Diagnosis

Test Diagnosis (T)	Gold Standard Diagnosis (R)		
	0 (negative)	1 (positive)	Total
0 (negative)	81	28	109
1 (positive)	19	122	141
Total	100	150	250

---

[5] If R is especially inaccurate, we call it an **imperfect gold standard**. When this is the case, disagreements between T and R are often adjudicated with the aid of a third method.

and conduct a trial to evaluate how well T agrees with them. In other words, in any case of disagreement between T and R, we say that the latter is correct and the former is erroneous.

Estimating T's accuracy is thus done by comparing its agreement with R at the subject level and involves looking at the data in the four inner cells of the table. There are several ways to look at these data and compute statistics from them. For the purpose of our example, we shall deal with two summary statistics only:

- **Specificity:** Of the total 100 true negatives—subjects diagnosed "healthy" by R—81 were also diagnosed negative by T. Thus, T detected 81 of 100 true negatives in the sample, which yields a proportion of 0.81. This proportion is termed *specificity* and is defined as the probability of T diagnosing an individual "negative" when the individual is in fact negative.
- **Sensitivity:** Of the total 150 true positives—subjects diagnosed "sick" by R—122 were also diagnosed positive by T. Thus, T detected 122 of 150 true positives, which yields a proportion of 0.81 as well. This figure is termed *sensitivity* and is defined as the probability of T diagnosing a person "positive" when the person is in fact positive.

We thus learn that your device has both specificity and sensitivity of 0.81, which may or may not be considered acceptable. Deciding whether or not a device is sufficiently accurate is between you and the regulator. And if the device is approved for use, the market will form its opinion as well. The following are two of the factors that determine whether a device's sensitivity and specificity are acceptable:

- The device's accuracy relative to those of similar products on the market.
- The relative advantages and disadvantages of your device compared to the gold standard. In this case, T is much more convenient than R and is also less expensive. On the other hand, T is less accurate in that it identifies only 81% of true positives and true negatives. In your report to the regulator, you will need to justify this tradeoff; in other words, you will need to explain why the greater convenience and lower cost of T are sufficiently advantageous to outweigh its relative inaccuracy. This is typically justified by **risk analysis**, a section in your clinical study report (CSR). Risk analysis is, essentially, a cost-benefit evaluation of your product.

Having completed your study and submitted the CSR, you now await the regulator's decision. The regulator, however, has asked for clarifications. One of her questions—a common one that should have been foreseen and preempted in the report—is whether your device performs similarly in different subgroups of your sample. In this example the regulator asks whether your product is equally accurate in both men and women.

Table 7.2 Outcome of Test Diagnosis by Reference Diagnosis by Gender

	Men				Women		
Test (T)	Gold Standard Diagnosis (R)		Total	Test (T)	Gold Standard Diagnosis (R)		Total
	0	1			0	1	
0	48	7	55	0	33	21	54
1	12	73	85	1	7	49	56
Total	60	80	140	Total	40	70	110

To answer this question, you reconstruct Table 7.1 to cover both men and women separately, and you come up with Table 7.2. Computing specificity and sensitivity of T within each of the subgroups yields the following:

- Specificity$_{men}$ = 48/60 = 0.80; Specificity$_{women}$ = 33/40 = 0.82
- Sensitivity$_{men}$ = 73/80 = 0.91; Sensitivity$_{women}$ = 49/70 = 0.70

Looking at these numbers, it appears that your device's accuracy in detecting negatives is about the same for men and women; specificity is 0.80 and 0.82 for the two groups, respectively. However, the sensitivity obtained for men (0.91) seems much higher than for women (0.70). Based on this result, you suspect that T's ability to detect True Positives is higher in men than in women.

I write "suspect" because a difference between two point estimates obtained from a sample does not necessarily reflect a true difference in the population. Recall that it is the truth in the population rather than outcomes in a specific trial that interests you. After all, another study would have yielded different results where the difference between the sexes may have been larger or smaller (or, perhaps, in the opposite direction altogether). And because you cannot know from a sample what the true sensitivities are, you cannot be certain that the difference you see reflects a true difference in the population.

The issue involved here is central in statistics and relates to how we distinguish between observed differences that are probably due to chance from those that are real. This is done by using formal statistical testing, where at the end you conclude whether or not the differences observed are **statistically significant**— that is, whether or not they are real (and not a result of sampling error).

Here I will compare the accuracy of your device between men and women using confidence intervals. There is in fact a more appropriate test, but I will use confidence intervals because they were explained in the preceding chapter and are intuitive.[6] Recall that in constructing a confidence interval around

---

[6] The relationship between statistical testing and comparison of confidence intervals is not straightforward, and the two are not interchangeable. However, for our modest purposes, this will do.

Table 7.3 Specificity and Sensitivity with Confidence Intervals by Gender

	Specificity			Sensitivity		
Subgroup	Value	Lower Confidence Limit	Upper Confidence Limit	Value	Lower Confidence Limit	Upper Confidence Limit
Men	0.80	0.67	0.89	0.91	0.83	0.96
Women	0.82	0.67	0.93	0.70	0.58	0.80

sample statistics, I provide a range of values within which I am fairly certain that the population parameter resides. Doing this for values obtained from your study for men and women separately, I obtain the results in Table 7.3.[7]

Before going on, I should point out that for all my examples in this section I construct 95% confidence intervals. This is the standard in clinical trials and therefore the most relevant. At the same time, you may recall from the preceding chapter that you can construct any size confidence intervals you choose— that is, those that provide greater or lesser likelihoods for presence of the true value between their upper and lower limits.

Let us now examine Table 7.3 and make some statements about it:

- Specificity of T in men was 0.80, and you can be 95% confident that the true specificity in the population is between 0.67 and 0.89.
- Specificity in women is 0.82, and you can be 95% certain that the true value in the population is between 0.67 and 0.93.
  - *Conclusion:* The confidence intervals overlap, so, for example, the value 0.78 is within both intervals. This means that two specificities might actually be similar or even identical in the population. In other words, you cannot say with 95% certainty that the device's specificity is different for men and women.[8]

Note that the confidence interval for women is wider than that for men. This is because there are more men than women in this study, enabling greater precision in estimating your device's accuracy in men.

---

[7] There are several methods for computing confidence intervals for proportions, which in most cases yield similar results. The confidence intervals in the table were computed using the Exact Binomial method.

[8] When confidence intervals do not overlap, the values compared always differ significantly. However, the reverse is not always true—that is, when confidence intervals do overlap, the respective values sometimes differ significantly. This is not the case here, and this particular issue is beyond the scope of this book. It does, however, point to the difference between statistical testing done correctly and that using confidence intervals (which can sometimes yield erroneous conclusions).

- Sensitivity of T in men is 0.91, and you can be 95% certain that the true value in the population is between 0.83 and 0.96.
- Sensitivity in women is 0.70, and you can be 95% certain that the true sensitivity in the population is between 0.58 and 0.80.
  - *Conclusion:* The confidence intervals do not overlap; you can be 95% certain that sensitivity in women is no higher than 0.80 and that in men it is no lower than 0.83. Consequently, you can say with 95% confidence that sensitivity of the device is higher in men than in women.

In statistical terminology, the difference in sensitivity between men and women is significant; it is real and not due to chance. Put a bit differently, you can now claim (with 95% confidence) that the difference observed between men and woman in sensitivity is not due to sampling error; it represents a true difference. The implication of this is that, in the context of my device's sensitivity, men and women belong to different populations. Understanding this logic is critical for understanding the concept of statistical testing (or hypothesis testing) and is as follows:

- In any given study, I do not believe the point estimates obtained, since they were computed on samples from the population and, as such, are subject to sampling error. In other words, the outcomes obtained in the study may or may not well represent the truth in the population.
- Because I do not believe that point estimates are perfectly representative of the truth, I cannot interpret differences observed in them directly. Thus, for example, if I observe greater accuracy in men than in women, I cannot say for certain whether this is true in the population or merely a chance occurrence in this particular study.
- Instead of taking point estimates at face value, I build 95% confidence intervals around them. Once I construct the confidence interval, I can say with 95% certainty that the true population parameter lies between its lower and upper limits.
- Looking at the confidence intervals of the two groups, I examine whether or not they overlap. If they do not, I conclude that the groups differ significantly—that I am 95% certain they differ—that is, they belong to different populations.
- The flip side of the preceding statement is that there is a 5% chance that I am wrong—that I happened to get an extreme result by chance (by sampling error). In other words, there is a 5% chance that the groups do not truly differ despite the results observed.
- Erroneously concluding that two groups differ is, in statistics, termed **Type I Error**. (**Type II Error** is concluding that two groups do not differ when, in truth, they do.)

Given the results obtained and the logic presented, you formally conclude that "my device's sensitivity is significantly higher in men than in women, and this conclusion has at most a 5% chance of being wrong." In statistical terminology, you conclude that sensitivity is higher in men than in women at $P \leq 0.05$—that is, there is a probability of 5% or less that your conclusion is in fact due to Type I Error.

Now just to remain on the right side of the law, I must emphasize once more that significance testing is not typically done with confidence intervals. Moreover, the result of testing with confidence intervals is not always in perfect agreement with more appropriate tests. Specifically, when a significant result is obtained, the correct test will also yield this. But there can be cases where looking at confidence intervals will not suggest a significant difference, and the appropriate statistical test will show otherwise. Still, I believe that significance testing is most conveniently understood in this context and thus, for the intuitive convenience of the non-statisticians among you, I present it.

There is a great deal more to be said about statistical significance, much of which is very technical. While I wish to keep the technical aspects to a minimum, I believe that a deeper understanding of the concepts presented is essential. My aim in the next chapter is to provide such an understanding.

It is time, then, to summarize the central points of this chapter:

- Descriptive statistics are meant to summarize data for the greater convenience of thinking.
- Data summaries are more accessible to our brain but necessarily lead to loss of information.
- Data summaries make sense when done on a single population; we should not, for example, compute the mean over two populations, since it will represent neither.
- Statistical testing, also termed hypothesis testing, is a method for determining whether groups of numbers represent the same population or different ones.

In the next chapter I shall take what we learned in this one on description and testing, and draw ever nearer to formalized hypothesis testing. And I will do this with no equations—and hope to get away with it.

CHAPTER 8

Statistical Significance, Explanation, and Prediction

"[The one] whom he took to be their captain came under the tree in which Ali Baba was concealed, and making his way through some shrubs, pronounced these words so distinctly: 'Open, Sesame,' that Ali Baba heard him. As soon as the captain of the robbers had uttered these words, a door opened in the rock...."

—*Arabian Nights*[1]

CONTENTS

- Statistical significance and clinical meaningfulness
- Using data to describe *what is*
- Using data to infer *why it is so*
- Measuring central tendency and spread in data
- Variance explained, correlation and causality
- Independent and dependent variables
- Dose response in autologous cell therapy
- The normal distribution
- Multiple views on hypothesis testing:
  - testing expectation with Null and Alternative hypotheses
  - explaining variance
  - assessing relationships
  - evaluating differences
  - identifying populations

---

[1] *The Arabian Nights: Their Best-Known Tales*, unknown author, from Project Gutenberg.

INTRODUCTION: OVERVIEW AND LIMITATIONS

In my own profession, the rock-tumbling words are "statistical significance." Earn the right to say them, and you win; otherwise, you lose. And while it is not always as simple as that, often enough it is.

When statistical testing yields significance, you conclude that the difference observed reflects the truth.[2] "Drug A," you say, "is more effective than B in the population." Adding that the result was significant at $P \leq 0.05$, you also caution that there is a 5% chance you have erred in this inference. Thus, statistical testing yields conclusions with probabilities attached to them. And while your confidence in these conclusions is usually high, uncertainty will remain until you assess the whole population. In other words, uncertainty will remain.

Here is an extreme example: It is generally acknowledged that death comes to all; that it is a certainty. But, based on this evidence alone we cannot say this for certain. While history tells us there has yet to be an individual born who did not die, the observation is based on a sample only. There are billions born who have yet to die and untold numbers yet unborn. Thus, the observation "all who live die" derives from a large sample, and we have great confidence in it. But it is not based on the whole population, so statistically there is some nonzero probability that it is incorrect (although I wouldn't get my hopes up).

Getting back to real life: Having conducted a clinical trial and achieved significance, your product will be nearer approval. There will be scientific publications and presentations, and a press release as well. If your results are not statistically significant, a postmortem begins.

At times I am somewhat puzzled by the absolute importance attached to "statistical significance." You see, it is a relative concept, and it depends on one's definition of it. Thus, what is significant with one definition may not be so with another. Moreover, significance in different contexts has varying implications for a product. For example, one will typically take more seriously a significant result in a preplanned analysis than one obtained post hoc (see Chapter 9).

So while statistical significance is typically viewed dichotomously—you either obtained it or you did not—there is a continuous scale underlying it. Thus, researchers will sometimes use phrases like "highly significant," "significant," "trend toward significance," and so on. Notwithstanding, statisticians are generally less fond of these "levels of significance" and would rather keep to the dichotomous "yes" or "no." This too will be discussed.

---

[2] I shall keep here to the common case where a statistical test aims to show the difference. While at times you may want to show similarity, the term *statistical significance* retains its meaning throughout.

Then there is this: Statistical significance does not necessarily imply **clinical significance** (or **clinical meaningfulness**). Formal statistical testing indicates whether an observed outcome is likely to reflect the truth in the population. Yet it remains silent on the importance of the phenomenon itself. For example, if one drug regularly reduces fever one minute faster than another, the difference between the two is statistically significant—that is, it is consistent and so not due to chance. But few physicians will consider a single minute sufficiently meaningful to influence their decision on which of two drugs to prescribe. In this particular instance, then, we have statistical but not clinical significance.

You see, statistical significance cares nothing for clinical utility. It is not just that it is heartless but because P values are computed quantities and so tend to detachment. Like all disciplines, statistics is designed to answer some questions and does not address itself to others. My own particular task is to determine if an observed result occurred by chance or reflects some truth in the population. The clinical interpretation of the outcome itself is left for others. Now this is the party line and is true. But really, statisticians will often have something to say about clinical utility as well. Having been exposed to numerous medical products, many of us have a sense for which effects are clinically meaningful and which are not. So while making clinical claims is outside our core competence, it is not outside our competence altogether. In the following sections I present some additional ways of looking at statistical significance that I hope will provide a deeper understanding of the concept.

DESCRIPTION, INFERENCE, AND TESTING

Give me a set of observations, and I will describe them. This is the statistician's basic attitude to data. I will compute summary statistics like the mean and present simple graphs "for the greater convenience of thinking." Examining these sample statistics, I will get a feel for the numbers and learn something about the population of interest. This, then, is one level of understanding, which entails describing the way things *are*. Yet, there is another, perhaps more interesting, level that concerns *why* things are as they are.

Let me explain. In statistics, as in everyday life, we differentiate *description* from *explanation*. Descriptive statistics provide snapshots of reality and make no effort to explain why the pictures turned out as they did. Observing these pictures, I simply state that this is what we see. It is like saying "What a beautiful day!" and no more. Yet, having said this, one might also add that "the sun is shining, pigeons are cooing, and Irish eyes are smiling" and so shift from the realm of description to explanation—from presenting the way things are to explaining *why* they are so. **Inferential statistics** is the subdiscipline concerned with discovering the "why."

Now the nature of statistical explanation has a very specific form that I will describe with examples. I suggest that throughout you relate these examples to everyday reasoning, and I suspect that you will find them similar. Indeed, you will discover that you have been doing statistics long before you ever heard the word. At the same time, statistics formalizes and quantifies, an activity not often done outside of science.

Suppose I have collected data on the Height of 100 children from some neighborhood A. Describing the data, I compute the following:

- **Central tendency**—the general *location* of the numbers obtained, which is a point on the 0 to ∞ centimeter scale. The most common measure of central tendency is the mean.
- **Spread**—the variation around this central location, which is most often described by the standard deviation.

In most cases these simple descriptors provide a good summary of the numbers and thus a reasonable starting point for getting a sense of the data. At the same time they remain silent on why the numbers are as they are. They do not, for example, answer questions like these:

- Why do these children differ in Height from one another?
- Do children in Neighborhood A differ in Height from those in, say, Neighborhood B?

Now looking at these questions, you might simply say, "Who cares?"—and you may have a point. However, my aim here is not merely answering these particular questions. Rather, I provide these examples to demonstrate the sort of questions scientists ask and that statisticians answer in terms of variation. It is a concept that for many of us will take some getting used to.

Inferential statistics—the second major subdiscipline of statistics—is designed to answer these questions and others using hypothesis testing (or statistical testing). The answers provided by inferential statistics are always of the same form and constitute "statistical explanation." Unless you are very familiar with the topic, the preceding statements may sound somewhat confusing. So I will now expand the example and see where this takes us.

For each of the 100 children whose Height I measured I also obtained the Heights of their mothers. I now have two **variables**: Height of Child and Height of Mother. I then relate the two variables using, say, **regression** and/ or **correlation**. As expected, I find there is a lawful relationship between these two variables such that the taller the mother, the taller the child. Conducting statistical testing on the data (the method for which is no concern of ours at the moment), I find the result significant. In other words, I conclude that there is a nonrandom relationship—a true relation—between the Height of the mother and the child emerging from the sample, and I specify that it is significant—it is pretty likely to be true in the general population as well.

Looking at this operation more formally yields the following:

- I measured the Height of Children in Neighborhood A and found there is variation in it—that is, the children differ from one another in Height.
- For each child, I measured the Height of his or her mother. As expected, I found that there is variation in Height of Mother as well—that mothers differ in Height from one another.
- I arranged Height in mother–child pairs, computed some statistical measure of association (e.g., correlation), and found a relatively consistent relationship between the pairs: Taller mothers tend to have taller children, and shorter mothers tend to have shorter children. I note, of course, that the relationship is not perfect; some tall mothers have short children and the opposite. Still, the relationship is there.
- I can now conclude that *variation in Child Height is explained by variation in Mother Height.*

Expounding on the last statement, I then say, "There is variation in Child Height. Some are shorter and others are taller. There is also variation in Mother Height. These variations are associated such that, in general, tall mothers have taller children and short mothers have shorter children. In other words, variation in Mother Height statistically *explains* variation in Child Height (and the opposite)." In statistics we use, and quantify, **explained variance** in one variable by another.

By simply collecting data and describing them, I learn something about the way things are. By relating variables to one another, I learn something about *why* they are this way. This, then, is the nature of statistical explanation: *showing that variation in one variable is related to variation in another.*[3]

It is critical to note that statistical explanation is simply a statement of a mathematical relationship between variables. As such, it makes no claim as to *cause*. Statistically, it is perfectly legitimate to say that "variation in Child Height explains variation in Mother Height," even though the statement may seem nonsensical. Inferential statistics is designed to detect relationships, and here its role ends. The underlying cause of the relationship—for example, heredity—is left to other disciplines.

---

[3] I can also explain variation in one variable using several others. For example, variation in Height of Child can be shown to be related to variation in Height of Mothers and Fathers. There are other "explanatory combinations" as well, and I will stick to the simple case where one variable explains another, single variable.

Summarizing so far, having collected data and related between variables, I have successfully explained why children vary in Height. It is so, I say, because their mothers vary in height as well.

At the same time, scientists are well aware that it is a rare phenomenon that can be fully explained by a single other phenomenon. Variation on Height is no different. Thus, Height of Mother is only one explanation for Height of Child, and there can be many other explanations, including Nutrition, Overall Health, Socioeconomic Status, Height of Father, and so on. Taking this into account, I state that my explanation is partial. And here is an additional strength of my discipline: It can quantify the degree to which any explanation is incomplete. For example, when the correlation between two variables is 0.90, I will say that my explanation is strong: "I have explained most of the variance in one parameter with another." When the correlation is lower, my explanation is weaker—that is, I have explained less of the variation in Y with X. Thus, statistics can provide *quantities* indicating just how well I have explained a given phenomenon using one or more others.

Recall that early in this section I asked two questions. The first was why children vary in Height. Well, I have provided one answer for it. The second was concerned with differences in Height between children from different locations. I will now show that my approach to the second question is identical to the first.

As before, I collected data on Height of children in Neighborhood A. I then also collected Height data from a sample of children in Neighborhood B. I now state the following, which should sound familiar:

- I measured Height of a sample of children from Neighborhood A and a sample from Neighborhood B. I found there to be variation in both groups.
- For the sake of convenience, I arbitrarily label Neighborhood A "0" and Neighborhood B "1." Thus, there is variation on the variable Neighborhood as well (some children receive the score 0 and others 1).
- For each child I now have two numbers: Height in centimeters and Neighborhood coded dichotomously.
- Arranging these numbers as pairs for each child, I compute the relationship between them. Recall that relating Mothers and Children also involved computing the relationship between pairs of numbers.

Let us assume that I have found a lawful and significant relationship between Height and Neighborhood such that "the 'higher the Neighborhood, the taller the child"; in other words, Neighborhood 1 is associated with taller children than Neighborhood 0—the mean height in Neighborhood 1 is greater than that in Neighborhood 0. I can now claim that variation in Neighborhood explains variation in Height.[4] Once more, I must caution you that statistics has only formalized the relationship and quantifies it; I might, for example, have obtained a correlation of 0.34 between the two variables, but this alone does not imply cause. To interpret this statistical/mathematical relationship, I shall need the help of other disciplines such as genetics, sociology, and economics.

Additionally, while I have explained variation *between* Neighborhood and Height, I have not explained why there is variation in child Height *within* Neighborhood.[5] So once again my explanation is partial. In sum, *understanding* in statistics entails relating variations to one another.

ON THE PARTIAL NATURE OF SCIENTIFIC EXPLANATIONS

Describing what we see is as essential in science as it is in our everyday lives. *Explaining* our observations—saying why things are as we see them—is no less important.

Here is another example: You visit your daughter's school and observe that "most of the kids in her class ride bicycles," which is a simple account of the way things are. Hypothesizing on the reason for it, you add that "many parents of the children in her class are members of the Bike for Betterment Club (BBC)." Now this is a reasonable explanation, and it may even be right. And in everyday conversation it is surely enough. But if you wish to be scientific, you need to test your hypothesis by collecting data and analyzing them. Specifically, you need to demonstrate a positive relationship between parents' membership in bicycle clubs and children's tendency to ride a bicycle.

There are several ways to assess this relationship analytically. One of these is by simply labeling each parent and each child as being a bike rider or not. This will yield one of two values (e.g., 0 or 1) for each individual. You can then relate these parent–child dichotomous values to each other. Using another method, you could compute the proportion of parents within each class that bicycle and the proportion of children. You will then relate these "proportion pairs" measured over many classes. There are other approaches as well and, generally, none is particularly superior to another in any absolute sense. Rather, different approaches answer slightly different questions and each is correct in its place.

---

[4] For those of you who are familiar with statistical tests, I should point out that using correlation to relate a continuous variable (Height) to a dichotomous variable (Neighborhood) is equivalent to conducting an independent group's t-test.

[5] In fact, this was partially done by relating children to their mothers previously.

Let us assume that you are right and children whose parents belong to bike clubs are more likely to bike themselves (however shown). Like most explanations, this one is partial at best. Thus, it is reasonable to expect that some children whose parents belong to BBC do not bike and vice versa. In other words, the model predicting children's behavior from that of parents does not completely explain the phenomenon in question. As one might expect, there are additional factors that come into play here that may include Family Income, Geographic Location, Child Age, Parent–Child Relationship, and others.

Virtually all of our explanations—in both life and science—are imperfect (partial). And being that it is a fact of existence, it should not be particularly troubling. As scientists we would, of course, wish it were otherwise, but this is the way it is. Thus, we cannot completely explain the causes of War or Weather or Psychotic Episodes, or perfectly predict how a medical intervention will turn out. But while virtually all of our explanations are partial, some are less so than others. Thus, for example, we can predict Weather better than we can Earthquakes.

Now scientists will not be completely happy until they explain a phenomenon of interest entirely. Statistically, their aim is to explain 100% of the variation in a phenomenon. And since explanations will always be partial, it follows that scientists cannot be completely happy—a point I shall not pursue.

Yet while we expect all of our explanations to be incomplete, on occasion they are especially so. And when we feel our understanding particularly lacking, we will seek additional or alternative explanations. Indeed, much of scientific activity is concerned with strengthening explanations—with increasing the ability to comprehend a phenomenon using others. For example, if I want to predict Outcome in a particular indication, I may appeal to several variables, including Drug received, Gender, and Age. Using all three, I may obtain a better prediction of Outcome. Moreover, I will be able to compare the degree to which each of the variables—or each combination of them—explains Outcome. In this way I can assess the relative contribution of each parameter to predicting efficacy. I might, for example, find that Age predicts clinical outcome better than Gender—that Age explains more variation in Outcome than does Gender. And I might also find that Drug—receiving one type rather than another—is more related to prognosis than the two other parameters combined. Statistics provides us with tools to both quantify explanations and assess their relative quality (completeness).

This, then, is the statistical path to enlightenment: Show that **independent variables** (also termed **explanatory variables**, such as Drug and Age) explain **dependent variables** (such as Quality of Life and Survival). You may have noticed that I used the words "explain" and "predict" interchangeably. Well, in this context they are in fact interchangeable. Using statistical modeling,

I relate between variables and obtain solutions. For example, I will demonstrate a relationship between taking a drug and recovering from pneumonia. Having done this, I can say that Drug "explains" Recovery, and I can also say that Drug "predicts" Recovery. The models themselves cannot tell you whether they are predicting, explaining, or merely relating. At the end of the day, it is *your* logic that will give meaning to statistical results. Equations cannot speak for themselves and are not meant to.

For example, global warming appears to be a fact of some periods in the twentieth century. It is also a fact that during this period humanity has released more CO_2 into the atmosphere than in previous eras. Some complex mathematical equations have related these parameters quantitatively. Yet, these equations do not by themselves prove that CO_2 *causes* global warming. This must be left for other types of scientific reasoning. Similarly, I can relate mathematically between Age and Height of children. Having done this, I can now partially predict Height from Age. But can Age be said to cause Height to change? This is not a question statistics can answer on its own.

PERSONALIZING MEDICINE

When reporting clinical study results, both the regulator and the scientific journal reviewers often expect information relating to **covariates**—variables such as Age, Ethnicity, and patient's General Medical Condition that may affect the outcomes of drug or device Treatment. For example, you might be required to assess whether your product affects females differently from males, Hispanics differently from Asians, and/or generally healthy people from those who have a chronic medical condition. Additionally, in multicenter trials you will likely be asked to compare outcomes between centers to assess whether Location/Center is related to a Treatment's effect. In this way those examining your overall results can learn whether or not they apply to identifiable subgroups equally. For example, knowing that a medication is more effective in warm climates than cold climates is relevant for making decisions about treatment.

In recent years responsiveness to Treatment has also been correlated with subjects' genetic characteristics. The area investigating these issues is called **pharmacogenomics**, which relates genetic variation with variation in Treatment efficacy. This particular branch of science is in its infancy, and one of its aims is to personalize medicine—that is, to tailor treatments to individual patients based on their genetic traits. In statistical terminology, pharmacogenomics investigates variation in genetic characteristics (covariates) that it hopes to use to explain/predict variation in Response to Treatment.

To summarize so far:

- The goal of inferential statistics is to understand phenomena by relating variation in them to variation in other phenomena.
- The stronger the relationship, the better the explanation.
- Whether the relationship is strong or weak, it is almost always incomplete. As such, prediction of parameters such as Response to Treatment cannot be perfect.

QUANTIFYING EXPLANATION

In the preceding section I noted that explanations can be strong or weak. They can, of course, be any point between as well. In everyday discourse I might, for example, say that "Sheldon will probably come to the party if I invite him." No one (other than the odd statistician), however, will ask me to provide the actual probability for it. But when doing science we must quantify our predictive/explanatory statements. Only then can we gauge their strength and completeness.

So the statistical path to enlightenment involves relating variables to one another. More important, statistics can quantify just how strong this relationship is or, if you will, just how good the explanation is. One such quantitative indication is **proportion of variance explained**.

Let me begin with an extreme example where distances between different locations are recorded in both Miles and Kilometers. Having done this, I now have two values for each distance. Relating the two (say, by correlation), I find that the relationship is perfect. In other words, 100% of variance in Miles is explained by Kilometers, and 100% of the proportion of variance in Miles is explained by Kilometers.

Now this, of course, is no explanation in the conventional sense. Miles and Kilometers are merely alternative ways of expressing distance, and being long in one does not cause you to be long in another. Recall, however, that statistical models are not concerned with *meaning*.

As a rule, percent of variance explained will be lower than 100%, and, more often than not, it will be much lower. Yet be it low or high, proportion of variance explained provides a quantitative indicator of the degree to which an explanation is complete.

Here are some examples:

- At a particular university, student's High School Grades explains about 10% of the variation in Grades at the University.
- Average Parental Height in one western country explains about 40% of the variance in Child's Height.
- In patients admitted to a hospital due to fever and neutropenia (low count of neutrophil, a type of white blood cell), about 30% of the variance in Length of Hospital Stay was explained by Monocyte Count (another type of white blood cell), Temperature at Admission, and Presence of Localized Infection. Thus, three parameters could be used to predict 30% of variation in Hospital Stay.

Proportion of variance explained can be affected by many factors such as the accuracy of measurement, range of values in the parameters measured, type and characteristics of the parameters used, and others. It is thus essential to remember that this quantitative indicator of the quality of explanation does not necessarily reflect the "truth." For example, we know there is a relationship between Height and Weight. But if the instruments we use are inaccurate, we may not discover this relationship. And if I fail to discover a relationship between Height and Weight—if the variance in one explains 0% of the variance in the other—it is because of an imperfect method rather than some truth of nature.

EXPLANATION AND INFERENCE IN CLINICAL TRIALS

Say your company has developed an **autologous cell therapy** VO-14C for venous ulcers, which are ulcerations in tissue caused by insufficient blood supply to veins. You are now planning a first trial in humans with the disease and wish to compare the safety and efficacy of your treatment with some standard of care (SOC), the currently accepted treatment.

This is your first trial in humans, and you do not know the optimal Treatment Duration for your drug. Your planned study will address this issue as well. After numerous discussions you decide on an 18-week trial with the following five groups:

1. SOC only (Control group)
2. SOC + 10 weeks treatment with VO-14C
3. SOC + 12 weeks treatment with VO-14C
4. SOC + 14 weeks treatment with VO-14C
5. SOC + 16 weeks treatment with VO-14C

The trial will include 150 patients, 30 of which will be randomly assigned to each treatment arm. Regardless of treatment duration, primary efficacy will be measured at 18 weeks.

You will collect many efficacy measures in this trial, the most important of which is whether or not a subject's ulcer has closed completely. Thus, Complete Closure, a dichotomous parameter taking on values of "yes" or "no," will be your primary efficacy endpoint. From your Company's view, the trial will be considered a success if the following occur:

a. At least one of the VO-14C groups shows a significantly higher proportion of Complete Closure at 18 weeks than SOC.
b. There is a discernable, and hopefully significant, relationship between Treatment Duration and Complete Closure. This will help determine the optimal Treatment Duration for the drug. In this analysis Treatment Duration with VO-14C in the SOC group is, of course, 0 weeks.

A NOTE ON CHOICES AND NONSIGNIFICANCE

When Treatment groups differ significantly, we conclude that what we see is real—that there is indeed a difference between them in the population. When differences seem "substantial" but are not significant, it is not clear what to think. First, the term *substantial* is open to interpretation, and what may seem a meaningful difference to one researcher may not be so for another. Second, as noted, it may not always be useful to view significance as an all or none concept, especially in the early stages of development. Clearly, in the trial described you would like at least one VO-14C group to be significantly superior to Control. But what if your result suggests you can be only 90% certain of a true difference instead of the traditional 95%? And what do you conclude when all drug arms show better numbers than SOC but none of the differences are significant?

At this stage I wish simply to point out that nonsignificant results must be approached with caution. Statistics has rules, and this is how it should be. But there is no harm in speculating, even optimistically. As human beings we have intuitions and should not forgo using them. Indeed, scientific knowledge will benefit if we find ways to combine its formal methods with our personal experience and hunches. And sometimes this might mean that when science points in one direction and your gut feeling points in another, you will put more faith in the latter. Willie Ashenden put it well when he said, "I was aware that the earth was round, but I *knew* it was flat."[6]

_____

[6]Maugham, S. Cakes and Ale. *New York: The Modern Library.*

Earlier in this section I wrote that primary efficacy in this trial is measured by the dichotomous Complete Closure. Yet, for the purpose of illustrating my point, I will use another parameter: Change in Ulcer Area from baseline to 18 weeks. This is computed by simply subtracting Ulcer Surface Area at 18 weeks from that measured at baseline. I will call this difference Delta, where larger deltas are associated with greater efficacy. In the case of Complete Closure, Delta = Area at baseline.

I noted that Complete Closure is the most clinically meaningful efficacy endpoint in a trial investigating treatment for venous ulcers. Both physicians and regulators will tell you so, and it is therefore specified as the trial's primary efficacy endpoint. But should we ignore patients whose Ulcer Size was reduced considerably but did not close? Clearly, two patients with open ulcers at the end of the trial cannot be said to be equally well off if one's ulcer was greatly reduced and the other's was not. Now some endpoints are more meaningful than others, and this is a fact. But it is a rare endpoint that encompasses all relevant information about a treatment. Consequently, almost all clinical trials specify numerous endpoints of interest. Judicious selection of these endpoints is an important factor in clinical trial study design and deserves its own chapter. (It will get it.)

So I have chosen the continuous endpoint Delta for my example as opposed to the dichotomous Complete Closure. Yet I could have just as easily chosen Percent Delta (% Delta), which also provides continuous data, as opposed to the dichotomous Complete Closure. In this way I could, for example, distinguish between an ulcer reduced from $10\,cm^2$ to $1\,cm^2$ from one reduced from $18\,cm^2$ to $9\,cm^2$; while both have equivalent Deltas, their % Deltas are very different.

As a statistician I can tell you which endpoints provide data that are *numerically* informative. And in measurement terms, the continuous variable Delta is generally more informative than Complete Closure, which has only two categories. However, the latter is more meaningful clinically, which is why it is the trial's primary endpoint.

It seems that as much as I try to stay the course, I find myself sidetracked by related issues. Getting back to the issue at hand, I focus here on the continuous Delta, of which the hypothetical outcome is described in Table 8.1 and Figure 8.1.

Having presented these results I have engaged the first stage of statistical analysis, which is concerned with describing. But while I have yet to interpret the data formally, I have some idea about what is going on just by looking at the graph. Specifically, there appears to be a dose-response relationship between Treatment Duration and Delta such that:

- Longer Treatment Duration is associated with greater Delta.
- The relationship between Treatment Duration and Delta is strongest between 0 and 14 weeks; there appears to be relatively little improvement between 14 and 16 weeks.

As noted in the preceding section, statistical explanation involves relating variables to one another. Well, this is precisely what I have done by observing the association between Treatment Duration and Delta. And in doing this I went beyond description to inference—addressing the "why" of your results. Variation in Ulcer Area, I tentatively say, is at least partially explained by Treatment Duration.

Table 8.1 Change in Ulcer Area (Delta) from Baseline to 18 Weeks by Treatment Period

| Treatment | N | Delta from Baseline to 18 Weeks | |
		Mean (cm²)	Standard Deviation
Standard of Care	30	2.2	0.9
10 Weeks	30	3.5	1.2
12 Weeks	30	4.3	1.6
14 Weeks	30	5.0	1.8
16 Weeks	30	5.1	1.7

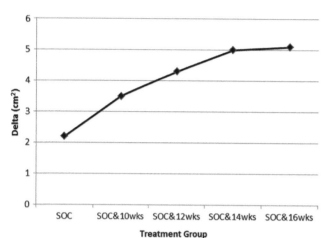

FIGURE 8.1

Change in Ulcer Area (Delta) from baseline to 18 weeks by Treatment group.

Now every discipline provides explanations in its particular language. A life scientist might explain outcomes based on chemical reactions, while the psychologist may point to the unconditional love patients receive from drugs and devices. Yet, neither the life scientist nor the psychologist should attempt an explanation before making certain that the relationship they are interpreting is in fact real. In science, as in life, it is good advice to remember that appearances can be deceiving—that data may reflect sampling error rather than truth. So the first order of business is for the statistician to conduct (inferential) statistical testing to assess whether the relationship observed is significant. An explanation of the results—in any language—should only follow once we know, or at least have a strong hunch, that what we see reflects some truth in the population and is not due to chance.

In this particular case there can be several statistical tests applied, and I will not trouble you with them. For my purposes it is enough that you know that interpretation of cause in clinical trials should follow statistical inference. Thus, the statistician's role in scientific explanation often precedes all other explanations and serves as the justification for them.

ON DESIGN AND ANALYSIS

When designing a clinical trial you should consider the statistical analyses planned for its data. In the current example you aim to assess the relationship between Efficacy and Treatment Duration. Clearly, you will not be able to do so unless your trial measures both parameters appropriately. To this end you include a Control group (Treatment Duration = 0 weeks) and four additional durations (10, 12, 14, and 16 weeks). Hopefully these will allow for the inference of interest. If, for example, the periods were more widely spaced, you might not be able to interpolate efficiently between them. If they were more narrowly spaced, there would be more of them, which would mean fewer subjects per group. Smaller sample sizes may in turn yield unreliable information for the effect of Treatment Duration on Delta.

As you can see, even in this relatively straightforward trial there are some nontrivial methodological issues to be addressed—issues that will have impact on the study's utility. Now while this certainly is obvious, it turns out that many studies are planned offhand with the expectation that once data are obtained, statistics will cause "answers to emerge." Well, this is not likely to happen. Statisticians, like comedians, can only work with the material they have. Sir Ronald Fisher put it best when he said, "To call in a statistician after the experiment is done may be no more than asking him to perform a postmortem examination: He may be able to say what the experiment died of."

To this point I have looked at inferential statistics from three related points of view:

1. Inferential statistics provides techniques that help *explain* phenomenon.
2. Statistical explanation—statistical inference—is done by relating variables to one another. Specifically, it is done by showing that variation in one variable is associated with variation in another.

3. Inferential statistics provides techniques that enable determining whether or not the differences observed between two or more samples reflect the *truth* in the population or are likely due to chance.

In the following section I present yet another view of inferential statistics.

MODELING

Rational thought and behavior are generally guided by *expectation*. For example, we do not cross a busy street when the light is green because we expect some unpleasantness if we do. And we plan our vacation expecting (hoping?) for a pleasant time. Similarly, we expect a good student to do well on any given test and believe that working hard generally begets positive results. Additional examples abound. Translating this idea into the more formal language we:

1. Construct **models** of reality. ("It is dangerous to cross a busy street when the light is green.")
2. Infer expectation from the model. ("If I cross this busy street, I could get hurt.")
3. Make decisions based on expectation. ("I will wait for the red light before I cross.")

Models are simplified versions of reality and in this sense are also stereotypes. They do not truly exist because the world we live in is much too complex for them to fit perfectly. A good student will not get good grades on every test, and crossing the street safely on a green light is not unheard of. But good models approximate the truth sufficiently "for the greater convenience of thinking."

Statistics makes use of numerous models. One of the more common ones is the **normal distribution**, which describes how some types of phenomenon behave. Many variables in nature are distributed more or less normally, like systolic blood pressure and the Height of some trees. Yet, before I show you how to use all of this, I shall first describe the characteristics of the normal distribution using Figure 8.2.

As you can see, and perhaps already know, the normal distribution is symmetric around the mean, and its particular shape is related to the standard deviation. It is a two-parameter model in that it is determined by the mean and standard deviation.

As an example, consider the Kubanga Forest in Angola, which has mature trees of which the mean Height (μ) is 648 cm, with a standard deviation (σ) of 62 cm. Given the characteristics of the normal distribution, we can state the following about Height of trees in Kubanga:

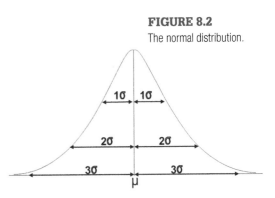

FIGURE 8.2
The normal distribution.

- The largest proportion (density) of tree Height is around the mean μ of 648 cm.
- The distribution is symmetric such that the greatest proportion of trees is near the mean, with decreasingly smaller proportions as we move away from the mean. Specifically, about:
  - 68% of the trees are within 1σ of either side of the mean. In other words, 68% of the trees in the Kubanga Forest are between 648 cm + 62 cm and 648 cm − 62 cm (586 cm–710 cm).
  - 95% of the trees are within 2σ of μ (524 cm–772 cm).
  - 99.7% of the trees are between 3σ of μ (462 cm–834 cm).

These are characteristics of the normal distribution as applied to Height of trees in Kubanga. It is also a model and is "about" right. Yet, like all models, it is a simplification and so not *completely* right.

After traveling treacherous roads and difficult trails, you finally arrive at a forest. You believe you are in Kubanga, but you do not know this for certain. It has been a long trek, the day is hot, and you are slightly disoriented. But while you may be unsure about your whereabouts, you have not forgotten the information in the preceding list.

After finishing off a canteen and resting for a few minutes, you select a tree at random and measure its Height (you have brought along your laser as well). The tree sampled is 835 cm tall. In other words, if you are indeed in Kubanga, the tree you have randomly selected is a rarity. In this particular forest there is only a 0.03% chance of randomly coming upon a tree shorter than 462 cm or taller than 834 cm.[7]

Before you did your calculations, there were only two possible answers to your question: (1) you are in Kubanga, and (2) you are not in Kubanga. And now, after having done your calculations, there are still the same possibilities. However, at this stage you are better placed to make an informed choice between them. Specifically you can reason either of the following:

- You are *in* Kubanga and have by chance stumbled upon a tree of which the Height is rare (about one-tenth of 1% of trees in Kubanga are this tall or taller).

or

- You are *not* in Kubanga, since the tree you randomly chose and measured is not typical for this forest. As a result, you conclude that you are in some other forest where the trees are generally taller than those in Kubanga.

---

[7] In computing the probability, I have used both tails of the distribution, saying that there is a 0.03% chance of randomly coming upon a tree below or above a particular Height. Alternatively, I could have said that the probability of randomly coming upon a tree over 834 cm in Kubanga is 0.015%. In the interest of avoiding the sometimes confusing issue of one-tailed and two-tailed tests, I ask that you accept the logic presented as is. As a rule (with some exceptions) we use two-tailed tests in clinical trials.

These were your two options, and now you must choose between them. Based on your computations, your chance of being in Kubanga is 0.015%. This is a very small chance, so you conclude that you are in the wrong forest. And in making this decision, you know there is about a one-tenth of 1% chance that you have erred—that is, that you are in Kubanga and have randomly come upon an atypically tall tree.

Now some of you might have found this reasoning simple, while others may have had to read it a couple of times. Be that as it may, I must point out that you have long been familiar with this sort of logic. As adults you have (implicit) models for most situations in which you find yourself—models that in great measure determine your expectations and conclusions. And when a chosen model does not seem to fit a particular circumstance, you consider modifying your conclusion. In this case you had an expectation of how "trees in Kubanga behave." You then compared observed data to this expectation and found a lack of fit. As a result, you concluded that you are probably not in Kubanga. In this way you continuously engage in (informal) hypothesis testing.

To discuss hypothesis testing formally, I will return to a simple clinical trial where you wish to show that Test drug (T) is better than a Reference drug (R). Translating this into formal statistical nomenclature, we specify competing hypotheses about reality:

1. **Null Hypothesis:** The Null Hypothesis is the "state of the world" until proven otherwise. In this case, you (and the regulator) assume that that T is about as good as R; until proven otherwise, you will not claim the new drug or device is more effective.
2. **Alternative Hypothesis:** The Alternative Hypothesis is what you would like to demonstrate in the clinical trial, which is that the initial assumption about the state of the world is incorrect. Specifically, you would like to show that T and R are not the same.

These translate into the following formal statements:

H_0: T = R (Null Hypothesis)
H_1: T ≠ R (Alternative Hypothesis)[8]

where H_0 is the Null Hypothesis and H_1 is the Alternative Hypothesis.

Now recall that even if the two medical products are equivalent, a given trial will show some difference between them. This is due to sampling error and

---

[8] Actually, you want to show that T > R, not only that they are different. After all, if T < R, they are indeed different, but it is of no interest to you as a drug developer. Once again, we encounter this issue of one- and two-tailed tests.

so is attributed to chance rather than reflecting a true difference. So to test the hypotheses, you do the following:

1. Specify the behavior of chance differences—that is, create a model that describes how sampling error behaves. For example, when you flip a coin 100 times, you know how it should behave if it were fair. Thus you know that even a fair coin has a decent chance of coming up 52 heads and 48 tails or, say, 54 tails and 46 heads. So if results such as these emerge, you will consider attributing them to sampling error rather than concluding that the coin is biased.
2. Conduct a clinical trial (or, in the example of testing a coin for fairness, flip it 100 times).
3. Compare the empirical result to the model, describing how chance behaves.
4. If the result obtained is very unlikely given the "chance model," you conclude that the difference is real (not due to chance)—that is, you conclude that the drugs differ significantly or that the coin is biased (differs significantly from "fairness"). If the result is likely given the chance model, you cannot conclude that the differences you observe are real rather than due to chance.

There are many nuances that can be added here and many technical details. As before, I refer those interested to standard texts. My point here is that significance testing, which is the tool of inferential statistics, simply formalizes the way we think: We construct models that lead to expectations, which we test using observed data. If the results are extreme enough given the (null) model—the initial expectation—we reject it. If they are not, we remain with our initially stated model. When we reject the Null Hypothesis, we say that we have obtained a *significant result*, and we infer that the Alternative Hypothesis is true.

ON INFERENCE AND POPULATIONS

Do men and women differ? Well, it depends on the attributes you consider. When looking at the attribute of being a Human, both are of the same population. When examining, say, Height, they differ on average—that is, each belongs to a different population, populations that differ in their mean Height.

Thus in statistics as in life, *population* is a matter of definition. Now there are times when the distinction between populations is obvious to us. But there are others, notably in clinical trials, where we do not know whether we have one population or two. For example, if T and R are equally effective, we say that while the products have different names, for the purpose of efficacy, subjects receiving either belong to the same population. If however they differ in effectiveness, we say that individuals receiving T belong to a different population from those receiving R.

I described how hypothesis testing is designed to assess whether T and R differ. Here is another way to say it:

H_0: Individuals receiving T and R belong to the same population.
H_1: Individuals receiving T belong to a different population than those receiving R.

Inasmuch as hypothesis testing is designed to assess differences between entities, it is a method for discovering whether we are dealing with one population or with more.

Remember Piaget and his concept of accommodation (Chapter 5)? When we encounter an entity that does not fit neatly into a ready-made category, we construct a specific category for it. Statistical testing is thus a formal procedure for creating such categories—for deciding whether something we see can be classified into an existing population (assimilated) or requires a new one (accommodated).

SUMMARY

Descriptive statistics provides techniques that help us to summarize data. Inferential statistics provides tools for all of the following:

- Explaining why the data are as they are.
- Assessing whether relationships between variables are real/true or likely due to chance.
- Discovering differences.
- Assisting in determining cause.
- Testing hypotheses.
- Discriminating between populations or, alternatively, indicating whether different sets of data were obtained from the same population.

CHAPTER 9

Exploratory and Confirmatory Clinical Trials

"Economists ... predicted eight of the last three depressions."

—Barry Asmus

CONTENTS

- Explanations: before and after the fact
- Example of statistical testing in reimbursement
- Secondary endpoints
- Statistical analysis plan (SAP)
- Inclusion criteria: clinical and statistical considerations in a stroke trial
- Post hoc analyses in a diagnostic device
- Modeling dose-response
- The difference between fitting lines to data and data to lines
- Simplicity, complexity, and robustness in modeling
- Cross-validation
- Guidance on confirmatory and exploratory clinical trials

INTRODUCTION: AN UNLIKELY STORY

Henri Delaunay played soccer in Paris at the turn of the last century. After he retired, he became a referee but then gave it up after being hit by a ball, breaking two teeth, and swallowing the whistle in the process. In 1906 Delaunay became president of the Paris team with which he had played and went on to become secretary general of the French Football Federation. In 1924 he joined football's governing body FIFA (Fédération Internationale de Football Association), where he served until 1928.

While in FIFA Delaunay proposed a European football tournament to decide the continent's champion. Thirty-one years later his idea bore fruit with the first European Nations Cup in 1958. The tournament's finals were held in France in 1960 where the Soviet Union was awarded the Henri Delaunay Trophy after defeating Yugoslavia 2–1.

The tournament has taken place every four years since and in 1968 it was renamed the European Football Championship. The cup is usually won by powerhouses like Germany, France, and Italy. But a few others have won as well and in 1992 something especially odd happened. The finals that year were held in Sweden, with eight teams participating the host and seven others advancing from the tournament's early stages. Among those taking part was the defending champion and favorite Germany, and a team not meant to be there in the first place.

Based on its performance in the qualifying round, Yugoslavia—which would soon be divided into component parts—had earned a place in the finals that year. But the country was embroiled in wars and was ultimately disqualified for political reasons. Denmark was the runner-up in Yugoslavia's group and received the ticket to Sweden instead. Thus it was no small surprise that Denmark made it to the final's championship game that year. And it was an even bigger surprise that the country went on to beat the heavily favored Germans.

Now every assessment is vulnerable to error and soccer matches are no exception. Each game is designed to measure which of two teams is better and while in a given game we expect the better team to win, upsets do happen. Was Denmark's victory over Germany an upset?

Before attempting an answer to this question, I should first define the term *better*. Recall that in statistics *truth* is the population parameter. Thus I conclude that team A is truly better than B if the former wins most of the games between the two in the (infinite) population of games. This is, of course, a theoretical concept because there could not have been an infinite number of games between Germany and Denmark either in 1992 or during any other period. Still, it is consistent with our statistical view where truth relates to the value in the population.

Viewed thus, each game in the European Championship is a sample of one from an infinite population. And while each game is meant to represent the population, it cannot do so perfectly because of error. At the same time we know that, on average, the larger the sample, the nearer its information to the truth—that is, the smaller the sampling error. Thus the tournament could have reduced error by increasing sample size. For example, it might have had the two teams in the finals compete in a best-of-three format. While even this would not *ensure* that the better team would be crowned champion, it would certainly increase the probability of its happening.

Using multiple measurements is common in many sports, including tennis, bicycling, and baseball. It is also applied in qualifying stages of soccer tournaments that are typically played over long periods of time. But the nature of the game makes it difficult for any team to play on consecutive days or even one day apart. Thus a multiple-game format for two teams reaching a tournament's final is impractical.

So it seems that football competitions are not necessarily conducted according to sound statistical principles. And given that upsets are most likely to occur in single games—and tend to get righted over repeated measurements "in the long run"—many in the soccer world wondered if Denmark was in fact the "best" team in Europe in 1992.

HINDSIGHT AND FORESIGHT

On June 27, 1992, a headline in the *Boston Globe* read:

"Denmark European champion, Germany loses in a shocker."

The article described Denmark's 2–0 win in the final and the ecstatic celebrations of its fans. The newspaper then pointed out that it was the first time in six years that the Danes had beaten Germany in soccer. Like virtually all who took an interest in such things, the writers concluded that an error had occurred, although they preferred the term "shocker."

Now let us suppose there was at least one person—a friend of yours—who disagreed with the conventional wisdom of the day. Allow me to offer alternative scenarios in which she shares her wisdom with you.

Scenario 1: After the final your friend tells you she knew all along that Denmark would beat Germany. Of the two teams reaching the final, she believes that Denmark was easily the better and adds that the Danes were the best in Europe that year. The surprise, she explains, was not that Denmark won the tournament but that the team had failed to qualify outright. This, rather than Denmark's victory in the final, was the glaring error.

Your friend justifies her conclusion by describing Denmark's performance in the early stages of the tournament and explaining how almost every one of its players is superior to Germany's in the parallel position. She adds that Denmark had the better coach as well. In short, she had known all along that Demark would be crowned European champion and that the team would win the final by at least two goals. She puts all of her thoughts in writing and asks you to look at it.

She is a good friend and you smile. Outside it is sunny and quiet—a restful Sunday afternoon. You go to the refrigerator and come back with a couple of beers. You hand her a bottle and, taking a seat on the couch, change the subject.

Allow me now to offer an alternative version of these events.

Scenario 2: On the Sunday before the games in Sweden your friend presents you with an analysis in writing. You read the typewritten document that explains why Denmark is the best team in Europe. The analysis is meticulous, and it is obvious that your friend has given a great deal of thought to the matter. She predicts that Demark and Germany will reach the finals and analyzes the strengths and weaknesses of each. She concludes that the Danes will win by two goals at least.

She is a good friend and you smile. You go to the refrigerator, take out a couple of beers, and change the subject.

The games begin and as the 16-day tournament progresses your opinion changes. It seems your friend has correctly analyzed Denmark's early group stage games. She had also predicted that there would be a difficult game against The Netherlands in the semifinals, in which the Danes would prevail (she wrote that The Netherlands are better than Germany that year). Finally there is her prediction for the final that "Denmark will win by at least two goals."

Despite your initial incredulity, you become convinced that Denmark was indeed the deserving winner of Europe. And you gain a measure of respect for your friend. Indeed, you consider asking for her hand in marriage but fear that she might predict *that* outcome as well.

Let us now examine the similarities and differences in these two scenarios. In both cases Denmark was crowned European champion. The team's performance in the final and the games leading up to it is a fact. And unless you believe that supernatural forces take the trouble to intervene in soccer, the tournament's events had nothing to do with your friend's opinion under either scenario. Thus the games' outcomes are identical under either of the scenarios. The difference, of course, is the timing of your friend's explanation of the results. In Scenario 1 she tells you that after the final she "knew all along" who would win and why. In Scenario 2 she had predicted the outcome outright. And your attitude toward the two explanations is completely different.

I am well aware that there is nothing here that is new to you. Yet I would like to emphasize again that in both scenarios the same events occurred on the field, and your friend provided the same explanation for both. The first scenario did little (perhaps nothing) to alter your opinion that Denmark's win was a fluke; in the second scenario you are pretty much convinced that Denmark was a deserving winner, if not *the* deserving winner. Now all of this may be very interesting (or not), but it is now time to relate all of this to biostatistics in clinical trials.

HYPOTHESES

Clinical studies involve comparisons. Depending on the design and indication, you will compare treatments, time points, doses, **routes of administration**, hospitals, ethnic groups, age groups, and more. Where possible you will also compare current outcomes with those obtained historically. And while there are endless variations on the "comparison theme," the most meaningful are those that are preplanned.

Suppose you are assessing an innovative surgical device and associated procedure relative to standard of care (SOC). Your device has already been approved by the regulator, and now you have to convince the insurance companies to cover the new procedure as they do the other; your trial is for **reimbursement** purposes.

In the pivotal study the regulator allowed you a single-arm trial with some performance goal requirement that you achieved. But these data did not provide direct comparison to SOC on Length of Hospital Stay, which is your primary endpoint in the upcoming trial. Your goal now is to convince insurance companies that your product is superior to SOC and, thus, less expensive overall. Stating this formally:

$$H_0: \text{Length-of-Stay}_T = \text{Length-of-Stay}_R$$
$$H_1: \text{Length-of-Stay}_T \neq \text{Length-of-Stay}_R$$

The alternative hypothesis claims that the two devices differ on the parameter of interest rather than stating your explicit goal of demonstrating a shorter Length-of-Stay. This is a two-tailed test, which is conventional and allows for rejecting the Null in either direction. If after having collected the data you reject the Null in the hoped-for direction, you declare superiority to SOC on Length-of-Stay.

If you had run your trial with no specific hypotheses and happened to achieve superiority on some parameter or other, you would be less convincing. After all, you will have collected many variables and conducted many tests; at least some can be expected to turn out in your favor by chance alone. It is like two teams playing many games against each other, with each match constituting a comparison. Even the weaker team will win every so often, and if you selectively present these wins only, you will "prove" the superiority of the weaker team.

To the degree possible, analyses of **secondary endpoints** should be specified in the protocol as well. Additionally, before the end of your trial, you should write a **statistical analysis plan** (SAP) in which you detail all the tests you plan to do. Between the Statistical Considerations section in the protocol and the SAP (and another element or two) you will convince others that your results reflect the truth in the population.

Invariably there will be analyses that you did not plan; statistical tests beget more tests in the same way that answers often lead to additional questions. There is no reason to avoid these analyses. Indeed, it would be a shame to waste any data. At the same time, these sorts of additional tests will be less than convincing.

Suppose you wish to conduct a late-stage clinical trial in **ischemic stroke**, where the brain's blood supply is reduced, causing brain damage. In the study you will compare between those receiving TYP-01, your new treatment, and Control. The study's central endpoints include established scales of physical and mental function in stroke such as the modified Rankin Scale (mRS) and the National Institutes of Health Stroke Scale (NIHSS). Your primary analyses call for comparing the two groups on these parameters three months after the stroke has occurred. Other endpoints for comparing the groups may include Amount of Brain Damage as measured by Computer Tomography (CT) and/or Magnetic Resonance Imaging (MRI).

The trial is done. Your chosen primary efficacy endpoint is mRS, a measure of patient physical function varying from 0 (fully functioning) to 6 (dead). Success or failure in this late-stage clinical trial will be determined by TYP-01's performance on the primary efficacy endpoint at three months. If you can demonstrate that your drug is superior to Control on mRS, you win; if you fail, you lose.

Like all such studies, your trial specified inclusion and exclusion criteria—parameters determining who is and is not eligible for the trial. Among the many criteria specified is that the NIHSS at baseline be between 7 and 22. You stipulated this range for the following reasons:

1. TYP-01 will be of little use to patients who have very high NIHSS, which is associated with severe strokes that cannot be treated effectively in any manner.
2. Your drug will be no more effective than Control in patients with low NIHSS, which is associated with mild strokes. These subjects will likely recover with treatment or without.

CONSTRAINTS

I said before that inclusion in your stroke study is determined in part by NIHSS, while primary efficacy is measured by mRS. Since both are measures of patient functioning, one would expect that the parameter determining the trial's success (mRS) would also be that used for trial eligibility. This is customary and recommended and, in this particular instance, impractical. For technical reasons it is difficult if not impossible to assess mRS at baseline. Thus, one measure will be used to assess patient function at baseline, and another, more meaningful parameter will be used to evaluate efficacy at three months.

Where possible you should measure critical endpoints at both trial entry and subsequent time points of interest. This will allow efficient assessment of patients' Change. But with a stroke, you cannot measure this change on mRS but can on NIHSS. This is unfortunate because "change endpoints" are typically more powerful than those measured at a single time only.

Be that as it may, you chose mRS at three months for primary efficacy. Did you make the right decision? Unfortunately, you will only know *after* your trial is done. The best you can do before the study is obtain the relevant information to make an informed decision. In this particular instance you must decide between the following:

a. The best clinical endpoint for measuring primary efficacy (mRS) but that cannot be measured at baseline.

b. An endpoint of lower quality that can be measured at both baseline and at three months (NIHSS).

There is something to be said statistically for the second option and clinically for the first. Yet, there may also be a third option in which you remain with the comparison described and statistically adjust the three-month mRS for baseline NIHSS.[1] This is not as good as having the same measure at both time points, but it might be a reasonable compromise given your options. It would appear, then, that statistical procedures can sometimes strengthen unavoidable weaknesses in design, and this is true. Yet, I say "unavoidable" because you should always specify the best design possible and only resort to statistical procedures for correcting design deficiencies. While useful, statistical adjustments for weaknesses in design are rarely as efficient (and convincing) as having a good design in the first place.

All the while you must keep in mind that the regulator will have something to say about this choice you face. For example, the agency may insist that mRS be your primary endpoint rather than NIHSS, in which case you have no choice in the matter.

---

[1] This approach is associated with a large family of procedures that are called *covariate analyses*. I will address this in greater detail later in this chapter.

Your study is completed and its data collected. At this stage your statistician compares the two groups as planned and finds that those receiving TYP-01 have slightly better (lower) mRS scores than Control. But the difference is not statistically significant. So it turns out that your study has failed to demonstrate TYP-01's efficacy, and everyone is disappointed. Naturally, you are reluctant to leave it at that.

Now clinical trials are costly affairs, and you are not about to ignore data that were so painstakingly collected, even if the overall conclusion is a failure. So you ask the statistician to look at the results in a variety of ways. In particular you request analyses of the primary endpoint in subsets of subjects. This is termed **subgroup analysis**, where you assess your drug's efficacy relative to Control in selected patients. In this particular case you decide to assess Treatment-Control differences in subgroups of subjects differing on baseline NIHSS, which is a measure of stroke severity at trial entry. Examining these analyses you discover a striking result: When you compare TYP-01 to Control only in those whose baseline NIHSS was between 11 and 16, your drug turns out to be far superior to Control—a difference that is statistically significant.

Now over 60% of the subjects in the trial had baseline NIHSS of 11 to 16, so this result is based on the majority of participants. In other words, the outcome of this post hoc analysis is not based on some small, obscure subgroup. Moreover, the difference observed is perfectly in line with your initial reasoning. Recall that you had specified a range of 7 to 22 on NIHSS for inclusion precisely because you felt that only patients with moderate strokes will benefit from TYP-01. To this end you excluded subjects who were either too severely disabled (NIHSS > 22) or not disabled enough (NIHSS < 7). Well, it turns out that you did not exclude enough and should have selected the 11 to 16 range, which you now do. Based on these results you conclude the following:

a. TYP-01 is superior to Control (SOC).
b. The intended use population for your drug includes patients with baseline NIHSS—with Severity of Stroke—of 11 to 16.

You report this to both the regulator and the investors, who reject your conclusions. The reason for this can be found in the preceding sections.

Here is another example: You conduct a trial to demonstrate the accuracy of a device that diagnoses significant cardiac disorders. You expect that your sensitivity and specificity will be 0.80 and 0.85, respectively, and you state this in the trial's protocol. Unfortunately, your actual results turn out to be weaker. On the face of it, your study is a bust. You then reanalyze the trial's data from different angles and discover that when assessing individuals less than 60 years of age, your sensitivity and specificity are both in the vicinity of 0.90. In other words, the device works well for younger subjects only. You consult with interventional cardiologists, who tell you there is a logical explanation for this. The device, they tell you, seems to be sensitive to the heart's disease status as well as to Age; older people's hearts are sufficiently weak that they appear disordered on your test regardless. In other words, the signal used by your device to diagnose disorders is indeed produced by cardiac problems, but it is also produced by shopworn hearts. Using this information you designate the product's intended use population as "younger than 60 years of age."

In both cases the outcomes obtained are fact. They were not *caused* by your analyses. When assessing TYP-01 in a subset of stroke patients and when examining your device in subjects younger than 60, you obtained statistically significant results. And in both cases your results are rejected. Given that your numbers actually occurred, the negative responses to them seem unfair. But they are not.

In both cases your results were a product of **post hoc analysis**—analyses *after* the fact. And because they were not anticipated before the trial, they are less trustworthy. So instead of accepting the new results outright, you will be asked to conduct another trial for each indication where the hypotheses stated in advance related to the following:

1. Stroke subjects with NIHSS at baseline of 11 to 16.
2. Subjects aged up to 60 for your diagnostic device.

The scientific approach to after-the-fact explanations, and with it the statistical approach, is no different from our natural attitude to the "Denmark explanation." In science we prove points by making predictions and *confirming* them rather than by observing outcomes and explaining them.

ON THE IMPORTANCE OF POST HOC ANALYSES

While post hoc analyses cannot be considered proof, they are nonetheless essential tools for generating hypotheses. Indeed, much scientific activity involves observing and hypothesizing. But the scientific method also requires replicating results, which in this case means demonstrating that observations-turned-hypotheses can be prespecified and tested successfully.

In practice, there is great temptation to make claims based on favorable post hoc results. This is especially true when there are good explanations for these outcomes. In my experience, unanticipated outcomes that can be explained *feel* predicted. And in reporting these results, as is often the case in scientific publications, researchers will often omit or "mildly conceal" the post hoc nature of such favorable findings. At the very least, this is scientifically wrong.

Like most statisticians, I frequently find myself in conflict with clients who want to believe favorable post hoc results and scientific principles that call for additional proof. Specifically, I will be asked (directly or indirectly) to report these outcomes as is without mentioning the manner in which they were obtained. This is not a comfortable place to be in. Years in the field have taught me that there is usually no conscious attempt at dishonesty here. Companies truly believe in their products and theories; they would not otherwise invest vast amounts of resources in them. Thus, they find it difficult to accept results that do not support the predictions. And when favorable post hoc results emerge, they embrace them.

It is part of the statistician's job description to restrain this particular nature of humans. But—despite some opinions to the contrary—statisticians are human too. As such we are subject to the same foibles as those we work with. I must admit that I have failed on this now and again, and I heartily recommend that you do as I say and not, alas, as I sometimes do.

THE ALL TOO HUMAN MODEL

There are times when I sit impatiently facing the computer monitor awaiting the Word in its contemporary form, called "output." Depending on the results I may praise or rail, but this does not trouble the machine. In moments of clarity, it does not trouble me either. On occasion even *I* realize that processors running statistical procedures are neither for nor against me; they simply go about their business, paying no personal heed to the hands that key.

The programs I use are set up to analyze data in fixed steps, and even the "decisions" they make—their choice of one routine or another within an analysis—are burned into their programs. They are, in this sense, unfeeling. But this does not necessarily mean that they are without bias. In fact, being extensions of our own reasoning, they are very much subject to the kind of human foibles I have been describing.

Figure 9.1 represents measurements of Engine Size (displacement in inches^3) and Acceleration (time in seconds from 0 to 60 miles) for 404 car models. As you might imagine, and as can be seen in the figure, the larger the engine, the greater the acceleration. Knowing this before having analyzed the data, and assuming the relationship will be adequately described by a straight line, I planned to fit a simple linear regression model to the data. This I did, and I present the line computed in the scatterplot as well.

The line in Figure 9.1 seems to fit the data, and I conclude that this simple linear model reasonably describes the relationship between Acceleration and Engine Size. Moreover, having prespecified the model *before* analyzing the data would seem to make this a confirmatory study and especially credible. Well, almost. Actually, I did prespecify that I would fit a simple linear model to the data, but I did not prespecify its specific parameters.

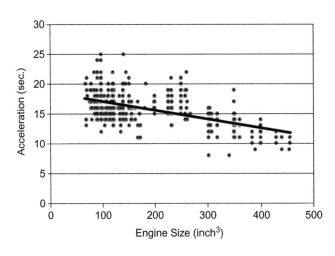

FIGURE 9.1
Relationship between Acceleration and Engine Size with a fitted first-order linear model.

Reach back to your high school algebra and recall that lines in two-dimensional space have the following general form:

$$y = c + b \times x \qquad (9.1)$$

In this particularly example:

  y = Acceleration
  x = Engine Size
  c = Constant (termed **intercept**, which is the point on the y-axis that the line intersects)
  b = Regression coefficient, which is the line's slope

On the technical side, the procedure requires that I provide the computer program with the model's (linear) form and data. It will then use the programmed procedure to compute the parameters "c" and "b" of the equation. Once done, I have a formula with which I can predict Acceleration from Engine Size. In this particular case it is the following equation:

$$\text{Acceleration} = 18.434 - 0.0150 \times (\text{Engine Size}) \qquad (9.2)$$

Plug in an Engine Size—one of the 404 models of which the data were already collected or another of your choice—and you will obtain the model's prediction for Acceleration. For example, estimating Acceleration for an engine of size 280 inch^3, I plug the number into the formula as follows:

$$\text{Acceleration} = 18.434 - 0.0150 \times 280 = 14.2$$

Thus, given the model, I expect an engine of size 280 inch^3 to provide a car's Acceleration from 0 to 60 miles of 14.2 seconds. Not too impressive.

Having posited a linear model before building it but not having prespecified the model's parameters, this "trial" is not purely confirmatory but rather:

■ Confirmatory with respect to testing whether a linear model fits the data.
■ Exploratory in that it uses an optimization procedure to determine the model's actual parameters after having "looked" at the data.

In a wholly confirmatory study, I would do the following:

1. Prespecify the model, complete with specific values for "c" and "b," which would have likely been developed on pilot data.[2]
2. Collect new data—obtain another random sample of cars from the population—and use Eq. (9.2) to estimate Acceleration given Engine Size.

---

[2] Models can, of course, be developed using theory as well. For example, I might test a model constructed by a mechanical engineer based on theoretical computations only.

3. Compare the results predicted by the model to the cars' actual acceleration values.

If the differences between observed and predicted Accelerations are sufficiently small, I have confirmed the model. If the differences are unacceptable, the model is disconfirmed. Thus, a confirmatory trial would test an existing model "as is" on data; it would not use the data to build or modify any part of Eq. (9.2).

The "partial-confirmatory" approach just described is common in research, and there is nothing wrong with it. Regardless, when building models we should distinguish between the confirmatory and exploratory elements in them. This will provide us information on the degree to which we can trust our results. In this particular example, I can be confident that a straight line is a reasonable way to model the data. After all, I specified the simple model in advance, and it fits the data. However, I am less trusting of the model's specific parameters; in other words, I am less certain that the constant (18.434) and the slope (−0.0150) are reasonable estimates of the true values in the population because they were not prespecified.

TESTING AND TRUSTING

Models are useful to the degree that they apply to the population in general. In this sense, their performance on the data used for building them provides limited information. So it is with a drug in an exploratory study that is shown to be effective; its utility must then be confirmed on a new sample of subjects—on another exemplar of the population. But confirming takes time and resources, and it would be nice to have some indication of the degree to which a model will perform in the future. Thus, the regression procedure provides **standard error** for c and b (constant and slope) that are quantitative indicators of how these parameters are likely to change when they are computed on a new sample. Other measures of model fit, such as **R-square and standard error of estimate**, relate to the distance of the points on the graph from the line. If the points, which represent actually observed cars, are far from the line, we say the linear model does not fit very well (R-square is low and standard error of estimate is high). If the points are near the line we say that our model fits well (R-square is high and standard error of estimate is low). Additional statistics abound, each of which provides some information on the degree to which you can trust a models' future performance before actually testing it (in the future).

I said before that a simple linear model fits the data reasonably well and the figure presented bears this out. Still, life is not mathematics—and neither are cars—and most of the points are off the line; in other words, the model does not fit perfectly, and there is no one-to-one correspondence between Acceleration and Engine Size. This too was expected. Examining the figure, I wonder if I can do better. I see, for example, that there are several relatively small engines (about 100 inch^3) of which the Acceleration is in the vicinity of 25 seconds, yet, according to the estimated model, they "should be" about 17 seconds. At the other end of the scale—when looking at the largest engines—all of the points are below the line. In other words, for all these engines the model predicts slower Acceleration than is actually the case. This is not optimal. Ideally a line will "pass through" the data throughout the range rather than be uniformly above or below in certain subranges.

Thus, the error in prediction of Acceleration from Engine Size produced by Eq. (9.2) is, at times, more than I would like. Hoping for a better model, I decide to fit a more complex equation to the data. Specifically I choose a model of which the form is a second-order polynomial—one that posits an element of nonlinearity in the relationship between Acceleration and Engine Size. The new equation (which you might also vaguely recall from high school algebra) has the following form:

$$y = c + b_1 \times x + b_2 \times x^2 \tag{9.3}$$

where:

x^2 = Engine Size squared (parabola, remember?)
b_2 = An additional coefficient to be estimated—the weight assigned to the nonlinear term (x^2) in predicting acceleration

Estimating the model using the optimization procedure mentioned yields the following:

$$\text{Acceleration} = 15.863 + 0.0139 \times (\text{Engine Size}) - 0.0001 \times (\text{Engine Size})^2 \tag{9.4}$$

If you are familiar with this procedure, fine. Otherwise, do not fret. It is enough to know that instead of using the simple model (Eq. (9.1)), I have fit a more complex model (Eq. (9.3)) to the data.

Having run the procedure, I obtain Eq. (9.4) and present the results of my efforts in Figure 9.2.

Looking at Figure 9.2, I see that the line is curved and appears to fit the data better than the line in Figure 9.1. There is a clear improvement at the high end of Engine Size, where the first-order model passed above the data points, while the second-order model passed through them. But there appears to be little or no improvement at the lower end of the Engine Size scale. As it turns out, the model in Figure 9.2 is statistically superior to the first in that its R^2 (R squared) is 0.36 as opposed to the first one's 0.32.[3] This is no dramatic improvement but

FIGURE 9.2
Relationship between Acceleration and Engine Size with fitted second-order linear model.

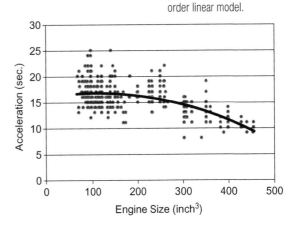

---

[3] R^2 is a measure of model fit. The higher it is, the better the fit.

is a step in the right direction. Moreover, the difference between the models is statistically significant. In other words, I can be pretty certain that the second model will fit in the population better than the first. Or can I?

I now have a better fit to the current data and, arguably, a better prediction of Acceleration from Engine Size. I write "arguably" because while the model fits the data at hand better, it is far from clear that its predictive prowess in the population will exceed that of the simpler model. Keep in mind that my more recent effort has two post hoc elements to it: the model's form *and* the parameters estimated. While in my first effort the model's form (linear) was prespecified, in my second effort I added a nonlinear term *after* looking at the numbers.

So I am once again in a situation where post hoc testing has provided me with apparently useful information. But how useful is it? This is no idle question, since in the future I will want to use *some* model to predict Acceleration from Engine Size on new data. This means that I must now choose between the two models computed. Based on fit alone, I should choose my second effort, while based on "planned versus post hoc analyses," I should choose the first. All the while I should remember there is a third option—namely, fitting an even more complex model to the data, since neither of my first two efforts yielded particularly impressive results. I will consider this third possibility soon.

The example described presents the statistician with a quandary: choosing between models to predict future events based on sample data. In one form or another, this issue arises continuously in clinical research.

Suppose you conduct a dose-response study testing five doses ranging from 0 mg to 60 mg in an indication where the stronger the response, the better. You start at 0 mg to make sure the kind of response you are trying to elicit does not occur naturally in the human body. And you choose 60 mg for your highest dose, expecting that your drug produces its maximal response at about 40 mg and weakens thereafter. This is what your early data have suggested and, judging by the limited research reported, what others have found as well. In fact, you could have probably forgone the 60 mg dose, but you had the resources and wanted to substantiate your earlier results and those reported in the literature. Figure 9.3 shows the results obtained in this trial.

Surprisingly, the 60 mg dose elicits a stronger response than 40 mg, and you must now to decide which should be used in your upcoming feasibility trial. Specifically, should you believe your expectation that 40 mg is optimal, or should you go with the apparently more effective dose of 60 mg observed?

As before, the preferred solution is to repeat the study and test whether these results replicate. But this is not an option. While your company has the monetary resources for another study, it cannot spare the time; its plan requires that the molecule move forward to a feasibility trial, and you have

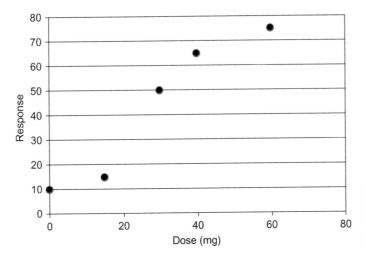

FIGURE 9.3
Relationship between
Medication Dose and
Subjects' Response.

no say in the matter. Discussing the issue with your superiors, they agree that another study is a good idea but that neither you nor they can make it happen. Given the results obtained, they say, any dose between 40 mg and 60 mg should do for now. They propose that you bring up the issue again after the drug is approved and starts generating income. Perhaps then, they say, the company will be open to considering tests of alternative doses.

So you have been given the authority to determine the dose, and decide on 40 mg. It is the safe option and probably not a bad one. But you are not completely comfortable with this route, and you review your results repeatedly to see whether more can be gleaned from them. In reassessing your results, you come up with Figure 9.4, in which two dose-response curves (models) have been fit to the data.

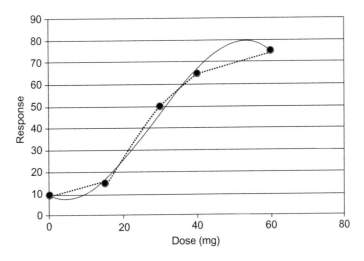

FIGURE 9.4
Relationship between
Medication Dose and
Subjects' Response with
fitted models.

Looking at the simpler, dotted-line curve, 60 mg is your best option; it produces the strongest response, which is preferred in this indication. In fact, you do not really need a model for this. The strongest response was observed at 60 mg, and that is that. At the same time, this result is at variance with your expectations. Specifically, the maximal response was expected at 40 mg, and pushing it up to 60 mg is sufficiently inconsistent to be questionable. Keeping this in mind, you fit the more complex, solid-line model. And although more complex, its form is often encountered in dose-response studies and thus may more accurately reflect this relationship than the simpler model. Examining the solid curve, the strongest response is slightly over 50 mg rather than 60 mg, which is situated on the curve's downward trend.

So it seems that repeated looks at the data have only complicated matters. You are now faced with three choices, each with advantages and disadvantages:

- The safest choice is 40 mg. It is consistent with expectation, yields an acceptable response, and no one will blame you for selecting it. Yet, you would not have conducted the study in the first place if you were completely sure of the 40 mg dose.
- Using a simple dose-response model, you ought to choose 60 mg. Of the doses tested, this provides the best response. Indeed, even if you had not used a model at all, you would have reached the same conclusion, which is also in 60 mg's favor.
- Given a more complex model of the type often fitted to dose-response data, the dose of choice for the feasibility trial should be in the vicinity of 50 mg.

Having dug into the data a bit deeper, you now have three options and no clear criterion to guide your choice. Now as a statistician I would really like to help you, but there is not much I can do. While the first argument might be the most powerful statistically, all three make sense. In this particular circumstance I would likely push (mildly) for the first option but would ask to discuss the matter further with clinicians.

Allow me another example—one that in one form or another I have encountered in the development of diagnostic tests. Suppose you have designed a device that produces a number for detecting some disorder. Let us call this number Score-X. Now Score-X is a product of theory, early testing, and intensive work by your company's algorithm experts. Applying it in a pilot yields reasonable, but not outstanding, accuracy: sensitivity and specificity of about 0.8 each. You are now planning your pivotal trial and writing a protocol in preparation for submission to the regulator. Once approved, you will go ahead with the trial, and if the results expected materialize, your device will likely be approved.[4] Meanwhile your company has added another algorithm expert to the staff, and she comes up with a modified diagnostic indicator that she calls Score-Y. Reanalyzing your pilot data with Score-Y, both sensitivity and specificity increase appreciably (to about 0.9 each). What should you do?

If this new expert came up with Score-Y after looking at the data, the solution is probably "post hoc enough" to be rejected. Indeed, chances are that your other experts would also have achieved better results if they were allowed to modify the algorithm based on available data. But this is not how it happened. The new person came up with the algorithm using the same information your other experts had *before* the pilot trial. She only used the more recently acquired data to test the model rather than to develop it. So here is what you have:

1. A post hoc study in the sense that Score-Y was computed after the pilot.
2. A planned study in that you assessed Score-Y on data that were not used in its development, which is certainly not post hoc.

The important moral of this story is that the difference between "planned" and "after-the-fact" is not necessarily a matter of chronology. To evaluate trustworthiness of outcomes, you must examine how these outcomes were obtained. When your model is fit to some data, these same data do not provide an optimal test of your model. However, if the model was built independently of a specific data set, this latter set provides an acceptable test of the model even if its numbers were collected before the model was constructed.

To address this issue, when developing algorithms, researchers often take existing data and divide them into two or three subsets. They use the first subset—usually the largest—for what is called "learning." Once the learning phase is completed, one has an algorithm that can be tested on "virgin" data—numbers that were not used in algorithm development (though collected at the same time). Whether you choose one or two data sets in addition to the first depends both on the amount of data at your disposal and your researcher's preferences. This is a technical issue that need not concern us. My point is this: Where possible, do not "waste" all your data on building a model. Select a random subset of them to be excluded from the model-building phase. Once your equation has been developed, use the data that have been set aside to test your accuracy. This way you have, for all practical purposes, conducted two trials, the first being exploratory and the second confirmatory.

---

[4] I write "likely" because even the regulator's preapproval of a protocol does not guarantee acceptance of the product after a successful study. At the same time, it certainly increases the likelihood for eventual marketing approval, so submitting your protocol to the regulator before going ahead with a pivotal study is highly recommended.

The examples described thus far involve "shades of gray" in decision making. Based on statistical "fit parameters" only, there are better results and worse. But statistical fit is not the only concern in choosing between models, and this makes your choice less than straightforward. Now all this might be an amusing intellectual exercise if the reality of biomedical development did not necessitate your deciding one way or the other. But you *must* decide, and at times the decision-making process feels a bit like gambling, which it is. You can collect information to increase your odds for success, but you will not know whether your choice has been a good one until the results are in.

ROBUSTNESS

Some creatures adapt to their environment so well that they are perpetually on the brink of extinction. Koestler[5] tells of the koala bear that is native to Australia and the last surviving member of its biological family. It feeds almost exclusively on eucalyptus leaves that are toxic for most animals and low in protein besides. The koala's liver neutralizes the toxins, and its gut extracts what little protein it needs. Lying motionless for up to 18 hours each day, its needs are modest. Thus, the creature has virtually no competition for its precious greens and has almost no natural enemies.

The koala and its environment are a perfect fit. But this is a precarious place to be. You see, when everything is "just right," it takes very little to make it wrong. In the case of the koala, you have an animal whose physiology is perfectly suited to its diet and its diet to its habitat. Thus, any tiny change in the supply of eucalyptus (due to climate, competition, disease, etc.) may render the animal extinct. So it seems that in some cases, when it fits like a glove, it fits *too* well.

This phenomenon has been termed an **evolutionary cul-de-sac**—a dead end brought about by evolving *too well* to a particular environment. Now there are those who suggest that this particular concept has had its day, and this may be so.[6] Yet, the concept is sufficiently intriguing and relevant to my statistical world that I find the tale worth telling. Moreover, it is but one example, albeit extreme, of the tension between generalization and specialization that is ubiquitous in both life and science. Examples abound, and the idea is sufficiently basic to have found its way into everyday language. Thus, you may deride the generalist as being a "Jack of all trades and master of none" or extol his virtues as a "Renaissance man." A sage once said some 2,000 years ago, "If you grab too much, you end up with nothing."[7] I suspect there have been others arguing

---

[5] Koestler, A. (1990). *The Ghost in the Machine*. London: Penguin.
[6] Erikkson, T. (2004). Evolutionary biology: Ferns reawakened. *Nature*, 428: 480–481.
[7] Babylonian Talmud, Yoma 80a.

this way or that. But, really, there can be no single rule about the advantages and disadvantages of specialization, and it depends on the circumstances.

At the same time, given the ever-increasing complexity of both our personal and professional lives, society seems to have come down on the side of the specialist. Yet as the koala's tale points out, it cannot be as simple as all that, and we will soon have our own statistical tale to back this up.

Closer to home—your kitchen, in fact—you likely have several types of knives, each for a special purpose. Thus, you may have one for butter, another for cheese, one or two for breads, and still others for steak and fruits and vegetables. Depending on your culinary propensities there may be more or fewer, but chances are there is at least some specialization there. Yet every once in a while you might change your environment and go camping, where there will be neither cabinets nor flank steak. For these occasions you will likely take a Swiss Army knife or some such compromise of a utensil—one that can perform a great deal, though none of it especially well (a generalist). Clearly, some situations call for specialization, while in others it presents more problems than solutions.

I shall now return to my Acceleration–Engine Size models with our newfound wisdom. Recall that our first model was a simple line. You might even call it "crude"—a simplistic, insensitive creature in our statistical arsenal of models. The second model was a bit more specialized—better fitted to the numbers in that it displayed a mild curvature in an attempt to better account for the data's scatter. But it was a relatively feeble attempt nonetheless, as evidenced by an R^2 that was only slightly superior to that of the straight line. In Figure 9.5, I present the most complex fitted model to this point.

Clearly, the line drawn in Figure 9.5 fits the data better than either of the models presented so far. This is so because the more complex polynomial allows it to fit better to local conditions in the graph (i.e., it can "squiggle" more as needed along the series of points).

Now all this would be well and good if my only task were to fit a line to observed data, where the greater the fit, the better. But in statistics I am rarely concerned with the data at hand. Rather, in analyzing sample data, my objective is to obtain information that will generalize to the population as a whole. And there is the rub.

The models and subsequent predictions/estimates I obtain from a sample data set must fit "in general" if they are to be of any use; they must be useful when assessing data that were not used

FIGURE 9.5

Relationship between Acceleration and Engine Size with fitted sixth-order linear model.

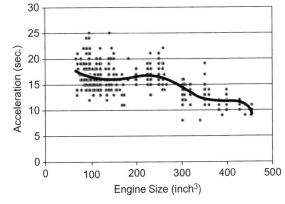

in building the model. If I wish to be practical, my "knife-model" should be nearer the Swiss Army sort than the one used by a chef for a specific task; it must be useful for predicting Acceleration from Engine Size *in general* and applicable to cars I have yet to observe. Because of sampling error—because the data I am fitting my function to do not perfectly represent all data of interest in the population—I had better construct a model that is sufficiently insensitive to peculiarities of a specific data set. In short, I had better not pay too much attention to "local curves" that are unlikely to repeat when obtaining another sample. So of the three models, which do I choose?

Well, there are no hard-and-fast rules here. But there *are* some principles that should be considered. One is that a model fit "overly well" to the environment at hand is unlikely to fit to other environments. In statistics we call this **overfitting**, which is adapting a model to local conditions to the point that it is not useful in other situations. In statistical terminology, an overfitted model will not generalize well to the population.

Now this idea of overfitting is very much related to post hoc testing. My overfitted model was made to fit a specific "data environment." It was not specified in advance without having seen the data. Thus, our mistrust of post hoc analyses springs from the same well as that of overfitted models, both being analogous to drawing the target after seeing where the arrow hit.

Long ago we were taught that the simplest explanation (in our case, a model) is preferable to all others (something about Occam and a razor). But this principle relates to models of which the explanatory power is equivalent; for example, if two models are equally efficient in explaining data, choose the simpler one. But in our case we have three models of increasing complexity, each explaining more of that observed. Which then should we choose—the simple and weak or the complex and strong?

As always, the answer is "It depends." I cannot tell you which is to be selected in any particular case. But here are some points you should consider when encountering this sort of situation:

- *Planned versus post hoc:* All else held equal, prefer a model you specified before evaluating the data to the one constructed after looking at them.
- *Sample size:* The larger the sample, the more likely it is to represent the population well, and thus the more I will trust the models fit to it. Thus, a post hoc model based on a large number of observations can be trusted more than one derived from fewer observations.
- *Complexity:* As a general rule, complex models are likely to be more efficient on the data at hand than simplistic ones. But the former are also likely to be more inefficient on future, yet-to-be-observed data. Thus, the optimal model is likely somewhere between the very simple and the very complex.

- *Statistical indicators:* When constructing models using statistics, outputs come complete with parameters describing how good they are for the data at hand (e.g., R^2) and how good they are likely to be in the populations (e.g., standard error or standard error of estimate). Use these statistics to evaluate the degree to which your model is likely to fit future data.
- *Intuition/logic:* A model that makes intuitive and/or scientific sense is more likely to be correct than one that makes less sense (even if the latter demonstrates superior fit in a particular data set). For example, if biology says that higher doses yield stronger effects within a certain range and a model says otherwise, be less trusting of the model (and, perhaps, repeat the study).
- *Cross-validation:* A model that has been cross-validated successfully—has been tested successfully on data not used to construct it—is preferable to one that has not been.

While there is no one principle that can determine your choice in every circumstance, the simpler the model, the more **robust** it is—that is, the more likely it is to be useful in different situations. A Swiss Army knife is robust in that it is moderately handy in a large variety of situations, while a steak knife is perfectly handy in only a few. If you know that all you will be doing is eating steak, stick to the latter. If you wish to generalize to camping trips and other situations, you should tend to the robust. In the following sections I will formalize the ideas presented with some quotations from the guidelines.

THE CONFIRMATORY TRIAL

A **confirmatory trial**, as its name suggests, is a study designed to confirm a prediction or hypothesis. The International Conference on Harmonization (ICH) guidance for statistical principles in clinical trials provides the following:

> A confirmatory trial is an adequately controlled trial in which the hypotheses are stated *in advance* [emphasis added] and evaluated. As a rule, confirmatory trials are necessary to provide firm evidence of efficacy or safety. In such trials the key hypothesis of interest follows directly from the trial's primary objective, is always predefined, and is the hypothesis that is subsequently tested when the trial is complete.[8]

Thus, when planning a confirmatory trial, you must do the following *in advance*:

1. Articulate your hypothesis clearly, as in the following:
   a. My innovative chemotherapy treatment will yield longer Survival than the standard treatment.

---

[8] International Conference on Harmonization. (2003). Guidance for industry: Statistical principles for clinical trials ICH topic E9.

    b. Subjects using my company's insulin pump will have fewer Hypoglycemic Events than when using their standard pump.

    c. My diagnostic device will yield greater Accuracy (sensitivity and specificity) versus the gold standard than the competitor's.

2. Indicate how you will test this hypothesis:

    a. Specify the endpoints.

    b. Specify the statistical tests to be applied.

3. Indicate what will constitute "success" or "failure"—for example:

    a. I will have demonstrated success if my therapy yields significantly more Cures than the comparator.

    b. I will have demonstrated success if both my Sensitivity and Specificity are significantly greater than 0.85.

Once you have specified your hypotheses—endpoints, statistical testing, and success criteria—your hands are more or less tied; you have taken away your freedom to conduct critical post hoc analyses. And this is precisely the point: When conducting a clinical trial, the data are yours, and there is nothing to stop you from analyzing them as you wish. But if you would like others to accept your outcomes as fact—if your objective is to have your results accepted by a jury of your peers—you will need to play by rigid rules. And one of the most important of these is that your product should not be judged definitively by post hoc analyses. It is for this reason that the confirmatory trial is "necessary to provide firm evidence of efficacy and safety." It, and not an **exploratory trial**, must be conducted to get your product approved.

THE EXPLORATORY TRIAL

The International Conference on Harmonization stated the following:

> The rationale and design of confirmatory trials nearly always rests on earlier clinical work carried out in a series of exploratory studies. Like all clinical trials, these exploratory studies should have clear and precise objectives. However, in contrast to confirmatory trials, their objectives may not always lead to simple tests of predefined hypotheses. In addition, exploratory trials may sometimes require a more flexible approach to design so that changes can be made in response to accumulating results. Their analysis may entail data exploration; tests of hypothesis may be carried out, but the choice of hypothesis may be data dependent. Such trials cannot be the basis of the formal proof of efficacy, although they may contribute to the total body of relevant evidence.[9]

---

[9] International Conference on Harmonization. (2003). Guidance for industry: Statistical principles for clinical trials ICH topic E9.

Thus, exploratory trials:

- Should have specific, well-articulated goals. It is highly inadvisable to go into a vaguely designed trial in the hopes that "data will speak for themselves."
- Can be flexible of design. You can look at your data as you go along and adjust the trial accordingly. For example, if you have a three-dose trial, and midway through it you find that one dose is completely ineffective, you should feel free (after serious consideration) to eliminate the offending dose and increase the size of the other arms.
- Involve data analyses that "may entail data exploration"; in other words, post hoc tests are both legitimate and expected.
- Are not luxuries. They are needed to move your product forward and will "nearly always" provide the basis for your confirmatory trials—those studies that will, ultimately, determine whether or not your product is marketable.

Helping you to determine the optimal mix of exploratory and confirmatory investigations in your development program is one of the statistician's central roles.

CHAPTER 10

One, Two, Three Testing: Hypothesis Testing and Multiplicity

"It's déjà vu all over again."

—Yogi Berra

CONTENTS

- Planning a drug trial in a neurological indication
  - design
  - selection of endpoints
  - relationship between logistics and data quality
- Challenges of collecting diary data
- Hypothesis testing for superiority step by step
- Type I Error
- Alpha
- P-value
- Type II Error
- Interpretation of nonsignificant outcomes
- Demonstrating similarity: equivalence and non-inferiority testing
- Interim analysis and multiple testing

INTRODUCTION: THE SHAKING PALSY

In 1817 an English physician and member of the Royal College of Surgeons published *An Essay on the Shaking Palsy*. In it he characterized individuals he believed suffered from a common ailment. Here is a description of one of them:

> It was a man sixty-two years of age; the greater part of whose life had been spent as an attendant at a magistrate's office. He had suffered from the disease about eight or ten years. All the extremities were

considerably agitated, the speech was very much interrupted, and the body much bowed and shaken.... He described the disease as having come on very gradually.[1]

In the essay James Parkinson provided the first systematic description of an illness that now carries his name. Parkinson's disease is a chronic and progressive illness in which the function of specific brain cells degenerates. The disease typically causes speech and motor difficulties.

Most patients who take medication for Parkinson's soon notice that their condition alternates between "On-Time," when the symptoms are milder, and "Off-Time," when the symptoms are more severe. Alternating between these two states is a reality for Parkinson's patients, who will often arrange their lives to accommodate the cycle. The principal aim of many Parkinson's drugs is reducing Off-Time and increasing On-Time, which is also the aim of your innovative molecule.

BY WAY OF INTRODUCTION

Many of the ideas described in this chapter have been mentioned in lesser detail in earlier chapters. Here I combine these sometimes disparate ideas to complete the puzzle of statistical testing in its various forms. I then add to it the problematic issue of multiple testing—of conducting a number of statistical tests on data collected in a single study, also termed **multiplicity**.

You may notice some repetition in this chapter because I approach similar concepts from diverging angles. This should assist the "minimally familiar" to gain a deeper understanding of the material. But it is also likely to bore others. One cannot, it seems, please all of the people all of the time. And you heard it here first.

A STUDY

Patients in later-stage Parkinson's take L-Dopa, a precursor of the actual neurotransmitter lacking in the disease. Once in the brain, L-Dopa gets converted into dopamine, a substance that is essential for proper functioning and that is not adequately produced in Parkinson's. Say your drug, Apparatone, is indicated in the ailment's early stages—before subjects begin taking L-Dopa. Aside from being designed to reduce Parkinson's symptoms, it also aims to delay the need for L-Dopa.

---

[1] Parkinson J. An essay on the shaking palsy. Published as a monograph in 1817, in *Journal of Neuropsychiatry Clinical Neuroscience*, 14: 223–236.

Preclinical studies have been completed with Apparatone, as have Phase I and a dose-response trial. Your company expects that the dose selected is good enough to take the drug through the remaining stages to marketing.

You are project manager for a late Phase II trial designed to confirm the selected dose's safety and efficacy. In it, Apparatone will be compared to what is considered the best drug now on the market, which will be its Reference (R, Control). Yours will be a simple design:

1. Each subject will be randomized to receive either Apparatone or R, using a 1:1 ratio—that is, there will be an equal number of subjects assigned to each of the groups.
2. The total number of subjects planned for the trial is 100 (50 per group).
3. The trial length is 24 weeks.
4. All through the study, subjects will complete daily diaries in which they record On-Time and Off-Time during waking hours.
5. Safety endpoints are adverse events, including a list of **anticipated Adverse Events** based on previous experience with the drug.
6. The trial's primary efficacy endpoint is Percent On-Time (POT) per day over the study period.
7. The trial's primary objectives are to demonstrate safety and efficacy, with the latter set up using formal hypotheses. You aim to show that Apparatone is:
   a. About as safe as R based on examination of descriptive data for each group.
   b. Superior to R on POT using formal statistical testing.

This particular trial will not test whether Apparatone delays future need for L-Dopa more than R. If it did, you might have:

a. Designed the first part of the trial as described and analyzed the data after all subjects have completed 24 weeks.
b. Added long-term follow-up to assess whether the two groups differ On-Time to L-Dopa therapy, which would be evaluated using **survival analysis**. The latter assess time-to-event parameters, such as, in this case, time to needing L-Dopa. This analytic technique is common in many indications and especially in terminal diseases, where treatments are related to time to death.

After an initial screening and baseline visit, subjects will see their physician every six weeks. At each of these visits they will hand in diaries and receive medication for the next six weeks. Other measures will be taken during these visits, including **laboratory parameters**, **vital signs**, Physician Overall Assessment, and self-reported Quality of Life (QoL). Adverse Events will be also solicited at six-week visits, but subjects are asked to report them as they occur between visits as well.

So to summarize: You have designed a two-arm, randomized trial of which the main aims are to show that Apparatone is safe and provides better POT than the standard of care (SOC) currently on the market.

DIARIES AND LOGISTICS

Our topic is multiple statistical comparisons, and I will get there. But in the tradition of "everything is connected to everything else," I should say a word on collecting diary data, which presents many challenges.

Diaries are self-report measures and thus are prone to patients' subjective perceptions. Now in many instances it is precisely subjectivity that interests you. This, for example, might be the case when evaluating Pain and QoL. But this is not so here where, if it were practical, On-Times and Off-Times would be measured by observation rather than by self-report. Being dependent on patients' perceptions, diaries are especially susceptible to measurement error.

The difficulties introduced by **measurement error** are typically less problematic in two-arm randomized trials than in single-arm trials. In the former you expect individuals of all groups to be about equally error-prone, canceling out one another's errors. You will then assume that any differences emerging between groups at the end of the trial reflect differences due to Treatment. At the same time, even errors that "more or less cancel out" introduce noise and weaken a study's power.

When collecting data with diaries, there is often a problem of compliance as well—of subjects not completing forms as instructed. In the Apparatone trial this could leave you with subjects who have no primary efficacy parameter, which effectively reduces your sample size.

My suggestion is that you avoid diaries where possible. And when you must use them, specify that their data should be secondary rather than primary. Yet avoiding diaries or specifying them as secondary are not always possible, and the current situation is a case in point. To test Apparatone you must estimate POT over 24 weeks, which can only be done by diary. So the best you can do is to make every effort that these data are collected reliably. For example, you might supply patients with fax machines with which to submit their diaries daily. This will provide you with a measure of oversight of the data. You might also consider calling subjects on a regular basis to remind them of the diary's importance, or even calling them for obtaining daily POT measurements. Here, then, is one of many examples where trial logistics affect data quality and, thus, a trial's outcome.

The moral of this particular story is that statisticians should make it their business to be aware of trial logistics in addition to understanding the measurement qualities of endpoints.

Your trial is almost finished, and all 100 subjects have completed the study and provided the required data. This sort of perfection rarely occurs in clinical trials, where missing data are the general rule. For the moment I shall keep things simple and deal with missing values later. It is now time to test your data, and in the sections that follow I describe several scenarios for it.

DATA ANALYSIS SCENARIO I

Scenario I is straightforward and is likely the one described in the study's protocol. The efficacy outcome of greatest interest is POT, which you compute and present separately for each of the two Treatments. Looking at the numbers, you find that this primary efficacy parameter is higher in Apparatone than

Control by 6%. Statistical testing comparing the two groups yields a significant result (P = 0.03). This is a good result, and based on this information, your Company is considering moving on to a pivotal trial with Apparatone. As for myself, I shall move on as well—to more complex data analytical scenarios. But before I do, some statistical background is in order.

POSSIBILITIES AND PROBABILITIES

Possibility 1: You conduct a clinical trial comparing some Test drug T to a Reference R. Having completed the study, you evaluate the results and find that T is more effective than R. You conclude that what you observe reflects the truth in the population and declare that T is superior to R. As when reaching conclusions in general, *you may be right or wrong.*

Possibility 2: You conduct a clinical trial comparing T and R. Formally comparing the two, you find the difference between them is not statistically significant. As a result, you conclude that there is no evidence that the drugs differ from each other. Once again, *you may be right or wrong.*

Now all of this is obvious. The trick, of course, is to ensure that whatever your conclusion turns out to be, it should be correct. Well, you cannot ensure this, and the familiar culprit is sampling error.[2] Even when drugs truly differ, sampling error can result in data suggesting they do not. Conversely, even when T and R are truly equivalent, a particular study may suggest that one is better than the other.

So it seems you will never be completely certain of any conclusion reached. But this is not as tragic as it sounds. It is in fact something you have long learned to live with. Every day you experience uncertainties in your life, but you do your best to deal with them and move on. Science is no different. And among the more important tools available to scientists for reducing uncertainty is statistics. Using the discipline's methods you can do the following:

1. Decrease the chance of reaching an erroneous conclusion.
2. For any given conclusion, specify your probability of being wrong.

In short, you cannot completely eliminate uncertainty, but you can keep it to a minimum. You have probably often said, "I'm pretty sure that ..." or "I'm guessing that ...," which is usually good enough to inform your listener. But this will not do in science, where you must quantify your terms with bolder statements like "I'm 95% certain that ..." or "There's about a 25% chance that I'm wrong." And statistics provides you with the tools to do that.

---

[2] There are other culprits that can mask the truth in a clinical trial, such as measurement error. For the moment we shall focus on sampling error.

DECISIONS, DECISIONS

During your lifetime, you buy new products, cross streets, and propose marriage. You bring a dog home, and you send your child to one school or another. Each of these involves risks and rewards. And at some point—perhaps long after you have made the decision and acted upon it—you will find yourself sitting in some armchair on a Monday morning wondering if you made the right decision. Alas, there is no Control group in life, so you can only speculate on "what might have been."

Certainty is rare. Yet the artificial environment of clinical trials enables designs that increase your chances for it; what is usually impossible in your everyday life—setting up a Control group—is usually possible in formal research. In this sense, scientific decision making is generally easier than it is in real life. Yet, the two have a great deal in common because they both:

1. Use empirical data.
2. Involve comparisons between results obtained under different circumstances. In real life, this is often done by speculation (e.g., "If I had done B instead of A, the results would probably have been …"). In science, you will specify a Control and compare your Treatment to it.

It seems, then, that the concepts of statistical decision making have been familiar to you long before you knew what science is. At the same time, I am not suggesting that all, or even most, real-life decisions parallel the scientific process. As human beings we have varied modes of thinking and numerous tools for reaching conclusions. We use "gut feelings," solicit others' opinions, and once in a while flip coins. I am simply pointing out that at least some of your daily decision making parallels the scientific method.

You may recall from Chapter 8 that statistical testing, also called hypothesis testing, follows some very specific reasoning. This in turn leads to a fixed sequence of analytical steps. To save you the trouble of rereading earlier material, I will summarize both logic and steps as they apply to the Apparatone study. For the moment, read the following without trying to make a connection to practical applications. View this simply as an intellectual exercise. Its value will emerge in time. The steps are as follows:

1. Until proven otherwise, Apparatone is assumed to be no better than R. For simplicity's sake we shall say they are about equal.
2. Given that the drugs are equally effective, you can predict the outcomes that would occur when comparing them over many studies. Specifically, an infinite repetition of a trial between Apparatone and an R equivalent to it will yield a distribution difference that has the following characteristics:
    a. A mean of 0. Since the drugs are equivalent and sampling error is random, observed differences will sometimes favor Apparatone and other times favor R. Necessarily, they will "average out" to 0.
    b. Most of the differences between Apparatone and R will be relatively small and on either side of 0. But sampling error can, by chance, also be large. So if you repeat a study comparing equivalent compounds many times, there will be the odd result where the drugs will *look* different even though they are not.

c. Entries a and b imply a normal distribution of differences of which the mean is 0—that is, a symmetrical distribution around 0 where most of the values are near the mean with a smattering of extreme values on either side.[3]

Now it would be good if we could end this little exercise here and actually construct the theoretical distribution of differences under the assumption of equivalence. Unfortunately, we do not yet have all the information required. You see, a normal distribution is determined by two parameters—the mean and spread—with the latter quantified by the standard deviation or its square: the **variance**. There is however no reason to fret, since the spread can be estimated from the actual data collected in the trial. So using the information available (mean = 0, shape = normal, variation estimated from trial), we can construct what is termed the **sampling distribution** of the mean. In our particular example, it is the distribution of expected outcomes when computing the difference between two equivalent compounds over an infinity of studies.

The reasoning outlined has determined that the mean of the distribution of differences must be 0 and that the spread will be "relatively small." But to actually construct this theoretical distribution, the phrase "relatively small" will not do; it must be quantified. To illustrate this, I present in Figure 10.1 two normal distributions with identical means (0) but different spreads, both of which you may choose to call "relatively small."

In B, for example, virtually all differences are between −5 and +5. In A there is still some nonnegligible chance of coming up with a difference within ±5. Translating this into probability: If I were to randomly select an observation from A, my chances of obtaining 5 and above (or −5 and below) are perhaps about 10%. If I were to randomly select an observation from distribution B, my chances of obtaining a value greater than 5 (or smaller than −5) are tiny and somewhere near 0%.

FIGURE 10.1

Normal distributions with different spreads.

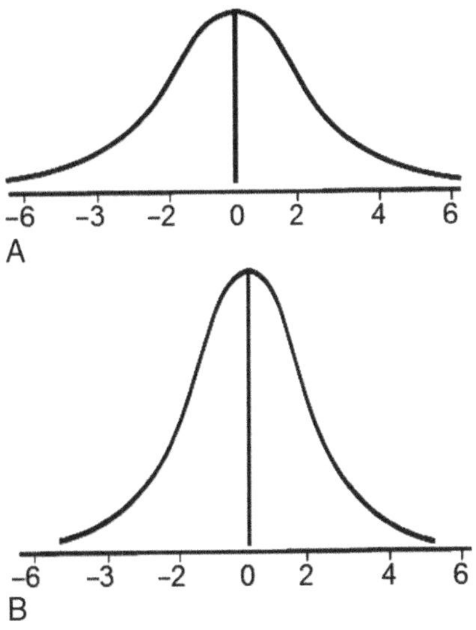

WHY IS THIS IMPORTANT?

Comparing Apparatone and Control in a clinical trial is, when the two are equivalent, like randomly selecting a single outcome from their theoretical distribution of differences. Once you obtain this outcome (in a trial), you can compute how likely this result is, given the assumption of equivalence—that is, given the distribution constructed assuming equivalence.

---

[3] I use the normal distribution here for illustration purposes. Hypothesis testing utilizes many other distributions, such as Chi-square, binomial, and Poisson. And when a specific distribution cannot be specified, we can use nonparametric techniques that assume none.

Please read the preceding paragraph as many times as necessary until it is clear to you. Now once you know what you *should* be getting when two compounds are equivalent, you go ahead and conduct your (single) trial. Having done so, you obtain an outcome—a difference between the two compounds. Finally, you compare this outcome to what is expected assuming the compounds are equivalent. If it is—if the difference is expected more than 5% of the time under the assumption of equivalence—you will not conclude that the compounds truly differ. The difference, you will say, is expected given sampling error alone; it should not be attributed to a real difference. But if the difference is very large— one that is expected 5% or less of the time assuming equivalence—you will conclude that the compounds are likely different. A large difference such as this, you will say, does not occur often with equivalent products. It is therefore likely that they truly differ.

As noted, the spread (standard deviation) of differences between T and R when they are equivalent and when the study is done repeatedly cannot be known exactly—at least not until the trial is repeated an infinite number of times, which it will not be. So, in practice, we estimate the spread of this distribution of differences from the results of the trial itself.

A final note: Constructing the distribution described is based on the central limit theorem, which states that the distribution's mean is 0, it is more or less normal, and it has a standard deviation termed *standard error*. According to this important theorem, the standard error is estimated from results observed in the trial by dividing the standard deviation obtained by the square root of the sample size.

GETTING SLIGHTLY MORE TECHNICAL

Suppose, for instance, that the standard error of my theoretical "equality distribution" is 3. Because the distribution is normal and I know the characteristics of the normal distribution, I can say the following:

1. About 67% of studies comparing equivalent drugs will yield a difference of up to 3. In other words, the chance of obtaining a difference between –3 and +3 when the drugs are truly equally effective in my trial is about 67%.
2. There is about a 95% chance that the trial's result (assuming equivalence) will be between minus and plus two standard errors of the mean—that is, between –6 and 6.
3. There is a one-third of 1% chance of getting a result that is either smaller than –9 or greater than 9.

Of course, you will only conduct a single study. But knowing all of the above, you can, *ahead of time*, design a method for making an inference from it.

For example, you might specify at the beginning of your trial that any difference of 1.96 standard errors or more will cause you to reject the H_0 of equivalence. This implies that any result that can only happen 5 of 100 times or fewer when the products are truly equivalent will bring you to conclude that "this result is too infrequent for equivalent products; I will therefore conclude that they are not equivalent."

There is, however, a critical point that I must add. Being, say, 95% certain that products truly differ is like saying that there is a 5% chance they do not—in other words, that the extreme result obtained was gotten by chance. After all, even equivalent products will, on occasion, differ greatly in a particular trial due to sampling error.

Using the information presented, you are now in a position to conduct a trial and make inferences. Moreover, you can attach the following probabilities to these conclusions:

- The probability that compounds truly differ.
- The probability of having erred in concluding a true difference.

The latter probability—that of erroneously concluding a difference—is termed **Type I Error**.

Here are two important points:

1. When doing statistical inference, it is certainly possible to erroneously *not* conclude that a true difference exists—that is, erroneously *not reject* the assumption of equality. This issue is related to power, which is central in all research, and its time will certainly come.
2. By convention, a significant difference is one expected to occur 5% of the time or less when the groups are truly equal. This Alpha = 0.05 is specified at the outset as the cutoff for inferring one way or the other. Obtain a probability > 0.05, and the result is nonsignificant; if it is ≤ 0.05, it is significant. Either way, you—or rather your computer program—will typically compute the actual probability of the observed result.[4] This probability is called the test's **P-value**. For example, if the difference observed was expected to occur only 12 of 10,000 times assuming equality, your P-value is 0.0012. The smaller the P-values, the more convincing the evidence for nonequality. However, significance is determined by one thing only: whether your P-value is larger or smaller than 0.05. The 0.05 cutoff was prespecified and so, formally, is the one that counts. This is consistent with the confirmatory approach described in the preceding chapter.

---

[4] Actually, the probability of the observed result or one more extreme.

FORMALIZING

I now return to our trial with Apparatone and describe how its hypotheses should be formalized in the trial protocol. We begin with the Null Hypothesis, which is the "state of the world until proven otherwise." In this case, you initially posit that Apparatone = R (in the population). You then specify the alternative, which is Apparatone ≠ Control in the population. Thus,

$$H_0: \mu_A = \mu_R$$
$$H_1: \mu_A \neq \mu_R$$

where:

H_0: Null Hypothesis (the "state of the world until proven otherwise")
H_1: Alternative Hypothesis (the "otherwise" you want to prove in the study; i.e., the study's objective)
μ: Mean Percent On-Time in the population
A: Apparatone
R: Reference compound or Control

Formal hypothesis testing works as follows:

1. Assume H_0 and specify H_1.
2. Specify the probability for rejecting H_0, which is usually 0.05. This value is denoted as **Alpha**, which is the chance for erroneously rejecting H_0.
3. Conduct the trial.
4. Compute the actual result and, using statistical testing, compute the probability (P) of its occurrence in a universe described by H_0— that is, in a distribution constructed based on the assumption of equivalence.
5. Reject H_0 or not based on the observed result.

The choice of 0.05 as the risk of erroneously rejecting the Null Hypothesis is that generally accepted. When a comparison is said to be "statistically significant," this almost always means the observed result was $P \leq 0.05$— in other words, that it had a 5% chance or less of occurring assuming the Null Hypothesis is true. This is also the figure typically expected by the regulator.

Rejecting H_0 erroneously—in our case, concluding there is a difference between Apparatone and Control when there is none—is termed Type I Error. And the chance for making a Type I Error (usually 5%) is termed Alpha. The probability of *not* concluding a difference when in fact there is one is naturally termed **beta**. No less naturally, we call it a **Type II Error**.

ON THE INABILITY TO PROVE THE NULL AND ITS IMPLICATIONS

Logic dictates that you can reject H_0 but not accept it. In other words, *the Null Hypothesis cannot be proven.* A great deal has been written about this topic, and I will not add to it. If this aspect of philosophy of science interests you, I suggest you pick up one of the many fine books on it. My concern here is rather with implications the principle has for product development. Specifically, the fact that you cannot accept H_0 creates at least two questions that must be addressed:

1. How are nonsignificant results to be interpreted?
2. Given that nonsignificance does not prove similarity, how are products to be shown similar?

The following sections deal with each of these.

INTERPRETING NONSIGNIFICANT RESULTS

Suppose you failed to show that Apparatone is significantly superior to Control. The obvious conclusion is that your drug is no better than the competitor. But this is technically incorrect, since all you can definitely say based on a nonsignificant result is that you cannot reject H_0. In other words, it may well be that Apparatone is truly better, but you happened to be unlucky in this particular trial. Now if you carry this reasoning to the extreme you will never reject a new product, which is clearly untenable. What then do you do?

Well as usual, it depends. For example, if your result was obtained in a large, well-designed trial, you will probably conclude, "I gave it my best shot, and now it's time to move on to something else." You will thus accept H_0 in deed if not in word. But if nonsignificance emerged in a small, exploratory trial, you might search through your data more deeply for any indication of a favorable result. Here, even a suggestion of your product's superiority may suffice to move on with it into a larger trial.

So while statistical significance is important, it is but one of many factors affecting decisions in drug and device development. The interpretation of nonsignificant results must depend on the circumstances. Following is a partial list of factors that will affect conclusions in the presence of inconclusive results:

- *Previous data:* A product that demonstrates especially strong results in earlier studies is more likely to survive a single failure than one that has a less successful history.
- *Actual P-value obtained in the study:* As a rule, all P-values larger than 0.05 are nonsignificant. At the same time, values near significance (e.g., $P = 0.08$)

are more likely to be looked upon favorably than those that are not (e.g., P = 0.42). A nonsignificant result that is near significance is called a **trend toward significance**, which is usually defined as P-values in the 0.05 to 0.10 range.

- *Overall direction of results.* Statistical analyses are typically conducted on a number of variables, many of which are related to one another. For example, when assessing an antibiotic, I might evaluate its effect on fever, bacterial count, and subject's self-reported health. When several tests of interest all point in a favorable direction, I will, even if the individual results are nonsignificant, tend to view the outcome favorably. But if outcomes across tests are inconsistent, I would be more skeptical.
- *Science:* A product that *should* work based on solid scientific reasoning (e.g., a known mechanism of action) will be given more benefit of the doubt than one where the science is shakier.
- *Finances:* The more resources at your disposal, the more likely you are to give a potential product additional chances after an apparent failure.
- *Pipeline:* The more products your company has in development, and/or waiting their turn, the less likely a product showing nonsignificant results will be pursued.
- *Stock prices:* Admitting failure will depress stock prices. Thus, even if a product deserves to be declared a failure, it may not be in a company's best interest to do so at a particular point in time. This is *not* a good reason for ignoring nonsignificance and trying again. In fact, this amounts to dishonesty. And where amounts are concerned—especially large ones—you will sometimes find dishonesty as well.

In sum, at times a nonsignificant result will sound the death-knell for a product. Other times it will not. Results of statistical testing, like that of all evidence, must be considered in the general context of a product's development.

STATISTICAL TESTING FOR NON-INFERIORITY AND EQUIVALENCE

Up to now I have explored studies where the Null Hypothesis states that two treatments are equivalent and the trial's objective is to reject this by showing T superior to R. But there are many scenarios in medicine where you wish to show that T and R are similar. One such occurrence is when a company wants to show that its generic version of a drug is just as good as a drug that has lost its patent protection. Another instance might involve a device that one wishes to show to be just as effective as the competitor, while having more advantages (e.g., price, safety, or convenience).

As mentioned in earlier chapters, demonstrating that two products are equivalent is tricky. First, the Null Hypothesis T = R is no longer appropriate, since this is what you would like to prove. Being that a product is guilty until proven innocent, the Null must reflect this, and if we assume T = R and remain with it when failing, we have defeated the whole purpose of scientific investigation. Clearly this is what we wish to prove rather than assume.

So the logical solution is reversing the hypotheses so that T ≠ R is the Null and T = R is the alternative. But this poses its own problem, since, as I have noted often, two products cannot be shown to be the same. Indeed, because of sampling error, even the same product will "come out different" when tested in two different groups.

In Chapter 4, I said that the statistical solution to these difficulties is showing that two products are *similar* rather than *the same*. This in turn entails defining the term *similar* in such a way that would allow for proving one's case using statistical methods while being acceptable clinically. Here is the reasoning followed for demonstrating similarity:

- T = R cannot be shown even if this is in fact the case.
- *Similarity* is then defined by selecting some small margin delta (Δ) for determining a range around R that T must meet. Specifically, we will say that T is:
    - Non-inferior to R if $T \geq R - \Delta$—that is, it is "no worse than R by some small margin."
    - Equivalent to R if $T \geq R - \Delta_1$ and $T \leq R + \Delta_2$—that is, it is "within an 'equivalence' range of R."

The quantity Δ must be clinically as well as statistically justified. Clinically, it must be sufficiently small to be "practically nonsignificant." In practice this means specifying by how much T can differ from R and still be considered *about the same*. At the same time, Δ must be large enough to allow for statistically rejecting the Null Hypothesis. Keep in mind that the smaller the Δ, the more difficult it is to reject the Null. At the extreme, when two products are truly the same and the Δ allowed is 0, it is nearly impossible to show equivalence.[5]

Specifically, you are required to determine some margin delta (Δ) within which T is allowed to differ from R and still be considered "equivalent" to it. For example, you might determine that if T is within ±10% of R, it is, for all

---

[5] "Near impossible" and not "impossible" because there is always an element of luck in statistical testing—good and bad—so there is some small chance for showing T > R (even when they are identical).

intents and purposes, clinically equivalent. Translating this into hypotheses, we specify the following:

$$H_0: T < R - 10\% \text{ or } T > R + 10\%$$
$$H_1: R - 10\% \leq T \leq R + 10\%$$

Translating these hypotheses into English, you:

1. Start out by assuming that T differs from R to a large extent—below R by more than 10% or above it by more than 10%.
2. Conduct the trial to show that R is within the $\pm$10% range.

This is the scenario in generics, where we aim to show the new product equivalent. In other cases we typically do not mind if T is better and only wish to ensure that it is not worse. These lead to a non-inferiority approach, where T is bounded on one side and not the other. Specifically:

$$H_0: T < R - \Delta$$
$$H_1: T \geq R - \Delta$$

Unless you are especially interested in the actual methods used for testing such hypotheses, the issue is best left to the statistician. At the same time, you should be aware that:

- There *are* statistical solutions for showing superiority, equivalence, and non-inferiority.
- When demonstrating equivalence and non-inferiority, you are showing similarity, not identity.

DATA ANALYSIS SCENARIO II

I began this chapter with an Apparatone-Control trial and described the simple scenario (Scenario I) where you conduct the trial and, as planned, analyze your data at the end of it. I then took a detour and dealt with implications of nonsignificant results and equivalence/non-inferiority testing. It is now time to continue with Apparatone where I left off and describe another common testing scenario.

Your Apparatone-Control trial is **double blind**: Physicians do not know which drug they are dispensing, and subjects do not know which they are receiving. Partway into the trial, several physicians in the study report that many subjects have shown relatively dramatic improvements. Since the effect of Control is known—your competitor has been on the market for years now—they believe it likely that these results are due to Apparatone. In other words, they are guessing that Apparatone is a good deal superior to Control.

By now about half of the subjects have completed the study's 24 weeks. Most of the remaining participants have already begun the trial, and a few have yet to be recruited. Given the length of the study, its logistics, and the necessary activities at trial's end, you estimate it will take another 10 months before you can conduct the planned, primary efficacy analysis on all subjects. Ten months is a long time, and your company would like to move forward with Apparatone as quickly as possible. The apparently positive results suggest it may be possible to statistically demonstrate Apparatone's superiority at this early stage.

Using the anecdotal information provided by the physicians, you decide to compare Apparatone to Control using those subjects who have already completed the trial—27 in one group and 26 in another. Analyzing these data you find that Apparatone patients have, on average, 11% more On-Time than those in Control (P < 0.05). You have thus obtained a statistically significant result in the right direction and so wish to stop the trial and declare success.

Well, you cannot. Indeed, unless you had planned this "halfway analysis" before the trial began, you should not have conducted it in the first place. Recall that before the trial began you did the following:

1. Planned a 24-week study, with the primary endpoint Percent-On-Time to be tested after trial completion.
2. Determined that when testing your study hypotheses, you are willing to accept a Type I Error of 5%; in other words, you are willing to live with a 5% chance of wrongly concluding that Apparatone is better than Control.

If you go ahead with your test as planned at the end of the trial and the results are significant, you will claim the following:

■   A 95% chance that your "superiority conclusion" is correct.
■   A 5% chance that it is incorrect (Type I Error).

But this 5% chance of erring is repeated every time you conduct a statistical test of which the criterion for significance is P ≤ 0.05. Thus the chance of error mounts the more tests you do. In fact, were you to conduct five statistical tests, there would be more than a 20% chance that at least one of your results would be significant by chance alone.[6] So conducting your interim test increases your chance for Type I Error beyond 5%. And this is unacceptable.

Now you might argue, "I have only conducted a single test, and it was significant. My chance for Type I Error on it was 5%, and I did not conduct another. Therefore, my Type I Error for the study remained 5%." Well, there are a couple of problems here. First, you chose to do the test based on physicians'

---

[6] This calculation assumes that the tests are independent as, for example, when testing five subgroups of patients.

observations, and so, in a sense, you conducted a post hoc analysis—one that was driven by results. And while the information that led you to the test was anecdotal, had you not been told that there is a good chance for favorable results, you would have not done this **interim analysis**. Second, it stands to reason that if your interim results had been unfavorable, the trial would have continued to its conclusion and the analysis repeated. This means that at the time of conducting the first test, you were already willing to accept a Type I Error larger than 5%. And this, as noted, is unacceptable.

Here, then, we have one example of **multiple testing** or, as it is sometimes called, multiplicity. The more tests you conduct, the greater your chances for erroneously obtaining favorable results. Thus, when planning your trial, you should always do the following:

1. Specify one test only with $P \leq 0.05$ the criterion for significance.

or

2. Specify several tests and make sure that all of them together have no more than a 5% chance of a Type I Error (more on this in a moment).

A NOTE ON BIAS

The trial was set up with both physicians and patients blinded. This was done to limit bias in the study, an issue that will be discussed at length in the chapter dealing with clinical trial design. Nevertheless, word sometimes gets out, and there is little that you can do about it. Thus, many "blinded" trials are not exactly that. In this case, report of dramatic improvements emerged, and both the physicians and you associated it with the new drug. Now you generally cannot help hearing what physicians are saying. But you *can* avoid acting upon it. Making interim decisions based on results already known (partially or fully) is akin to post hoc analysis. And in the preceding chapter I noted how problematic this is. Additionally, and perhaps more importantly, knowing results while a study is ongoing is likely to influence the study's conduct. It might, for instance, affect the type of patients physicians decide to recruit to the study and their conduct with them. This will introduce bias in that the sample is no longer completely random and physician evaluation of results is likely affected by expectation; in other words, they are less objective and so, by definition, biased. Conversely, when results are unfavorable, the pace of recruitment may slow and the type of patients selected for study may change. Evaluations will likely be more unfavorable as well.

Thus, to the degree possible, you should set up your trial so its results remain unknown until all of the data have been collected. And if by chance you come across information on outcome while the trial is ongoing, make every effort not to advertise it and/or act upon it.

DATA ANALYSIS SCENARIO III

Another frequent scenario is, in principle, statistically not so different from the one just described. For the purposes of Scenario III, I shall modify the Apparatone-Control trial to include three arms:

- Apparatone 25 mg
- Apparatone 50 mg
- Control

The trial is done and the numbers look fine. Apparatone 25 mg shows an increase of 7% in On-Time relative to Control, while 50 mg yields an increase of 3%. You compare each of these groups separately to Control and find that the lower dose is significantly superior to the competitor, but the higher dose is not (tests 1 and 2). When combining the two Apparatone arms together and comparing the combined group to Control, your result is significant as well (test 3). Finally, when comparing the two Apparatone arms to each other, the statistical test is nonsignificant (test 4). You conclude the following:

- Apparatone is superior to Control.
- If there is a difference between the two Apparatone doses, 25 mg is likely better. But there is no statistical testing result to back this up, and you did not expect one. The trial was powered to compare Apparatone to Control; it was not designed to detect a significant difference between Apparatone doses.

Well, in terms of multiple testing we have quite a mess here. Because you conducted four tests, your chance for a Type I Error is certainly greater than 5%. And since this is the case, you cannot be completely certain how to interpret your results. The solution is, as always, to plan the statistical tests you will conduct at the end of the trial—their type and number—*before you begin the trial*. You would then ask the statistician to set up the planned tests so their combined chance for Type I Error is no greater than 5%.

SUMMARY AND SOLUTION

In the preceding sections I provided two examples that result in multiple testing. There are many others, and a partial list follows:

- *Multiple comparisons between treatment groups:* This was the case in the preceding section, where three treatment groups led to four comparisons of interest.
- *Repeated testing at different points in time:* In most clinical trials, measurements are taken over time. Repeating the same comparison at different time points—even if done at the end of the trial after results for all of the time points are in—entails multiplicity.
- *Interim analyses:* This involves analyzing data before the trial has been completed, as described in Scenario II. Keep in mind that planned interim analyses are possible and permissible. This will be discussed later.
- *Testing different endpoints:* Virtually all clinical trials have more than one endpoint of interest. Indeed, the number of endpoints in a typical clinical trial often seems endless. Comparing groups on many endpoints entails multiplicity. And multiple testing is likely to yield a significant result here and there, even when this is not the truth in the population.

- *Conducting different statistical tests on the same data:* Different statistical tests can at times be appropriately applied to the same comparison. Applying more than one procedure to a particular comparison constitutes multiplicity as well.

As noted in both of the preceding sections, the solution for an increase in the chance for Type I Error resulting from multiplicity is to make sure that your *overall Type I Error* remains no more than 5%—that all of the critical tests in your trial do not, together, have more than a 0.05 chance of yielding a chance significant result.

While the statistics of multiple testing should be left to the statistician, the principles are sufficiently straightforward that it would be useful for you to be aware of them when designing a study:

1. Plan all primary analyses in advance and specify them in the trial protocol.
2. Make sure that your chance for a Type I Error for all primary tests combined—overall Type I Error—is no greater than 5%. This is done by adjusting the acceptable Type I Error for each test to be less than 5% so that when all tests are considered, the overall chance for Type I Error is 5%. One simple, and overly conservative, way to do this is to divide 0.05 by the number of tests you plan to do and use the new value as the criterion for significance. For example, if you plan to conduct five tests, specify in advance that a result will be considered significant only if $P \leq 0.01$. I mention this to provide you with some idea of how multiplicity can be accounted for. At the same time, I also noted that this is an overly conservative method—one that will reduce your chances for justifiably rejecting the Null. It seems, then, that you will have no choice but to consult with your statistician on this. Recommendation: Where possible—and this is usually possible— specify a single primary analysis in your trial. All other tests are then specified "exploratory" and you do not need to control Type I Error for them. But you must keep in mind that there is a price to paid here, and it is this: Be your secondary analyses what may, they will be viewed as providing weaker evidence than if you had controlled Type I Error for them as well.

Finally, I should note that it is certainly legitimate to conduct multiple tests without controlling for Type I Error. Collecting data via clinical trials is an arduous and costly endeavor, and you should feel free to obtain all the information possible from these data. Statistics should not dictate what you can or cannot do with your data. It will, however, have a great deal to say about the certainty associated with results. Specifically, when you controlled for Type I Error—when you controlled for multiple testing—you can be fairly certain that significant results represent the truth in the population (in fact, 95% certain). Conversely, outcomes of testing where multiplicity was not controlled are more tenuous and are unlikely to be accepted by regulators, companies, or individuals contemplating investing in your product.

COST AND BENEFIT

Setting overall Type I Error at 5% ensures that your chance of erring by incorrectly rejecting H_0 is acceptable. But you obtain this at the price of having a trial that is less sensitive to discovering a new phenomenon—that is, you reduce your chance for rejecting H_1 when it ought to be rejected—you reduce your study's *power*. In other words, the more you protect yourself from Type I Error, the more you are likely to commit a Type II Error (not rejecting H_0 when it should be rejected).

Allow me to illustrate this using an extreme and unrealistic example. Suppose you conduct a study and decide in advance that under no circumstances will you reject the Null Hypothesis. In this case you have ensured that you will not make a Type I Error; because you will never reject H_0, you will also never reject it incorrectly. But when this is the case, H_0 will not be rejected even when it *should* be. In other words, by perfectly protecting yourself from Type I Error, you reduced your study's power to 0. Conversely, deciding in advance to reject H_0 regardless, will ensure that you will not make a Type II Error; you will always reject H_0 when it should be rejected and have 100% power. But then, of course, your chances for rejecting it incorrectly (Type I Error) are high as well. In any study planned, you must balance between:

- Caution—avoidance of incorrectly rejecting the Null

and

- Power—the wish to discover something new by correctly rejecting the Null

And finding the optimal balance must be done via informed interactions among clinicians, R&D managers, and statisticians.

CHAPTER 11

Elements of Clinical Trial Design I: Putting It Together

CONTENTS

- Adapting methodology to objectives
- Blinding and randomization
- On the difference between "less rigorous" design and "shoddy"
- Questions to ask when designing a clinical trial:
  - questions relating directly to design
  - questions relating indirectly to design
- Case study: designing trial in psoriasis
- Independent groups versus paired design
  - power
  - clinical and logistical issues
- The principle underlying correct design
- Random error and bias in testing an antidepressant
- Missing data, bias, and imputation
- Sensitivity analysis
- Analysis sets (intent to treat, per protocol, etc.)

INTRODUCTION: THE FIRST STEPS

A clinical trial is designed to meet specific objectives. It is your job to ensure that there will be a good chance for it. So before all else you must articulate your aims clearly. In Chapter 2 I noted that in any study the basic question is *"What do I want to show?"* This leads to the distinction between a trial's primary *attributes of interest* and its *analytic aims*. Combining these two dimensions generated Table 11.1, which covers most trials' objectives.

Table 11.1 Clinical Trial Aims and Attributes

Analytic Aim	Attribute of Interest			
	Efficacy	Safety	Performance	Pharmacokinetics
Superiority	A	B	C	D
Equivalence	E	F	G	H
Non-inferiority	I	J	K	L

In Chapter 10, we wanted to demonstrate that Apparatone Percent On-Time is better than Reference over 24 weeks. This primary objective lands you in cell "A," where the aim is to show superiority on efficacy. Yet, virtually all trials are concerned also with safety, which puts you in "J" as well.

Unlike efficacy, demonstrating that your product is safe is typically done informally by comparing descriptive statistics between study arms; unless a trial has a very high frequency of product-related safety events—and fortunately most do not—hypothesis testing on these parameters is neither practical nor meaningful. Thus, in most trials, safety will be evaluated by examination of descriptive statistics relating to proportions of adverse events (AEs) in study arms, their severities, and their relationship to Treatment. These semiformal comparisons will be supplemented by biological knowledge, where AEs will be related to what may or may not be expected in the indication. For example, we are more likely to attribute an occurrence of stroke to Treatment in a cardiology trial than in gynecology, even if in both cases there may have been no apparent causal connection. Either way, statistical testing on infrequent serious AEs (SAEs) is unfeasible. For example, observing "only" 1 death in 100 due to study Treatment should certainly be enough to be rid of it (assuming, of course, that a safer alternative exists). At the same time, formally comparing 1/100 to 0/100 will not yield statistical significance.

Be that as it may, there certainly *are* cases where safety is tested formally. One might, for example, require a heart valve replacement procedure to yield significantly less than, say, 5% major adverse cardiac events (MACE), such as heart attack and death.

Like most activities, trials are conducted under multiple constraints, the most common of which are time and money. But whatever the limitations, your resources must be sufficient for a trial's informational needs, including the following:

1. Type of information required (efficacy, safety, etc.).
2. Amount of information required (number of subjects, length of follow-up period, etc.).
3. Level of certainty in the information obtained—that is, the degree to which you will be confident of the results obtained.

It goes without saying that companies prefer more information to less and wish to have great confidence in it. And they would also like to have all this within timeline and budget requirements. Well it is generally impossible to maximize everything and, personally, I know of no bakery that provides cakes that can be both had and eaten. More importantly, maximizing everything—if at all possible—is usually unnecessary, since the amount of data collected and confidence in a study's conclusions should correspond to the intended audience's needs and no more. Moreover, investing more resources in a trial than are needed may be unethical as well as wasteful (see Chapter 14).

A study's informational needs are addressed by the question *"Whom do I want to show my results to?"* (see Chapter 2). This refers to the study's intended audience, which may include regulators, investors, management, physicians, the scientific community, and others—individuals who typically have different "evidentiary requirements" from a trial. Consequently, pinpointing the audience for your study's results is central to design.

For example, regulatory agencies are likely to require extensive information that was collected using precisely defined procedures before granting marketing approval. This is not the case, however, with companies that are assessing feasibility, where a relatively informal trial aimed at providing "some idea" of safety and efficacy will suffice. Physicians, on the other hand, are generally more impressed by articles in leading scientific journals than by FDA approval. Thus, for example, when submitting to the regulator, you might go for a non-inferiority trial to increase the likelihood of formal success. Once regulatory approval is "out of the way," you will design another study that may only get into a leading journal if it results in superiority.[1] Conversely, when information is for internal company use only, a trend (rather than significance) might suffice. Specifying more modest goals will allow for using more modest resources. Thus some objectives and audiences will require rigorous trials, while others will get by with less.

Rigorousness of design is very much what this chapter is about. We will examine how to achieve it and look at some of the more common techniques for "rigor by design," such as **blinding** and **randomization**. Some of the elements that were discussed in the preceding chapters will make an appearance, as well as some new ones. Taken together, these will provide you with general principles of trial design. At the same time, what makes most clinical trials fascinating (and difficult) are the elements that are unique to them. Indeed, I have rarely encountered a study—simple as it may have seemed at

---

[1] Or, more commonly (and not completely kosher), write a non-inferiority protocol that obligates you with the regulator, and if superiority emerges, publish it (omitting to mention the initial hypothesis).

first glance—that did not present distinctive challenges. And while it is always advisable to apply common principles of correct design, stock solutions will usually only get you partway there.

So some studies are less thorough than others, and this is fine. But it is important to distinguish between "less rigorous" and "shoddy." It is one thing to knowingly design a less-than-ideal trial, optimizing resources to coincide with objectives, and it is quite another to use resources inefficiently. In short, your study should be as sound as possible given the means available. To ensure that this happens, you should do the following:

- State your goals clearly, and delineate the consumers for your data.
- Correctly apply the principles of experimental design.
- Consult with experts where you feel your knowledge is lacking.
- Think!

And when resources are limited, you must be also courageous enough to forgo a study that has little chance of achieving its objectives.

CLASSIFYING DESIGN PRINCIPLES

When doing science one's natural tendency is to classify. In this frame of mind I have often tried to come up with a classification system for issues relating to clinical trial design. At times I thought I had met with success, only to find novel permutations that cannot be fit neatly into any predefined category. So instead of forcing my questions into an artificial classification system, I shall present them in two very general categories: questions relating *directly* to trial design and those relating *indirectly*. And even here you will find that some distinctions are artificial. Regardless, my goal here is to present and overview only. If you are especially interested in trial design principles, I suggest you pick up one or two books on that topic.[2]

QUESTIONS REVISITED

Following are some questions that experience has taught me are important when designing clinical studies. They relate to practical issues, and I suspect that you have encountered at least some of them yourself. Where possible I suggest you recall the situations in which you were faced with them and the solutions applied.

---

[2] Pocock, S. J. (1991). Clinical trials: A practical approach, New York: Wiley and Sons; Piantadosi, S. (2005). Clinical trials: A methodologic perspective, **Hoboken, NJ:** Wiley and Sons.

Questions Relating Directly to Trial Design

- What are your primary objectives? Do you aim to show superiority, non-inferiority, and so on? This is the study's most basic element—that on which its very purpose hangs. It comes under the heading *Analytic Aim* in Table 11.1.
- Which primary characteristics do you wish to test? This too is basic and appears in Table 11.1 under *Attribute of Interest*.
- What are the endpoints that will best address your study's objectives? In other words, how will you translate attributes such as safety and efficacy into actual measures to be evaluated at trial's end? This issue of endpoints—their choice, measurement properties, and number—is sufficiently important to warrant its own chapter and will get it soon.
- For whom is the study's information meant?
- How many arms will the study have, and, most important, will one of them be a Control group?
- What is the most appropriate comparison group for your study? In most cases you will have more than one option. For example, you might choose a Placebo, a Predicate, or, perhaps, another Dose of your own medication. In some cases you may forgo a Control group altogether in favor of, for example, comparison to historical data. An alternative may be a one-arm trial where each subject is compared at the end of the trial to his or her condition at baseline.
- How many subjects will participate in the trial? This relates to sample size and will naturally be honored with a chapter of its own.
- If the study is to have more than one arm, how will subjects be divided among them? This relates to both:
  - Randomization technique used, if any.
  - Ratio of assignment of subjects to groups. For example, you might decide to assign subjects in equal proportions to study arms (i.e., a 1:1 ratio) or apply a 2:1 ratio in favor of the experimental product. Assigning a larger number of subjects to Treatment than Control is typically done for obtaining more precise information about the effects of the experimental product—that is, the new product for which there is usually less information than the Comparator.
- Is blinding possible in the trial? If it is, will both patients and physicians be blinded or only one of these? Will the statistician be blinded as well? What specific procedures will you put in place to ensure that those who should not be aware of subject assignment to Treatment and overall study results will, in fact, be unaware of them?
- How many study centers and treating physicians will there be?
- Will there be decision points during the trial in the form of **interim analysis**, or will all formal analyses be done once the trial is done and all the data collected?

Questions Relating Indirectly to Trial Design

- What is the intended use population for your product in general? How will you increase the likelihood for your drug working in the population selected? For example, you may want to exclude those with:
  - Very severe forms of the disease, because they will probably not be helped by your treatment.
  - Especially mild forms, since they will often recover spontaneously without an intervention.
- Will the current study represent the whole of the intended use population or a subgroup of it only? For example, when your primary aim is to demonstrate feasibility—to show your drug has some "promising potential"—you might include only that subgroup with the greatest likelihood of benefiting from the product. This sort of limited trial will typically require a smaller sample size than one assessing the whole of the intended use population.
- Are the study's goals primarily exploratory or confirmatory? If the trial will have elements of both, what are they? Which of the study endpoints will be confirmatory and which exploratory?
- Where will the study be conducted? This refers to centers, regions, and countries, as well as to actual physical surroundings (hospital, outpatient clinic, home, etc.).
- Who will conduct the trial? Specifically, you must make sure that the health care personnel participating will represent those who will be using the product once it is on the market. For example, when evaluating a device for detecting skin cancer, will the device be intended for physicians in general or dermatologists only?
- How will you ensure that participating centers adequately represent those in which the product will be used once it is approved?
- What are the resources available for the trial?
- How does this particular study fit into the company's overall development plan? For instance, if this is a Phase II study, will its primary endpoint be the same as that planned for the pivotal trial?
- How are missing values to be addressed when analyzing study results? This relates directly to statistical analysis of data rather than study design. At the same time, a trial's procedures and logistics must be planned to minimize the occurrence of missing data. For example, specifying few visits and measures in a short trial is likely to provide more complete information than planning a longer trial with many visits and measurements.

The questions listed, and the many others that are not, overlap to some degree or another. You would do well to raise as many questions as possible and answer them as best you can with the resources at your disposal. There is no need to be concerned about this. Asking questions is cheap and answering them is often inexpensive as well.

COMPLICATIONS

The topics described in the preceding section were raised freely. In the sections that follow, I will describe more systematic principles for optimizing trial design. But before getting there I must emphasize again that planning a clinical study is far from an orderly process. As much as you might like it otherwise, you will likely be sidetracked in study design as well.

Here is an example: Say you are evaluating a topical agent for psoriasis. The preceding trial was a dose-response study that identified what the Company believes is the optimal dose. It now wishes to test this dose in a small- to medium-size trial to confirm the finding and, hopefully, justify moving on to pivotal Phase III testing. The primary efficacy endpoint in the current study is—as it will be in Phase III if you get there—Change in Affected Area on the skin from baseline to end of trial (or Change in Lesion Size).

You initially plan a simple two-arm study in which one group receives R (standard of care) and another T (Company's innovative ointment). Subjects will be randomized using a 1:1 ratio, meaning there will be an equal number per group. You consult with the statistician, who asks you a few questions and comes back with a recommendation for 123 subjects per group, for a total of 246.

Your regulatory affairs manager then reminds you that for market approval in this indication, the regulator typically requires that at least 1,500 subjects in total be exposed to a drug (over all phases). The regulator's concern is safety, anticipating that a sample of 1,500 subjects can reveal relatively rare adverse events if any exist. The regulator could, of course, have chosen a larger or smaller number. While to some degree arbitrary, the specific "overall exposure" requirement determined by the agency is based on risk analysis in the indication, experience with similar drugs, and the burden that can be reasonably placed on companies in the process of a **new drug application** (NDA) process. Be that as it may, if 1,500 subjects must be exposed to the product before approval, you must make sure this will be the case.

So while your focus on the current Phase II trial has not changed, you are now also thinking about future trials as well. Specifically, you wonder whether more subjects should be getting T in this trial, which will get you nearer to the 1,500 required at the end of the day.

Now thinking ahead is generally a good idea. Yet it can, like thinking in general, complicate matters. Here it leads you to consider exposing more subjects to your new medication. You now contemplate a 2:1 ratio assignment for the current study—two subjects assigned to T for every one to R. Keeping the number of subjects planned constant at 246, 164 will be randomized to T and 82 to R.

Now all this would be good and well if it were not for the issue of free lunches—or rather, the lack of them. Specifically, trial power—its chance for correctly rejecting the Null—is optimal when sample sizes are equal in treatment arms. Having changed your trial's treatment allocation, you will also need to increase sample size to obtain the original power planned.

One option is to remain with your 1:1 trial and worry about the pivotal trial later. You reason that if the drug does well in the upcoming study, there will surely be enough resources for larger pivotal studies—such that would yield the 1,500 exposed to T over all phases. This might in fact be your best alternative. Still, you do not want to give up on what, after internal Company discussions, seems a good option: a 2:1 assignment ratio. Yet choosing this alternative requires going back to management for more resources, which you are loathe to do. So what *do* you do?

Well, all things considered, what you want to do is the *right* thing. But you have now complicated matters sufficiently that you are no longer certain what that is. Then some little articulate bird whispers "statistician" in your ear, and you reluctantly pick up the phone.

You tell the statistician that you wish to treat more subjects with the new medication, given the fixed budget allotted to a two-arm trial; is it possible, you ask, with the same budget to design a trial with a larger number of subjects receiving the new medication? The statistician says there might be and suggests a **paired design**—one in which each subject receives both medications. For this trial you would choose subjects with at least two skin lesions and randomly assign T to one lesion and R to the other. At study's end you will do the following:

1. Compute Change in Affected Area for each lesion separately.
2. For each subject, compute the difference between T-treated and R-treated lesions on Change in Affected Area.
3. Average the differences computed in step 2 over all subjects.
4. Test whether the average computed in step 2 is sufficiently different from 0 to indicate that T and R truly differ.

Note that if T = R, the average difference between Change in Affected Area between them should be about 0. Thus, statistical testing in this trial aims to show that T – R is significantly greater than 0; in other words, Change is greater with the new ointment compared to standard of care. In principle this is no different than a trial in two independent groups, where your objective is demonstrating that Reduction in T is greater than that in R (or T – R > 0).

Using this design, you have a 1:1 assignment ratio, except that now each subject receives both T and R—that is, a subject is his or her own Control, and this way, you have cut the initial sample size by half. You can now go on to add to this number and obtain the total of 164 you aimed for with the 2:1 design, except that with this design the number of subjects receiving T and R is equal. This provides better power relative to the uneven ratio. Moreover, the statistician tells you that this setup is likely to be *much* more powerful than the other because comparisons are paired.

PAIRED DESIGNS AND POWER

I mentioned that paired designs, where each subject receives both treatments, are more powerful than **independent group designs**, where each subject gets one of the treatments. There are some exceptions, but when the paired design is logistically practical and clinically relevant, they are few.

I will now present some hypothetical numbers that should help understand why paired designs can be especially powerful:

1. In Table 11.2, **A** represents a design with six subjects: three whose lesions are treated with R and the remaining three with T; therefore, the study has six subjects and six lesions.
2. **B** represents a design with three subjects. Each has one lesion treated with T and the other with R;

therefore, the study has three subjects and six lesions.

Table 11.2 describes hypothetical results of these two studies for each individual lesion. Each outcome represents a reduction in Lesion Size from baseline to the end of the trial. Thus, the larger the value the better.

The following can be said of the similarities in outcome in the two studies:

- The three values for lesions treated with R in A and the three for R in B are identical. The same can be said for lesions treated with T. Consequently:
  - Mean R_A = Mean R_B = 31.3
  - Mean T_A = Mean T_B = 28.0
  - Mean difference of R and T is 3.3 in both groups

Table 11.2 Reduction in Lesion Size in mm² From Baseline to End of Trial, for Each Subject by Type of Study (Independent or Paired) by Treatment (Reference or Treatment)

A: Independent Groups Design[a]		B: Paired Design[b]				
Group			Group			
	R (mm²)	T (mm²)	Subject	R (mm²)	T (mm²)	Delta
	6 (subject 1)	13 (subject 4)	1	6	4	2
	71 (subject 2)	4 (subject 5)	2	17	13	4
	17 (subject 3)	67 (subject 6)	3	71	67	4
Mean	31.3	28.0		31.3	28.0	3.3
SD	34.8	34.1		34.8	34.1	1.2

[a]*Each of six subjects has one lesion chosen and is treated with either R or T on it.*
[b]*Each of three subjects has two lesions chosen, one randomly assigned to treatment with R and the other to T.*

Continued

PAIRED DESIGNS AND POWER— CONT'D

Note that the mean difference in A was computed by subtracting 28.0 from 31.3, which is the mean of all R subjects taken from the mean of A subjects. In B, I first computed the difference for each subject, then computed the mean of the differences. Since the operations of addition and subtraction are transitive, I obtained the same result: The difference between means equals the mean of differences.

But while the numbers are the same in the two studies, there is a crucial difference between the two setups with regard to statistical testing. To understand why this is so, you must remember that when we do statistical testing we must give meaning to numbers, since by themselves they have none. For example, 100 miles may be nothing to a truck driver, but it is a great distance to one who commutes 2.3 miles to work every day. In statistics we have an elegant way of demonstrating this formally, which works as follows:

1. Observe all distances covered daily by the truck driver and the commuter.
2. Compute the mean of distances for each separately.
3. For each, compute standard deviation (SD) of these distances using the following formula:

$$SD = \sqrt{\frac{(X_i - \overline{X})^2}{N}}$$

Now the formula for SD is one of those few revealing formulas that provides insight into statistical thinking. It is for this reason that I present it here. Let us now attempt to tease out its meaning. In the formula:

- The overall mean is subtracted from each individual value. In our case, we have a commuter who, say, has a mean of 2.3 miles per day computed over 200 commuting days.
- The differences are squared. For example, if on a particular day the commuter drove 1.2 miles, the deviation from the mean is –1.1, which we square and obtain 1.21. If on another day the commute was 5.3 miles, the difference from the mean is +2 miles and its square is 4. We do this for all distances

observed, divide by N,[3] and take the square root of the result. In slow, more meaningful motion we do the following:

- Subtract each trip from the mean of all trips. This provides a deviation—the commuter's deviation on that day from her typical commute, where "typical is represented by the mean over all trips."
- Square each individual deviation so that all differences are positive.
- Sum all the squared differences and divide by N. This yields the "typical squared deviation" from the typical trip. If you will, it is the average squared deviation.
- Take the square root, which returns the numbers to their original units in miles (they are no longer squared).
- The final result is something like the average deviation of all the trips from their mean. Since we have some squaring and square roots here, the final result is not exactly an average. It is therefore termed a *standard deviation* rather than an *average deviation*. But while technically it is not precisely an average, this is its meaning; in other words, the SD is, more or less, the average deviation of values from the mean in a given distribution.

The SD provides us with an excellent tool for putting numbers into context—for giving them meaning. For example, let us suppose that on a particular day our erstwhile commuter traveled 4 miles and that her mean over all days is 2.3 and SD is 3.4. Now while 4 miles is 1.7 miles more than her usual commute, it is well within her typical deviation from her average. In fact, it is half her usual deviation:

---

[3] *Or N – 1, depending on whether we are computing a sample or population standard deviation. But this need not concern us here because (a) I wish to present the concept and not detain you with more mathematical issues and (b) when N – the number of observations is large, the difference between dividing by N or N – 1 is near meaningless. For example, divide 10 by 200 and you get 0.05, and divide 10 by 199 and you get 0.0502512.*

PAIRED DESIGNS AND POWER— CONT'D

(4.0 − 2.3)/3.4 = 0.5. In other words, this 4-mile trip can be said to be "typical" and "about average" for her (even though her actual average is 2.3 miles).

Once more in slow motion: To evaluate whether a distance such as 4 is greater or small, I subtracted it from the mean of 2.3 and obtained 1.7. Now 1.7 may be very little or very much; recall that distances by themselves tell you next to nothing. So I put this 1.7 into the context of 3.4, the "average distances from the average" for this commuter. And this turned out to be half the typical deviation from her mean trip (not very much).

On the other hand, a truck driver whose mean may be 80 miles and SD 20 miles is only one SD from the mean when driving 100 miles. In other words, this is his "typical" deviation—a "regular" trip for him. Thus, 100 miles for the truck driver is about the same as 5.6 miles for our commuter; these respective distances are, relatively speaking, the same for both.

What is the moral of this story? In statistics we evaluate differences (and ratios and other measures of disparities between numbers). Based on the values (of distance) that we obtain, we must decide:

- This distance is really large—"T and R truly differ."

or

- This distance is not really large—"T and R cannot be said to be different."

To evaluate distance, we compute an SD, which serves as our reference, our context. If the distance we obtain is very large in SD terms, it is large. If the distance between T and R is very small relative to SD, it is small. In short, we look at a distance relative to its context that we term SD; we do not look at the distance by itself.

- Back to our independent and paired designs: Paired designs usually (but not always) yield much smaller references/contexts/standard deviations and with them, a much greater chance to conclude that T and R are significantly different. The SD in our paired design is 1.2, and the distance between T and R

is 3.3. The SD in the independent design is about 50,[4] and the distance between T and R is 3.3 as well. Using the reasoning presented, the same "raw difference" (3.3) in the two groups has a completely different meaning in terms of magnitude. It is a great magnitude in the paired design and a small one in the independent design; it is a significant difference in the paired design and a nonsignificant difference in the independent design.

- A challenging exercise might be to look at Table 11.2 and figure out how this sort of magic occurred—where the same distance in the context of the same T and R can have very divergent meanings. Regardless of whether or not you figure this out, it is important to remember that paired designs can, when appropriate, provide very powerful tools for getting at the truth (in the population). Unfortunately, they are often inappropriate—impossible even—which will be discussed.

Just a final note: The statistical test described here involved subtracting one value from another and dividing by some measure of variation, such as SD.[5] This is typical of the most common statistical tests, which are classified under the heading of the general linear model (GLM, including t-test, analysis of variance, regression, mixed linear models, and others). Now in statistics there are many different types of tests, depending on the data available; GLM can be used in many cases but not all. But the principle is always the same: Evaluate divergence (by difference or ratio or whatever) relative to some context. If the divergence is great, we conclude a real/true difference in the population between the groups tested in the trial, and the result is significant. If the divergence is not great, we hold our peace.

---

[4] The formula for computing the common standard deviation for two groups—in this case, for computing the standard deviation of their differences—can be found in any basic statistics book, and we shall just leave it at that.

[5] Actually, we use the standard error (SE) rather than standard deviation (SD) for very important reasons but it is not sufficiently important for our purposes to dwell on them here. For general information SE is typically much smaller than SD and is computed by $SD / \sqrt{N}$ where N is the number of subjects in the trial.

Paired designs can, however, have drawbacks. Indeed, in some cases they are impossible. For example, you may want to compare the relative efficacy of mastectomy and lumpectomy as treatments for breast cancer, where a paired design is impossible for obvious reasons. There can be other, more subtle difficulties with the paired design, and our particular psoriasis study illustrates them:

- Both medications are topical, so you expect their effect to be mostly, if not exclusively, local. This is good and suggests you can in fact treat two lesions on the same subject with different medications. At the same time, enough of each drug may enter the bloodstream so that, to some degree, each lesion gets treated by both medications. This will bias your results in that the estimated effect of one drug will be confounded by the effect of the other. Thus, before embarking on a paired design, you will need to make sure that treating two lesions on the same subject with different medications will be indeed that.
- Now, even if the medications do not enter the blood (which is something you should already know from Phase I), a paired design introduces another problem. Specifically, if your Test drug is in fact more effective than the Reference, subjects are likely to notice it. And if they do, they may apply your medication to both lesions, which is understandable. After all, their personal comfort is of greater priority than scientific knowledge. In other words, at least some of your subjects may not comply with the trial's protocol. This will weaken the difference between lesions and so bias the trial's results. And if many subjects choose to do this, your outcome may be invalid altogether.

I will leave you to address these different options—to think about what might be an optimal design under varying considerations of time, money, and compliance. My point in this section is to show the kind of back and forth inherent in clinical trials that makes it often difficult to "work by the book." And yet despite what I have written in this section, we will now move on to "the book."

THE PRINCIPLE

A clinical trial is planned, run, and analyzed to provide information on a product of interest. As such, *its data must reflect on the product*. This, as the U.S. Constitution would have it, should be self-evident. Stating the idea analytically in the context of a simple study, we have something like the following:

- In your trial, groups T and R have a similar makeup of subjects who will have been treated the same in all respects but one: One group will receive the Test drug and the other will receive the Reference.
- When this is the case, (nonrandom) differences that emerge from the two groups will necessarily be attributed to the drug received—to the fact that the *only* difference between the groups was the type of treatment dispensed.

This, then, in its simplest form is how to ensure that your trial will provide information on the product of interest:

1. Equate groups on all but the parameter or parameters of interest.
2. Run your trial—treat each group differently in a controlled manner.
3. Assess whether or not the groups provide "about equal" results.

Putting it the other way around, a clinical study's outcome should not reflect factors extraneous to the information you seek. For example, if subjects in T are generally younger than those in R, you will not know if any group differences that emerge are due to Treatment, Age, or both.

While the principle is obvious, and we have likely known it long before doing science, it turns out that factors *other* than Treatment often come into play in clinical studies. As you might imagine, it cannot be otherwise since it is impossible to equate groups completely on all but Treatment. And this means that you must be very careful in both designing clinical studies and reaching conclusions from them.

RANDOM ERROR

Statisticians distinguish between two types of error that can influence study results. One is **random error**, which is so called because it can go either way about equally. For example, suppose your trial's primary endpoint is Systolic Blood Pressure. Random error may occur because:

- Physicians vary in ability to measure blood pressure. Some may provide higher values, others lower, and some will usually be about accurate. Moreover, each physician will vary in measurement accuracy from one occasion to another.
- Some devices are more accurate than others, and here too, a given device is likely to vary in accuracy from one occasion to another.
- Some subjects may have exerted themselves more and others less before being measured. And since subjects vary in the behavior on different occasions, so will the accuracy of measurements obtained from them.

These errors in measurement are likely to increase or decrease Blood Pressure values about equally in the different study arms. As such, they are random and will add noise to a study's outcome but are not expected to *bias* results in one direction or another—that is, the resulting error is not expected to provide a consistent advantage to one group or the other. For example, random physician error is expected to be about the same in both groups, so neither group will be disadvantaged by it. However, overall measurement will be "noisier," making results less reliable and the study less powerful—less likely to detect true differences between T and R, since they are at least partially masked by noise. Hence when designing a trial, you should make every effort to reduce random error. In the specific case of Blood Pressure, you might, for example, do the following:

- Provide physicians with standard and explicit instructions on the procedure to be used (e.g., subject must have rested five minutes before being evaluated, and actual measurement should be done when subject is in a sitting position in a chair with backrest, etc.).
- Provide physicians with uniform training of procedures.
- Use devices of the same make in all clinics and calibrate them regularly.
- Monitor the data as they are being collected, investigate erroneous/ suspicious results, and take corrective action if needed.

Now all this will not solve your random error problem completely. But it *will* reduce it. So first you design all technical elements of your trial to minimize error (e.g., select accurate instruments and train participants to measure correctly). Once done, specify a sufficiently large sample size to reduce the remaining error to the point that reliable conclusions can be reached.

Random error is a fact of both sampling and measurement. In the long run (on average), it tends to even out, leaving you with outcomes that are unbiased estimates of T-R differences. But you can imagine that in small samples even randomness may not help, since it has not gotten its "long run" chance. Here is a simple example related to sampling: You assign subjects to groups T or R in an indication where males and females are equally likely to have the disorder. If your study has only four subjects per group, imbalances in gender makeup can happen easily. For example, in one group 75% of those assigned will happen to be women and in the other 75% will be men. So while sampling error is indeed random (when sampling is done correctly), it may still yield groups that differ appreciably and bias results.

In this example, any differences (or lack thereof) at the end of the trial may be due to Gender rather than to the medication of interest. However, this sort of imbalance is unlikely to happen with 100 subjects per group. When the numbers are large, imbalances in sampling are expected to be relatively small.

Similarly, measurement error tends to even out in the long run. For example, if you have only a few subjects in each Treatment arm, a large error in the blood pressure values of one subject may have a major effect on group comparisons. However, when the sample is large, this sort of error will likely occur in both groups about equally, and a single subject's erroneous outcome is less apt to affect the study's results overall.

So to summarize thus far:

- Random error in sampling and measurement is a fact we must live with.
- Random error will add noise to data but will not bias in one direction or another (it is, by definition, random).
- Good design reduces random error.
- Larger samples reduce the effect of random error.

The last bullet deserves emphasizing. Many who plan clinical studies feel that a large sample size will "take care of business." Well, it often will. Yet, it is both wasteful and unethical to increase sample size to solve problems that can be dealt with by designing a better trial. So first design a good trial, and only then resort to the "sample size solution."

BIAS

What I said in the preceding section is unfortunately not true for **bias**, the second type of error statisticians talk about. Bias, as the word implies, *misleads*. An example of potential bias was described earlier where subjects in one group were younger than in the other. As long as this remains, increasing sample size will not help you; whether your sample size per group is 20 or 200, as long as subjects in the two groups differ on Age, the result may be due to this parameter rather than the different treatments administered. The solution, then, is designing a study where this bias will not occur.

The moral of this story is that there will always be at least some superfluous influences on your trial's outcome. This in turn will make it impossible to attribute *all* T-R differences to the treatments administered. Studies are done *by* people and *with* people and in real-world environments. As such, their outcomes will be affected by other than Treatment differences. These include differences among physicians, subjects, centers, equipment, laboratories, and so on. But as long as these "contributors to error" are random—as long as they influence the results in all groups randomly and so, we expect, about equally—your results may be weaker than you wish, but the weakness can be overcome. But if your study is biased, its results will *deceive* and so may be invalid altogether.

Here is another example: Suppose you are testing an innovative antidepressant using a simple two-arm study in which half the subjects are assigned to receive a placebo and half will receive your drug. The study is planned for four weeks, at the end of which you will compare the two groups.[6] While you expect results

---

[6] The comparison will usually be done on the difference between baseline and end-of-trial values on some measure of depression. However, the actual endpoint chosen is not particularly relevant for the moral of this particular story.

to reflect the difference in efficacy between T and R, let us explore why this may not be the only reason for group differences:

- Subjects recruited for studying depression are naturally depressed. In fact, they are likely to be even more depressed than the general population of depressed individuals. This is so because a trial in this indication typically specifies a minimal depression score for inclusion in the trial—one indicating an abnormally high level of disease. This is reasonable. After all, your drug is meant to treat people who are ill, and you want to make sure that those participating are sufficiently so to be helped by your drug. At the same time, depression is known to wax and wane. On average, those with high levels will tend to improve over time and those with low levels will tend to worsen. And this waxing and waning is unrelated to Treatment. Since you have included especially depressed people in your trial, you can expect that, on average, more will improve than worsen regardless of Treatment.

- Depression has known neurological causes. But to a great degree it is also under psychological control. Consequently, you can expect a sizeable **placebo effect**—improvements that have nothing to do with the chemical makeup of treatments. This too will cause the study's actual results to inaccurately reflect the effect you wish to study.[7] In fact, the differences you obtain in this particular trial may be smaller than the true, "long run" difference between the two treatments. This takes us to the next bullet.

- Your trial is relatively short—shorter than most in an indication where study periods are typically 12 weeks or more. Your study's length (or rather, the lack of it) may yield a relatively large placebo effect masking your drug's effect. This is because placebo effects tend to decrease over time, and your planned study provides little opportunity for this to happen.

As study designs go, this one is straightforward. And in it I have identified reasons that it may produce outcomes reflecting something other than Treatment differences. As you can imagine, there are several solutions for the difficulties described, although none are perfect.

The bottom line is that bias is generally a more serious problem than random error.[8] While the latter can be overcome by large samples, bias cannot

---

[7] If the placebo effect is equal in the two groups and the drug's effect is "on top" of the placebo effect your results will not be biased. Whether this is or is not the case should be discussed with clinicians familiar with the indication.

[8] As with most rules, here too there are exceptions. For example, a slightly biased trial providing a slight underestimation of a treatment effect is preferable to one in which random error is so great that the effect goes undetected.

and must be addressed directly. Thus, a central principal of clinical study design is:

Identify bias and eliminate it!

Read this sentence a few times and burn it into your brain. It cannot be overemphasized.

In the following sections I present common examples of potential sources of bias in clinical trials. Some of these have been mentioned in passing, some not, and many others are not on the list. Virtually every trial has the potential for its own, specific brand of bias. It is pointless to attempt an exhaustive list. Here I merely intend to point you in a few directions when looking to reduce bias in clinical trials. In general, however, you will have to seek your own unique trouble in any particular trial.

Missing Data

In virtually every trial some of the subjects drop out at one point or another. The number of **dropouts** can be quite large, especially in longer trials and/or studies of which the procedures are particularly burdensome for participants. In many cases the reasons for individual dropout are unknown. But the potential for the bias they introduce can be substantial and must be considered. In point of fact, missing data can lead to random error and/or bias. The difficulty, of course, is that since the data are missing, you cannot know. ICH guidelines state the following:

> If all subjects randomized into a clinical trial satisfied all entry criteria, followed all trial procedures perfectly with no losses to follow-up, and provided complete data records, then the set of subjects to be included in the analysis would be self-evident. The design and conduct of a trial should aim to approach this ideal as closely as possible, but in practice, it is doubtful if it can ever be fully achieved.

It goes without saying that the preferred way to deal with the problem is to not have missing data in the first place. And to the degree possible, efforts should be made in this direction. At the same time, missing data are generally inevitable and must be dealt with. One way to address the problem in statistical analyses is to make "intelligent assumptions" on why subjects dropped out. Based on these assumptions we then **impute** (attribute) outcomes to them. We will then conduct analyses under different "missing data scenarios." This is termed **sensitivity analysis**, and its goal is to assess the degree to which outcomes are sensitive to different assumptions about (1) why data are missing and (2) what results may have looked like had the data not been missing.

For example, in acute indications such as bacterial infections, subjects dropping out might tend to be those whose disease was treated successfully. Once treated, their problem is resolved and they feel no need to return for follow-up evaluation. If your drug is particularly effective, this sort of "dropout tendency" will weaken efficacy. This is because more subjects will have dropped out due to success. And if Treatment is indeed superior to Control, more can be expected to drop out from the former. But keep in mind that this is an assumption and that you do not really know whether it is the case; the subjects who dropped out are long gone. You can, however, make reasonable assumptions about the causes of dropout, impute missing values accordingly, and assess outcomes under different imputation scenarios. In the example described, you might assign success to all dropouts—in both Treatment and Control—reanalyze the data, and see how this affects your results. If in both analyses—that using only observed data and that including imputed "success" to dropouts—your Treatment emerges superior to Control, you may be in the clear; your data are insensitive (robust) to different, reasonable assumptions about missing data. But what if the following are true?

1. Analyses on observed data show no difference between Treatment and Control.
2. Analyses on data where missing values have been imputed produce superiority of Treatment to Control.

Well, it is not clear.

Moreover, there is always the possibility that subjects dropping out from each of the groups do so for different reasons. For example, those who dropped out from Treatment may have done so because their problems were solved, and those who dropped out from Control may have done so because their problems were not solved. If this were the case, the appropriate imputation would be "success" to those dropping out from Treatment and "failure" to those leaving Control. This in turn would strengthen your results.

Depending on the pattern of missing data and the imputations chosen, many results are possible. And these outcomes may be inconsistent with one another, which may introduce uncertainty into any conclusions you wish to reach.

In chronic indications, for example, it is reasonable to assume that subjects are more likely to drop out when their treatment is ineffective; had the treatment been effective, they would return because their disease requires continual attention. Having only successful subjects remain in the study may increase observed success in *both* Control and Treatment. Here, too, reasonable imputations should be made and sensitivity analyses conducted. For example, you might assign failure to missing subjects in both groups. And if there are more of them in Control than in Treatment, the latter will profit. Indeed, as part of your exploration of the possible effects of missing data, you should assess their pattern across study arms—explore whether their numbers and types differed across groups. For example, you might ask if more dropped out of R than T or if those who dropped out differed in any way (e.g., Age) from those who stayed. There can, as you can imagine, be many more questions such as these, the answers of which are likely to help you better interpret study outcome.

Missing data can occur for reasons other than patient dropout—for example, when a physician forgets to assess a certain parameter or a measuring instrument has malfunctioned. In these cases, a particular measurement has been lost but not the subject. The degree to which this can be a serious problem depends, of course, on the number and type of such missing values. As a rule, this sort of lost data presents less difficulty than subject dropout for the following reasons:

1. The magnitude of lost data is usually smaller.
2. It is generally safe to assume that phenomena such as device malfunction and physician forgetfulness occur randomly. This may definitely not be the case for subject dropout.

There are many other possibilities. For example, in some cases, it is reasonable to assign a subject's last observed value to his or her missing measurement. This is called **last observation carried forward** (LOCF). There are, however, instances where this sort of imputation will bias your results. For example, when assessing a disease in which patient's condition deteriorates over time (e.g., Alzheimer's), LOCF is inappropriate. This is because LOCF keeps measurements constant over time, which is not appropriate in diseases where measurements are expected to change over the course of a trial. Thus, using LOCF in Alzheimer's—substituting later measurements with earlier ones—is likely to bias outcomes upward.

The issue of missing data is as difficult to deal with as it is common. While there are general rules for addressing the problem, missing values must ultimately be dealt with in the context of the specific trial.[9] Most important, *methods for addressing missing data should be specified in the protocol*. In this way you will avoid the potential bias of specifying imputations and analyses after already having information about a trial's results.

---

[9] For additional (readable) information, see European Agency for Evaluation of Medicinal Products (EMEA). (2001). Points to consider on missing values. London: European Medicines Agency.

The analytic approaches described are designed to overcome possible biases attributable to missing data. Yet, as noted, it is best to avoid missing data in the first place. Good design and logistics will help. Here are some examples:

- Shorter trials will generally have fewer missing data than longer ones.
- Measurement procedures that are easy on subjects are more likely to have fewer missing data than those that are more difficult.
- Measurements taken at the clinic are less likely to be missing than those collected by having subjects record data at home.
- Good study monitoring and data management will identify problems early.
- Centers with a favorable history of conducting clinical trials are likely to do a better job collecting complete data than those with an inferior track record.

Unblinding

Say you are a nice person (as you already know), and your physicians like you a lot. Additionally, your company is paying them well for conducting research. If the trial is not blinded—if physicians know which subjects receive T and which R—they may unconsciously report better results than warranted for the drug relative to the placebo. Similarly, subject reporting of their condition may be biased when the Treatment received is known. The solution, of course, is to blind both physician and subjects to Treatment. This is not always possible and will be discussed in the next chapter.

In many instances, despite a trial's "blinding by design," physicians (and sometimes subjects) can pretty well guess which arm is which. For example, a medication given intravenously may cause a rash at the site of entry, while the placebo will not. This "unofficial unblinding" is common and as much a threat to trial validity as a lack of blinding by design. Indeed, it may cause even greater bias than the usual unblinded trial. This is because you have assumed blinding and will have taken no measures to prevent bias from that particular quarter.

Compliance

A drug may be effective, but if the subjects do not take it as prescribed, the results will be unfavorable. At the same time, this bias will relate to the chemical properties of the treatment but not to the "Treatment as a whole." Allow me to explain: Suppose you have developed an effective molecule but one of which the pill is large and difficult to swallow (literally). Thus, you have an effective molecule and, despite this, an ineffective Treatment; people simply do not take it. In this instance, lack of compliance will bias the estimate of the molecule's efficacy.

It will not, however, bias the estimate of your Treatment's efficacy in real life. This is because "real-life" efficacy—of the Treatment rather than the chemical—is also associated with the degree to which the pill is taken as prescribed.

In late-stage clinical trials, the effect of the molecule is less important relative to the effect of (real-life) Treatment overall. Late-stage clinical trials are designed to assess a drug's performance in the marketplace and are less concerned with its "chemical efficacy." And if this is the stage you are in, lack of compliance cannot be said to bias your results; it is part and parcel of Treatment outcome and evaluation. However, in early stages you may be more interested in the molecule's efficacy, leaving open the option for modifying the product (e.g., making the pill smaller, coating it differently, etc.). When this is the case, lack of compliance will indeed bias the outcome of interest. The moral of this particular tale is that the definition of bias itself may depend on the circumstances. Belaboring the point, while you must be aware of the general principles of study design, this should not exempt you from actually thinking. And in this case, thinking should lead you to ensure that the Treatment your company has devised enables good compliance.

Some Additional Sources of Bias

- *Nonrepresentative subjects:* If trial participants do not well represent the population of interest, the study may provide biased estimates of effects in the intended use population.[10] The solution for this is straightforward and involves sampling correctly.
- *Nonrepresentative physicians and/or medical centers:* This, like biased sampling of subjects, must be avoided. And this too is done by using appropriate sampling methodology.
- *Baseline difference between subjects in Treatment and comparator groups:* For example, if subjects in your Treatment group are older and more infirm than those in Control, you will likely underestimate Treatment efficacy. Indeed, when this occurs, your anticipated effect may disappear altogether. Randomizing subjects to a study group will typically take care of this potential problem. When by chance it does not, there are statistical methods designed to overcome the difficulty (e.g., **analysis of covariance**; ANCOVA). Still, it is always preferable to trust good design rather than statistical corrections after the fact.

---

[10] Note the difference between nonrepresentative sampling, which is incorrect sampling and leads to bias, and sampling error, which does not. For example, you might sample more women than men in a disease where males outnumber females. This will produce a biased sample. On the other hand, even if you sampled correctly (randomly from a representative sample), your sample is likely to be an imperfect representation of the population due to random sampling error. Being random, sampling error is not biased.

Intent to Treat (ITT)

I have mentioned now and again that clinical trials will often turn out differently than planned. This is not necessarily a result of inadequate planning but often simply due to their complexity and their dependence on large numbers of people. As stated, one nontrivial consequence is missing data that can be missing for numerous reasons and can affect results in unexpected ways, most of which are difficult to evaluate properly.

Imputing missing data is one method for addressing the problem. But there is an even more basic issue, and it is this: *Whom do I analyze?* Now, the answer to this seems obvious enough: all who participate in the trial. Yet, even this seemingly straightforward statement is far from sufficient. What, for example, do you do with the following subjects?

- Those who dropped out in the first week of a 12-month trial.
- Those who came to all the planned appointments but never took any of the medications given to them.
- Those who consented to participate in the trial, were randomized to one of the arms, and then never returned.
- Those who were randomized to R but mistakenly given T.
- Those who took trial medications incorrectly throughout the trial—for example, took one pill a day instead of three.
- Those who should never have been included in the first place because they did not meet all of the inclusion or exclusion criteria—for example, women who participated in a trial for excessive menstrual bleeding but did not meet the criterion for "excessive."

Now it is a rare trial in which one or more of the preceding, or other **protocol violations**, do not occur. And when it does, we have on our hands subjects who did not participate in the trial as planned. To deal with such situations, we define **analysis sets**, which specify the data that will be included in an analysis. Any given study may have various analysis sets. Thus, for example, we may define one that includes only measured data and another that will include missing data as well (dealt with using one of the many methods developed for it). One common analysis set is called **intention to treat** (ITT) and is described in the ICH guidelines as follows:

> The intention-to-treat (ITT) principle implies that the primary analysis should include all randomized subjects. Compliance with this principle would necessitate complete follow-up of all randomized subjects for study outcomes. In practice this ideal may be difficult to achieve, for reasons to be described. In this document the term "full analysis set" is used to describe the analysis set which is as complete as possible and as close as possible to the intention-to-treat ideal of including

all randomized subjects. Preservation of the initial randomization in analysis is important in preventing bias and in providing a secure foundation for statistical tests. In many clinical trials the use of the full analysis set provides a conservative strategy. Under many circumstances it may also provide estimates of treatment effects which are more likely to mirror those observed in subsequent practice.

The guidelines then go on to describe what the **full analysis set** might be. The details are less important for us, especially when we consider that the same methods applied to different studies may have different implications. But the principle is clear: Once you eliminate subjects for *any* reason, you are in danger of biasing a trial's results. A comparative trial is based on random assignment and the consequent assumptions that the groups will thus be equal on all but Treatment type. This and this alone allows you to reach definitive conclusions about the effect of T versus R. Once you violated this principle—have eliminated subjects from the trial who were randomized to it—you will potentially cause bias. Fisher and colleagues (1990)[11] define the ITT analysis set as follows:

Includes all randomized patients in the groups to which they were randomly assigned, regardless of their adherence with entry criteria, regardless of the treatment they actually received, and regardless of the subsequent withdrawal from treatment or deviation from the protocol.

Well, the ITT principle is often very difficult to apply and in some cases has the potential for causing more bias if applied than if not. Still, it is the ideal, and this is where one should begin. In practice, analysis sets—the types of subjects who will or will not be analyzed—must be specified in the protocol. Specifying whom you will analyze ahead of time will eliminate the potential bias of picking and choosing at the end of the trial after some or all results are known. Here are some general rules (that, as usual, have exceptions):

- When assessing safety you should analyze anyone who received treatment whether or not they violated the protocol.
- An individual who provides no data after receipt of treatment (postbaseline data) can usually be excluded from the trial.
- Subjects with major entry violations—such that have the potential to affect their outcome—can be eliminated if:
  - The decision to include or exclude them from the analysis is done blind to outcome.
  - The decision can be made objectively and for all groups equally.

---

[11] Fisher, L. D., Dixon, D. O., Herson, J., Frankowski, R. K., Hearron, M. S., & Peace, K. E. (1990). Intention-to-treat in clinical trials. In K. E. Peace (Ed.), *Statistical Issues in Drug Research and Development* (pp. 331–350.) New York: Marcel Dekker.

And, as always, use your head. If elimination of data has the potential for causing bias, avoid it. And if you feel that at least some subject should be excluded from the trial, then you must:

a. Explain why eliminating them will not bias trial results, and/or
b. Provide additional (sensitivity) analyses that demonstrate that leaving these subjects out will minimally affects trial results.

SUMMARY

In this chapter I emphasized the importance of rigorous design customized to a study's goals. However solid your design and well planned the trial, the data yielded will be imperfect; they will be influenced by random error and, if you are not careful, by bias as well. Random error can be addressed relatively easily. Bias can easily ruin your trial. Keep your eyes open to where it might occur and eliminate it to the degree possible.

CHAPTER 12

Elements of Clinical Trial Design II

CONTENTS

- Blinding in clinical trial design
  - Potential effects on subjects, physicians, study monitors, and administrators
- Randomization in clinical trial design
  - The centrality of randomization to statistical inference
  - Stratified randomization
  - Dynamic randomization
- The Intent to Treat (ITT) principle
- Control groups
  - The need for Control groups and exceptions
  - Performance goals in lieu of Control groups: spinal cord injury and diagnosing preeclampsia
- Interim analysis: logistics and potential bias
- Data monitoring committees
- Interim analysis goals:
  - futility
  - superiority, non-inferiority, and equivalence
- Interim analysis methods:
  - classic ("standard")
  - adaptive: classic and Bayesian designs
- Adjusting sample size by counting events during a trial

INTRODUCTION: METHODS FOR AVOIDING BIAS

When describing methods for avoiding bias, I can do no better than begin with the International Conference on Harmonization (ICH) guidelines:

> The most important design techniques for avoiding bias in clinical trials are **blinding** and **randomization** [emphasis added], and these should be normal features of most controlled clinical trials intended to be included in a marketing application. Most such trials follow a double-blind approach in which treatments are prepacked in accordance with a suitable randomization schedule and supplied to the trial center(s) labeled only with the subject number and the treatment period so that no one involved in the conduct of the trial is aware of the specific treatment allocated to any particular subject, not even as a code letter.[1]

Blinding and randomization are the major tools for preventing bias in trial design, and I shall now discuss each in turn.

Blinding

In a double-blind trial neither physician nor subject knows the Treatment administered. This is meant to eliminate potential sources of bias such as the following:

- *Recruitment and allocation of subjects to Treatment:* Physicians, knowing the treatment that a particular subject is about to receive may, consciously or not, decide to keep the subject out of the trial. Alternatively, they may manipulate allocation to ensure that specific subjects receive a selected Treatment. They might do this, for instance, based on her or his assumptions on who can best benefit from each of the treatments. This would lead to nonrandom differences in composition of trial groups and bias—that is, between-group differences at the end of the trial may be due to group composition rather than to Treatment. In statistical terminology, subject differences between study groups may **confound** the Treatment effect.
- *Physician and subject behavior during the trial:* I just described a situation where the physician may bias allocation through knowledge of it. But even if allocation is completely blind, unblinding during the study (e.g., the "informal type" noted in the preceding chapter) may affect study results by:
    - Physicians providing different care based on what they believe is necessary for the different treatments.
    - Physicians recruiting subsequent subjects for the trial based on the results of those recruited earlier. For example, if the physicians, based

---

[1] International Conference on Harmonization (ICH). (1998). *Statistical Principles for Clinical Trials.*

on early results, believe Treatment to be ineffective they will be less keen on recruiting subjects to the study. And when they do recruit, they may decide to avoid placing subjects in special need of care in the Test drug group.

- Subjects who know their Treatment allocation at any stage in the study may drop out of it as a result.

- *Assessment during and after the trial:* Subjects suspecting they receive a new drug may subjectively report better results than those believing they are taking a placebo. This applies to physicians as well, who are no less susceptible to bias than trial participants.

- *Handling of withdrawals:* In most trials there is subject dropout that companies are committed to minimize. At the same time, study personnel may be more or less "committed," depending on observed results and group allocation. For example, the sponsor's personnel may be keener to recover a Control failure than their innovative drug's failure.

A QUANDARY

Physicians must provide patients with the best care possible. There is even a Greek oath involved here. Now life is not mathematics and neither oaths nor meticulous planning can ensure that all patient care is dispensed as it should be. Moreover, in any particular indication, the conception of "best care" typically varies among professionals. This means that the doctor—or any other caregiver—usually has some flexibility when treating patients. For example, a physician can decide how often to see patients and select the diagnostic tests and medications for them.

But in clinical trials this changes dramatically. A health care professional participating in a clinical study is also signing on to a protocol—that is, to the manner in which patients will be treated, including number of visits, diagnostic tests, and medications. And while all protocols provide some flexibility depending on patient condition and reaction to treatment, they also introduce inflexibility as well. Thus, physicians in clinical trials give up at least some autonomy—and often, a great deal of it—when choosing how to treat their patients. While it cannot be otherwise, it is also reflexively difficult for health care professionals.

The ethics of restricting physicians' flexibility when treating in clinical studies have been discussed extensively and are continually being discussed in specific contexts and indications.

This is an important issue that we shall leave for others. In this context, however, it is critical for me to point out that clinical trials are often difficult environments for physicians. Giving up one's autonomy to a protocol (as must be done in a well-controlled trial) often goes against the very basic instincts of caregivers. And I suspect that it is no less difficult for them to be blind to the treatment they are dispensing.

Now this does not change the fact that those participating in studies agree to relinquish at least some authority to a document. It does however mean that physicians' reflexive actions may, inadvertently, be at variance with the protocol and so undermine study design. Consequently, when planning and monitoring studies, you should be aware of this and make sure that those signing on to protocols are well aware of what they are committing to. Moreover, your trial's monitoring should pay special attention to protocol violation by physicians.

As much as we would like clinical trials to represent the real world, they do not. And it is no surprise that medications' performance in clinical trials often differs in meaningful ways from their performance in the more flexible, and less controlled, environment of everyday treatment. Remembering this will go a long way to preserving a trial's integrity and, most important, will guide correct interpretation of study data.

I just presented a partial list of negative effects associated with an unblinded trial. Clearly, trials should be blinded where possible, but sometimes they cannot be. For example, when comparing a surgical technique to pharmaceutical intervention, it is impossible for either physician or subject *not* to know the treatment received. Here you will need to come up with methods other than blinding to minimize bias, such as the following:

- To the degre possible, make use of objective assessments such as imaging— assessments that both patient and treating physician have little influence over.
- Ensure that those evaluating patients are unaware of the Treatment received—that is, that Treatment and assessment are separated where possible.
- When there is little risk to the subject, consider sham surgery for those being treated with medication. In this way, both groups will undergo surgery and receive medication, with those in the sham group receiving the active medication. While this will not blind the physician conducting the surgery, it *will* blind the patient.

In other cases blinding is possible, but it requires some additional logistics or sleight of hand. Imagine, for instance, that you are comparing two drugs, one given twice a day and one given three times a day. In this case you might specify that both groups will take three pills a day, with the first taking two with the active drug and one with a placebo. Here, then, is one more example of where a potential source of bias has been identified and eliminated.

As you can imagine, the number of potential biases is about as large as the number of clinical trials; only a small fraction of them can be covered in any book. The implication for those designing clinical studies, then, is (and I repeat) to identify potential biases and eliminate them in any given instance.

RANDOMIZATION

I said before that "a clinical trial is planned, run, and analyzed to provide information on a product of interest. As such, *its data must reflect on the product.*[2] And while the principle is not new to you, some of its implications may be.

To allow for definitive conclusions about Treatment, you must compare its results with Reference subjects who are "about similar." This similarity relates to **prognostic factors** such as Age that are deemed predictive of outcome. In

---

[2] As opposed to reflecting imperfect design, such as all those receiving Treatment A being from San Francisco and those receiving Treatment B being from Kuala Lumpur.

short, subjects in groups you plan to compare had better be similar in their chances for Cure or some other clinical effect studied. Without this similarity you cannot definitively attribute differences in outcome between groups to the Treatment of interest.

I use the phrase "about similar" because it is impossible to match groups perfectly on all subject characteristics and trial procedures. First, trial participants differ on factors that we know about and usually measure such as Age. Being known, these are relatively easy to deal with. For example, we might compare the groups on them to demonstrate equality. And when inequality arises, statistical techniques such as analysis of covariance (ANCOVA) can go at least part of the way to addressing potential difficulties in statistical inference.

At the same time there are variables potentially related to outcome that we typically do not measure, such as Emotional Strength and Social Support. And since they have not been measured, you cannot compare the groups in regards to them. Finally, there are numerous, potentially prognostic factors that we do not even know about and so do not contemplate measuring. Such variables might include relatively esoteric variables like Churchgoing, Hair Color, and Number of First-Order Relatives under Age 10.

Yet all this does not change the fact that subjects in study arms must be matched if we are to reach unbiased conclusions when comparing them. And in an imperfect world we settle for "about equal," which we hope to achieve with randomization. Consequently, randomization provides the basis for meaningful comparisons between study arms and no less.

Now this is the general principle, the permutations on which can be many. To take an example, the extent of recovery from stroke is related to subject and stroke characteristics such as History of Previous Strokes or Near Strokes,[3] Area of Brain Affected, and Physical Function prior to stroke and immediately after. Since these are strongly related to prognosis—with or without Treatment—you will want to ensure that the groups are more or less equivalent on them by "helping the randomization out." You can do this by using **stratified randomization**, where subjects are randomized within strata (class, category). For example, you might divide all subjects into three prognostic strata such as "favorable," "average," and "unfavorable." Once classified, you will randomize subjects *within each prognostic stratum* to either Treatment or Control. Doing so will ensure that, at least with respect to the prognostic factors you know about, study arms are matched.

---

[3] Transient ischemic attacks (TIAs) are "ministrokes" that typically leave no measurable damage and are often predictive of more serious ischemic events to come.

INTENT TO TREAT

I have noted throughout that clinical trials are imperfect affairs. There are many reasons for it, not least of which is that subjects are humans and behave accordingly. For example, some comply with Treatment, while others do not. This, then, can make it problematic to decide which subjects to include in any trial's definitive (primary) statistical analyses. For example, should subjects who are taking only 60% of the pills prescribed be included in the analysis? Should those who drop out before receiving *any* treatment be included? And if so, how is it to be done? For instance how are you to analyze a subject's outcome when he or she has not provided you with any outcome data?

To address this issue, we begin with the principle that clinical trials are meant to simulate real-world performance. And given that real-world medicine is usually even messier than that in clinical trials, we should include all subjects we planned to treat in the trial—all intent to treat (ITT) subjects regardless of their behavior or that of those treating them. In this way we will best simulate our treatments' safety and effectiveness in the wild.

Thus one reason for analyzing all ITT subjects is our aim that, to the degree possible, trials must represent real-world therapeutics. But there is also a fundamental statistical principle associated with ITT analysis, and it is this: Including all ITT subjects means *preserving randomization*, which is the basis for reaching unbiased conclusions from statistical comparisons. ITT subjects include all randomized patients, whereas excluding randomized patients for any reason impairs randomization. And impaired randomization undercuts the theoretical justification for reaching conclusions from group comparisons.

As noted in the preceding chapter, Fisher and colleagues[4] stated that the ITT analyses set (or population)—the data of all ITT subjects—includes "all randomized patients in the groups to which they were randomly assigned, regardless of their adherence with the entry criteria, regardless of the treatment they actually received, and regardless of sub-

sequent withdrawal from treatment or deviation from the protocol." Now this definition is extreme, as are its implications. For example, it necessitates including subjects in the group to which they were randomized, regardless of treatment received. Suppose, for instance, that a subject was randomized to Control but erroneously received Treatment. The ITT principle dictates that she or he will be analyzed as belonging to Control. Only then will initial randomization be maintained and with it, the justification for inferring differences between groups. In fact, there are many complications that arise from adhering to the ITT principle. But these are usually fewer than those resulting from not adhering to it.

So here is the bottom line:

- Reaching definitive conclusions about a product from comparing groups A and B is only justified if A and B are "about the same" on all but product use.
- Randomization is designed to ensure this "about sameness."
- Using the ITT principle maintains randomization and, with it, allows for meaningful comparisons between A and B.
- The ITT principle—using all randomized subjects when comparing groups—is straightforward in principle but can be problematic to apply.

If you wish to explore the complexities of the ITT issue in clinical trials—and there are many—I suggest you begin with the relevant guidelines.[5]

---

[4] Fisher, L. D., Dixon, D. O., Herson, J., Frankowski, R. K., Hearron, M. S., & Peace, K. E. (1990). Intention-to-treat in clinical trials. In K. E. Peace (Ed.), *Statistical Issues in Drug Research and Development (pp. 331–350.)* New York: Marcel Dekker.
[5] *International Conference on Harmonization (ICH) (1998), Step 5.* Statistical principles in clinical trials. *European Medicines Agency (EMEA), London.*

Here are just a few notes on randomization techniques:

- Simple and stratified randomization are just two of many randomization methods of assigning subjects to treatment. There are others such as **dynamic randomization**, which adjusts randomization along the way to increase the likelihood that groups are balanced on critical parameters.

In other words, dynamic randomization continually evaluates the quality of randomization and makes corrections as required. Suppose, for example, that Gender is an important prognostic factor in a particular indication, and you wish to ensure that Treatment groups have about equal proportions of males and females. A dynamic randomization scheme will monitor male/female proportions as you go along, and when it detects an imbalance, it will alter the odds accordingly. For example, if more females have been randomized to B relative to A, subsequent females may be randomized with a 60% chance of A rather than the usual 50%. In this way randomization is maintained technically, while its odds have been adjusted to increase the likelihood of ultimate equality between groups (on Gender).

- Thus, if you fear that simple randomization may not adequately match groups, consult with a statistician. She should be able to help you achieve this "about equality" of groups that is so important for your trial.

- Straightforward randomization is not always simple logistically, and stratified randomization can be a logistic nightmare. Dynamic randomization is more difficult than either. Consequently, in any particular trial you must weigh the risks and benefits of various randomization approaches. While the principle of randomization is the basis for unbiased statistical comparisons, we must not allow statistical principles to be a tail wagging the trial dog.

- Fair coins—or computer randomization programs for that matter—do not have a deep understanding of probability theory. As such, they will sometimes deviate greatly from what is expected. For example, even a fair coin will, on occasion, come up "heads" 10 times in a row. It happens. Thus, every so often, group imbalances will arise *despite* randomization. And if you detect such imbalances at the end of the trial, statistical techniques can often address them.

- Infrequently, randomization itself may *lead* to bias. This may occur when patients cannot be blinded to treatment, as when comparing surgical and pharmaceutical interventions. In these circumstances subjects randomized to their preferred treatment are more likely to remain in the study than those not. At the very least, subjects' motivation will vary depending on whether or not they have received their preferred treatment. The effect of patient preference on outcome is not straightforward and inconsistent results have been obtained across studies. Indeed, the effect of patient preference may very well depend on the indication in question with no "one rule fits all." One proposed solution to this potential bias is the **partially randomized patient preference design**. In the design, patients with strong preferences are allocated to their treatment of choice while those with no strong preference are randomized in the usual manner. Intriguingly, this may be one situation where random assignment causes bias and non-random assignment reduces it. For those interested in the topic, McPherson et al.[6] is a good place to start.

AN INTERIM SUMMARY

The preceding two sections can best be summed up by the following quote from ICH's Statistical Principles in Clinical Trials:

> Randomization introduces a deliberate element of chance into the assignment of treatments to subjects in a clinical trial. During subsequent analysis of the trial data, it provides a sound statistical basis for the quantitative evaluation of the evidence relating to treatment effects. It also tends to produce treatment groups in which the distributions of prognostic factors, known and unknown, are similar. In combination with blinding, randomization helps to avoid possible bias in the selection and allocation of subjects arising from the predictability of treatment assignments.

THE CONTROL GROUP

With some exceptions, Control groups are necessary for arriving at definitive conclusions from clinical trials. Without them you cannot obtain a good estimate of your product's effect (versus Control, of course), which will naturally limit information about your product and claims for it.

Yet, despite the importance of having a Control group, there are instances where you will choose not to have one. This is fine. But when going this route, you must be aware of the ramifications and weigh the costs and benefits carefully. If you decide to forgo a Control group, your trial will be logistically simpler and cheaper, but the data from it will be more limited. All the while, you should keep in mind that with or without Control, *every clinical trial involves comparisons*. These may be implicit, explicit, or both.

Let us look at an example: Suppose you are testing an innovative heart valve meant for replacing a defective original, which is implanted by catheterization rather than the standard open-heart surgery. While this is currently an experimental procedure, it will likely become common in the future. Be that as it may,

---

[6] McPherson K., Britton A., Wennberg J. E., (1997). Are randomised controlled trials controlled? Patient preferences and unblind trials. *The Journal of the Royal Society of Medicine*, 90, 652–656.

because this is an experimental procedure, you will only be permitted to do it on those who cannot undergo the standard, open-heart surgery. Typically, these are patients whom surgeons consider too infirm to undergo a major procedure such as open-heart surgery. Thus, it would make no sense to compare between the two techniques—replacement by catheterization and open-heart surgery—since subjects in the two groups are likely to be very different. Specifically, those in the open-heart arm will probably be in better medical condition overall, thus biasing any subsequent comparison to the catheterization arm.

Another, more appropriate option would be to compare subjects undergoing your procedure, with similar subjects receiving noninvasive—pharmaceutical—standard of care only. Doing this will provide you with a Control group, and so with a Reference to compare to at the end of the trial. This comparison is reasonable, but due to budgetary reasons, you choose a single-arm trial nevertheless. What few resources you have, you wish to invest in assessing the innovative product only. First, there is currently no clinical information about your procedure, so you would like to maximize the number of people exposed to it in your trial. Second, at this stage you are interested in technical performance more than you are in efficacy. A Control group of subjects receiving standard of care will allow a formal comparison on efficacy but not performance. After all, those undergoing noninvasive standard of care receive no surgical procedure at all.

So this is your first study in humans, and you feel that having fewer than 20 subjects in Treatment will not provide enough information on the product. Truth be told, even 20 subjects is not a great deal, yet you have little choice but to keep to the budget. Thus after extensive discussions, you decide to go with a single-arm trial.

Having no Control, there will be no perfectly suitable comparison to your Treatment's outcome. Regardless, you will make several comparisons, since this is the only way to estimate your product's worth. For example, you will contrast your procedure's technical success with some figure you believe is acceptable. Additionally, you may ask participating physicians to evaluate the procedure's technical aspects by questionnaire. Their answers will necessarily depend on procedures they are familiar with, so they too will be comparative in nature. You might also contrast your trial's outcomes with those typically observed in similar patients who received a noninvasive standard of care. This will provide you an estimate of efficacy relative to historical data that can be had from patient files and/or scientific publications. In the absence of a Control group, this is the best you can do and is likely sufficient at an early stage of product development.

I will now go back to an earlier statement that in some circumstances a Control group is unnecessary. There are at least two instances where this can occur, one more frequent than the other.

Existing Reference

When developing a new medical device, you might be required to compare it with some existing *Reference value* rather than to some *Reference test*. Your goal would be to demonstrate either similarity or superiority to the Reference value. This happens when the regulator sets a performance goal, obviating the need for a Control group.

Suppose, for example, that you have developed a diagnostic kit for predicting preeclampsia (pregnancy-induced high blood pressure with, perhaps, other symptoms) in late pregnancy from a first-trimester blood test. In this indication you may be required to show that your sensitivity and specificity values are above some threshold like 0.70. Here there is no other choice, since another test for predicting preeclampsia does not exist;[7] in other words, there can be no Control even if you wish to have one.

I just described a situation in which there can be no Control. However comparison to a Reference value, rather than to Control, is also appropriate when there is a well-established Reference—that is, when the results of alternative procedures are known with a fair certainty.

Known Outcome

In some infrequent cases the outcome of standard of Treatment is definitively or almost definitively known. For example, a particular late-stage cancer may be associated with no more than a three-month survival rate in virtually all cases regardless of Treatment. Suppose you have developed an innovative drug and believe your product can extend this period considerably for all subjects. Given the natural history of the disease, you know that any Control group will yield a three-month survival at most. As such, your study need only show that survival with your treatment exceeds this three-month period; there is no reason to include a Control group in it.

Here is another example: You have developed a treatment for generating nerve growth following complete spinal cord injury. When a spinal cord injury is truly complete, there is also complete paralysis from some location in the body downward. At present there is no treatment that can restore movement after complete injury. This implies that any Control group in this indication will yield 100% failure in restoring movement. Thus in the

---

[7] There are some known risk factors for the disease, but their predictive power is very low, identifying only about 25% of cases.

trial you plan, there is no need for Control because its outcome is known in advance.[8] In general, where outcomes of standard of care are known with near certainty, you can forgo a Control group with little or no loss of information.

To conclude, an ideal design will include both Treatment and Control. Yet there are circumstances where you reluctantly make do with a one-arm trial due to monetary and/or logistical considerations. And there are still other instances where a two-arm trial is unnecessary or minimally informing. Yet regardless of trial design, all studies entail some sort of comparison. Depending on the design selected and the indication, some of these will be more informative than others. Following is a list of trial designs and their consequent comparisons from most informative to least. Note that the list is not exhaustive and is meant only to provide some idea on the relative merits of various designs.

- Parallel groups, randomized:
  - There is a Control group.
  - Subjects are randomized to one group or the other.
  - The two arms—Treatment and Control—are run parallel in time.

The comparisons in this trial are straightforward, as are the conclusions from them.

- Parallel groups, nonrandomized:
  - There is a Control group.
  - Subjects are assigned to groups based on nonrandom criteria—typically associated with clinical and/or logistic considerations.
  - The two arms—Treatment and Control—are run in parallel.

Comparisons here are suspect because differences in Treatment may be confounded by differences between subjects in the two groups. At the same time, in some indications a trial like this may better simulate clinical practice by enabling subjects to select their preferred treatment.

- Nonparallel groups:
  - The trial includes both Treatment and Control, the assignment to which may or may not be random.
  - The groups are not run in parallel. For example, all subjects in Treatment are recruited first, and only after the Treatment arm is completed, Control initiated.

---

[8] I have made things a bit more simplistic here than they ought to be, since there *are* reports of (partial) movement restoration after complete spinal cord injury. It is not clear if they occurred due to some nerve regeneration or, perhaps, because the initial diagnosis of "completeness" was wrong. Regardless, even in cases such as these, you must carefully weigh your design options and be ready to defend the one selected.

Here, too, your results may be biased. This is because any differences between the groups may be due to difference in Time of Treatment. In other words, Treatment may be confounded by Time of Treatment.

- Baseline Control:
  - There is only a single arm: Treatment.
  - Subjects are compared to themselves—that is, outcomes following treatment are compared to baseline values.[9]

Single-arm differences from baseline are especially problematic to interpret for various reasons, including possible placebo effects.

- Historical Control:
  - There is only a single arm: Treatment.
  - Outcomes are compared to available data from other sources. Ideally, this "other source" will be individual data obtained from subjects treated in the same center. Less ideally, your comparison will be to summary statistics from published data on subjects as similar as possible to yours.

Because Control here is nonrandomized, chances are that the subjects in your trial differ in meaningful ways from those in others (or in hospital records). Thus while historical controls can be useful to some extent, they are far from ideal. Where there is no choice but to use them, statistical techniques to minimize bias, such as **propensity analysis**, can be used.

- No explicit Control or accepted Reference value:
  - There is only a single arm: Treatment.
  - There is no specified comparison group—that is, no historical, concurrent, or baseline control.

In this, as in all, trials there will be comparisons. But they will be informal and will likely involve contrasting your outcome with some "best guess" expectation.

LOOKING AT DATA DURING THE TRIAL

Efficacy

Blinding is mostly mentioned in the context of subject assignment to Treatment, where to the degree possible you should keep this information concealed from both the physician and the subject. But this rule is just one special case of the general principle: *Any* data that might potentially bias the trial outcome should be hidden from those they may unduly influence.

---

[9] This should not be confused with trials in which each subject undergoes both Treatment and Control as, for example, in crossover trials. When designed appropriately, such trials provide comparisons that are as meaningful as randomized, parallel group studies.

Now let us look at the potentially distorting effects of interim analysis—of analyzing outcome data before a trial is completed. Suppose you accrued complete data for about half the planned number of subjects in a study. And suppose further that you analyze these data and find Treatment to be only marginally effective relative to Control. Now you have no idea whether this state of affairs will continue. But for the moment you do know that your product does not appear particularly useful. If you choose to make these data known to physicians, you may bias their behavior and with it, trial results. They may, for example, now begin to recruit difficult subjects only—such that standard therapy holds little hope for them ("If the patient will be helped by standard treatment," reasons the physician, "why should I enroll him or her in a trial where one of two treatments is relatively ineffective?"). These newly recruited subjects are likely to show low rates of recovery in both arms, weakening study results in general. Moreover, anticipating weak outcomes, physician evaluations may become biased. Patients will then pick up on the doctors' nonverbal messages and report their own condition more negatively. Finally, the study's sponsor might give up on the trial or, at the very least, allocate fewer resources to it. This will reduce study quality and subsequent data from it.

Of course, bias can also occur when favorable results emerge and are made known. And while the potential distortions will differ from those just described, they will nonetheless have an impact. Thus, *the greatest threat to trial validity associated with interim analysis is potential bias.* Statisticians in particular should be reminded of this, since for many, problems related to interim analysis are statistical in nature only. As such, they can be solved statistically. Well, it is indeed the case that interim analyses have statistical aspects that must be addressed. And it is also true that in most cases the statistician can address them properly. Regardless, the greatest threat to a trial's validity posed by analyzing data along the way is bias.

BLURRED VISION

Even in the land of the blind there will be some who see, be it with one eye or two. Trial data simply cannot remain hidden from all. There are too many people and processes involved, and at least some of these require knowledge of group assignment. Moreover, even in well-blinded studies physicians know the state of their subjects, and subjects know how they personally feel. While neither knows precisely the Treatment group involved, each will speculate, and at least some are bound to be right. Additionally, **clinical research associates**—personnel monitoring the study—regularly review a study's **case research forms** (forms on which trial data are recorded; CRFs). Thus, trial monitors are privy to trial results, which they pass along to those managing the data. In sum, there are those who will do their best to guess about blinded data and others who cannot, for logistical reasons, be blinded in the first place.

Yet there is a vast difference between exposing trial personnel to locally collected numbers—as is normally the case with physicians, subjects, and monitors—and revealing the results of aggregate data. The former are often blinded and, even when not, are merely local snapshots that may not reflect the trial as a whole. They can provide a sort of blurred vision of the trial's status but no more. However, the results of interim analysis constitute information on the current status of a product and so have great potential to influence trial participants and procedures.

Interim Analysis of Safety

To this point I have emphasized biases arising from interim analysis of efficacy data. This can be expected from a statistician, since some of our most interesting work is associated with these data. For example, power analyses determining sample size are typically based on efficacy, and our most sophisticated techniques are generally applied in the service of efficacy analyses.

But clinical trials often collect other types of information as well, and in all instances they *must* obtain safety data. In fact, safety is arguably more important than efficacy, since the first tenet of treatment is "safety first." Before you attempt a cure, make sure you are doing no harm. So as a rule you will proceed to demonstrate efficacy only after having showed your product to be reasonably safe. And because it is safety first, you can expect our attitude to making safety data known to differ from that of efficacy. This is indeed the case.

In the first place, every clinical trial must have a mechanism for informing relevant bodies and personnel of major safety events as they occur. In other words, there is continuous "interim analysis" of at least some safety information throughout a trial. It would be unethical otherwise. Additionally, some trials—especially those in relatively risky indications and lasting longer—establish **data monitoring committees** (DMCs) of which the main task is to look at accumulated safety data along the way. The mandates of a DMC will differ depending on trial needs, but the committee is almost always charged with reviewing safety data at specified intervals. In an article titled "Role of Independent Data-Monitoring Committees in Randomized Clinical Trials Sponsored by the National Cancer Institute,"[10] the authors state the following:

> DMCs ... provide a body able to protect patient safety, to protect the integrity of the clinical experiments on which patients have consented to participate, and to assure the public that conflicts of interest do not compromise either patient safety or trial integrity.

Thus, unlike efficacy data, the following is true:

- Critical safety data such as unexpected **serious adverse events** (SAEs) must be routinely reported and, if even remotely related to Treatment, must be revealed to trial participants.
- Less serious adverse events (AEs)—even if they are **expected adverse events**—are often analyzed in the aggregate. This is typically done for DMCs or other types of safety monitoring bodies. And while these bodies are generally independent,[11] their conclusions may need to be revealed, depending on the circumstances.

[10] Smith M. A., Ungerleider R. S., Korn E. L., et al. (1997). Role of independent data-monitoring committees in randomized clinical trials sponsored by the National Cancer Institute. *Journal of Clinical Oncology*, 15, 2736–2743.
[11] Independent in the sense that they are not associated with the day-to-day running of the trial and are not beholden to special interests associated with the study.

At the same time, and like most issues in clinical trials, relating to unblinding of safety data is far from straightforward. For example, some DMCs regularly receive AE data by arm but are not told which arm is which. This is a sort of "partial blinding" meant to reduce members' bias in deciding whether or not to discontinue a trial for safety reasons. Moreover, some DMCs are charged with evaluating efficacy as well and will incorporate the information into decisions on whether or not to continue a study. Thus, an innovative drug that causes many AEs may, in some indications, be considered useful if it is sufficiently effective.

DMCs are independent bodies, and data provided to them need not be revealed to trial participants. At the same time, study information is hard to keep secret. And in any case, a DMC's decision on whether or not to continue a trial must be made public. In fact, you will often find early-stage companies releasing statements to the press on a DMC decision to allow the trial to continue. Of course this is not much of an accomplishment. If it were not expected, the trial would not have been run in the first place. But it may sound sufficiently impressive to the uninitiated, who might then foolishly invest their money based on press releases such as this. Yet expected or not, public pronouncements of DMC decisions constitute information in the aggregate on an ongoing clinical trial. As such, they have the potential for biasing outcome.

Another potential problem occurs in cases where it is virtually impossible to separate efficacy from safety. Suppose, for example, that you are testing the efficacy/performance of an insulin pump—a device designed to provide diabetics with appropriate quantities of insulin under different conditions. Such conditions might include patient's current level of blood sugar, sensitivity to insulin, and the amount of carbohydrates the patient plans to consume at his next meal. An ineffective pump will cause inappropriate quantities of insulin to be pumped into the body, causing adverse events such as hypo- and hyperglycemia. This will also happen when the device clogs. In other words, the product's performance is directly related to safety, so knowledge of the latter will necessarily provide information on the former. And since safety data are often made known, here this may amount to providing efficacy information as well.[12]

I will not delve more deeply into this topic. While clearly related to statistics, it is not purely statistical, and solutions for it must be found outside the realm of statistics.

---

[12] While the relationship between AEs and device malfunction is more direct here than in most indications, it is far from being "one-to-one." Hypo- and hyperglycemia can be caused by factors other than the device, so reporting these AEs does not necessarily reflect on the product. But it reflects enough on the device to potentially bias the trial.

STATISTICAL CONSIDERATIONS IN INTERIM ANALYSIS: MULTIPLICITY

I said before that unless you have sufficient reason for it, efficacy should be analyzed only after all study data have been collected. Doing otherwise may introduce unnecessary bias into an ongoing trial. And for the record, *curiosity* is not a sufficient reason. Yet potential bias is not the only reason for avoiding data analysis along the way. Let us look at the statistical issues involved, which relate primarily to Type I Error. I previously dealt with this topic in Chapter 10. If you do not require a review, feel free to skip this section. For those of you who remain, I will proceed gingerly through this minor statistical minefield.

Conclusions from statistical testing are probabilistic in nature. For example, obtaining a significantly superior effect of T over R implies that you are 95% certain that T > R. And by stating this you acknowledge that there is a 5% chance you have erred—have mistakenly concluded that T is better. Statistically speaking, you have allowed yourself a 5% chance of committing Type I Error, which is rejecting the Null Hypothesis when it should not be rejected.

Formally, then, Type I Error is incorrectly rejecting the Null Hypothesis— whatever it may happen to be; contingent on your study's objectives, it can take on several different forms. For the sake of simplicity, I shall deal here with the fairly common case where you wish to show some T superior to R and specify the Null and Alternative hypotheses as follows:

$$H_0: T = R$$
$$H_1: T \neq R$$

Now, when comparing two entities there is always the chance that one will emerge superior to the other by chance alone. On occasion, for example, even a weak dueler will eliminate a stronger one. So when measuring "superiority" in a single duel, results can go either way. And while the chance of the better shot killing the poorer is greater than the reverse, the latter can happen as well. Now it is generally impossible to eliminate the chance of Type I Error—in this case, of concluding that the truly weaker dueler is stronger. But it is possible to reduce the chance of this happening. For example, you might require that the comparison consists of a "best of 5" series as opposed to a single duel. Increasing sample size increases the chance of the truth emerging, and consequently it reduces the chances of a Type I Error. Thus, while the possibility of committing a Type I Error will always be a cloud hovering above any comparison you make, you have some control over its size.

The Type I Error rate generally accepted in science (and by regulators) is 5%—that is, when you wish to reject the Null Hypothesis, journals and regulators will require that you be 95% certain of your rejection. And while exceptions exist—cases where higher or lower probabilities for rejecting H_0 are allowed—they are few and far between.

Getting back to clinical trials, you can keep the probability for Type I Error manageable by determining what must happen in order to "prove" superiority. The more stringent you set the criteria for success, the lower your chance of a Type I Error. For example, before a study you might state that only if T's efficacy is at least twice R's in a sample of 400 subjects will you conclude that T > R. Conversely, you can set more liberal criteria and, for example, accept an 8% difference obtained on 30 subjects as sufficient evidence for superiority.

In sum, your statistical decision-making game is, with respect to Type I Error, played between the following goalposts on either side of the field:

a. Choose lenient criteria for rejection → greater chance of rejection → greater chance of incorrect rejection → greater chance of Type I Error.
b. Choose harsh criteria of rejection → smaller chance of rejection → smaller chance of incorrect rejection → smaller chance of Type I Error.

Now, statisticians know how to calculate your chances of error in a trial (and given there is Type I, you can safely assume there is a Type II as well). Computations are typically based on various assumptions, statistical and clinical in nature, and range from "fairly simple" to "bafflingly complex." For the moment it is enough that you know that statisticians know how to do this, and I recommend that you leave it to them.

In conclusion, the chance of a "false positive"—of erroneously claiming success—occurs every time you compare two groups statistically. And since it happens with every comparison, the more comparisons you make, the greater the chance of it happening. This, then, is the statistical problem with interim analyses: On each comparison your chance of this sort of error is 5%. Thus when you multiply such analyses, you also increase the chance of Type I Error beyond the permissible 5%.

In my own particular discipline, this issue is called multiple testing or multiplicity. If, for instance, your drug is truly ineffective and you conduct five separate comparisons with it (say, you compare T and R on five endpoints), you have more than a 20% chance of obtaining at least one false positive result.

A more intuitive example might be flipping a coin that, when done often enough, will eventually yield the hoped-for result, even if not justified. Using this analogy, statistical testing is akin to flipping a coin of which the chance of coming up false positive is 5% on each flip. Flip often enough, and even if your product is not superior, you are bound to get lucky and obtain a favorable result by chance alone.

Now getting lucky is highly recommended, especially when the luck happens to be good. But when you seek the truth, you had better avoid both good and bad luck and stick to the facts. In clinical trials we ask that your overall chance of Type I Error—regardless of the number of comparisons you make—remain no higher than 5%.

TYPE I ERROR IN PRACTICE

Increasing the chance of wrongly concluding success would seem to be a bad thing. And it is. Yet, setting stringent criteria for success also means that your chance of detecting a true effect is reduced as well. Allow me to demonstrate this with an extreme (and unrealistic) example.

Suppose you conduct a trial in which you decide in advance that you will *never conclude success* regardless of the results. Having made the decision, you have also effectively reduced the chance of Type I Error to 0; since you will never conclude success, you will also never conclude success erroneously (a good thing). However, by playing it safe you have also eliminated any chance of detecting true success (a bad thing). Let us now take the opposite and equally unrealistic example.

Before proceeding with a trial, you decide that you will declare superiority irrespective of trial results. Here, you will always conclude success. Thus, you will always conclude success if warranted (good), but you will also always conclude success when it is not warranted; in other words, you will have a high probability of Type I Error (bad).

Thus we have here a typical tradeoff between risk and caution: Protect yourself from Type I Error, and you reduce your chance of detecting true effects; increase your chance to detect favorable effects, and you also increase your chance of "detecting" them erroneously. In formal statistical terminology, you cannot have your cake and eat it, too.

Using even more formal terminology, the more you defend from Type I Error, the greater your chances to commit a Type II Error, which is *not* detecting superiority when you should. On the other hand, the less cautious you are—the less you defend from Type I Error—the greater your trial's power for finding a (true) favorable effect. Yet, by doing this you have also increased your chance of accepting a chance favorable effect.

I said before that the generally accepted Type I Error rate is 5%. And this is true. At the same time, statistical procedures and criteria must be subservient to study goals and not the other way around. If, for example, you are running a pivotal trial for regulatory approval, you will need to go with the 5% Type I Error rate. This is what the regulator demands, and satisfying the regulator is, along with a few other goals, your trial's aim. Thus determining an acceptable Type I Error rate cannot be determined in mathematical isolation. Here is another example: In an exploratory trial you are typically more concerned with detecting efficacy than with protecting yourself from making a false positive. At this stage of development you reason as follows: "My primary aim is to discover some hint of effectiveness if it is truly there. If obtained, I will conduct a confirmatory trial with the customary chance of Type I Error (5%). Thus the truth will emerge at the end of the day even if I am a bit lax with it early on. And if I am not lax with it at the exploratory stage, I might just pass up a good product—not detect its effect for lack of power or simply bad luck—and the opportunity will likely not return." In other words, incorrectly embrace a product and you will eventually discard it; incorrectly discard a product and it is usually gone for good.

Consequently, in feasibility studies you might allow for a 10% Type I Error rate and so increase your study's power—its chance of detecting a true effect—while increasing the probability of Type I Error. Indeed, in the early stages of trials, companies and statisticians often ignore Type I Error altogether. Instead, they will make go/no-go decisions based on informal examination data. For example, if most of a trial's results point in the hoped-for direction, you will decide to continue development even if none of the individual tests was actually significant. As noted, at this stage of development you are more fearful of discarding an effective product than with keeping an ineffective one.

To conclude, there is no single Type I Error rate that is correct in all circumstances. Statistical testing, like trial design itself, must meet study objectives.

REASONS FOR INTERIM ANALYSES AND SOME STATISTICAL SOLUTIONS

While looking at data along the way is not recommended, there *are* exceptions—cases where for one reason or another you must make decisions before the trial is completed. And to make these decisions you will require comparative data—that is, you will have to conduct a statistical test on the data available. Adding tests along the way—like adding tests in general—will increase your chance of reaching conclusions based on chance alone (rather than truth).

Imagine you are planning a study of 200 patients per group, and you chose this sample size "to be on the safe side." You suspect that fewer subjects will do, but you are not completely sure. You therefore plan a larger—perhaps too large—study.[13]

---

[13] In fact, conducting a larger-than-needed clinical trial is usually unethical; after all, you are needlessly exposing a certain number of subjects to unproven treatment. This, then, is one additional reason for making T – R comparisons along the way to assess whether the number of participants can be reduced. Saving money is also a not unheard of reason for preferring smaller trials over larger ones.

In this sort of trial it would be very helpful to have some mechanism to allow for testing results before all 200 subjects have completed the trial. This mechanism should enable you to stop the trial earlier than planned while maintaining the Type I Error rate at 5% (despite the fact that you may end up testing at least twice—once in the interim and, if the results are not sufficiently favorable, once again at the end of the trial).

Well, formal interim analysis is a mechanism for this. Statistically the term *interim analysis* is quite general and can refer to any one of several scenarios of analyzing data while the trial is ongoing. The specific statistical technique applied for interim analysis depends on various factors, including the following:

- The reason for wanting to analyze partial data in the first place.
- The point or points in the trial at which these analyses will be conducted.

As an aside, I should note that the issue of multiplicity can be very technical and is not limited to analyzing interim data (see Chapter 10). It also applies to cases where you wish to analyze multiple endpoints or apply multiple statistical tests to a single endpoint. In each of these cases the more tests you conduct, the greater your chances of (unjustifiably) obtaining a favorable result. I noted that the technical statistical aspects of multiplicity are beyond the scope of this book. At the same time, the nonstatistician should be aware of the following:

- There can be some very good reasons for wanting to analyze data while a trial is ongoing, and doing so (correctly) is perfectly legitimate.
- Analyzing interim data is statistically problematic.
- There are both statistical and logistical solutions for difficulties arising from interim analyses.

I mention that there can be some "very good reasons" for interim analysis, and I elaborate on some of these in the following sections.

Futility

Futility analysis is designed to evaluate whether or not to continue a trial—that is, whether keeping to the trial's planned sample size is or is not worthwhile. For example, when interim results (after, say, half the subjects have been completed and analyzed) are such that the chance of success at the end of the trial is tiny or nil, you may want to declare the trial "futile"; there is simply no point in going on with it.

Futility analysis permits stopping the trial for failure but does not allow stopping for success. Thus, if your planned futility analysis actually obtained significant T > R, you are not permitted to stop the trial and claim success. This relates to the idea that conclusions based on statistical analyses are convincing only when the analyses have been specified in advance (see Chapter 9). And since in this case you did not specify in advance that success is an option—

you specified a futility analysis that allows stopping for failure only—if you happen to unexpectedly come up with a favorably significant result, you will not be able to claim it.

"Standard" Interim Analysis

As it is most commonly used, the term *interim analysis* refers to analysis of partial data for the purpose of making one of the following decisions:

a. Declare success and stop trial, which will happen if you obtain significant results in the hoped-for direction.
b. Continue with the trial as planned, when interim results are sufficiently favorably to continue but not so favorable as to allow for declaring success.
c. Stop the trial for futility when the results are so unfavorable that it is pointless to go on.

Now this "conventional" option includes futility, so you might rightly wonder why futility analysis exists as a stand-alone option. Well there is good reason for it: When testing futility, you do not give yourself the option for success. As such, you are also not increasing the probability of a Type I Error. After all, if you will never claim success, you will never claim success mistakenly. Thus, futility analysis does not require any adjustment for an increase in Type I Error. And not adjusting the Type I Error rate can make it easier to obtain success in later stages. Specifically, multiple comparisons (for success) require that the overall Type I Error rate—what we term α—must be 5% for all tests. This means that for each individual test, α must be lower than 5%; only thus will overall α remain at 5% or lower. This also means that each individual test now has a more stringent criterion for success and so is less powerful for showing $T > R$.[14]

There are numerous variations on these themes of futility and conventional interim analyses. For example, you might set up a trial with three arms: two dose groups and one placebo. If an interim analysis suggests that one dose is better than another, you will have the subjects who have been receiving the less effective dose switch to the more effective one and continue the trial as planned. And from this point on, you will recruit patients into two arms rather than to three. This will increase your sample size in the remaining arms and with it, the power for detecting differences between them.

---

[14] When adjusting for overall comparisons correctly, your overall chance of success—for rejecting H_0—remains the same when considering the trial as a whole. At the same time, the chance of each individual analysis obtaining the hoped-for result is smaller. In many cases a Company wishes to have a high probability of success in a particular analysis (say, at the end of the trial). And to achieve this in the presence of multiple analyses, the Company will have no choice but to increase the sample size.

Additional reasons for looking at data as you go along include:

- Determining the ultimate trial sample size needed.
- Determining the most appropriate inclusion/exclusion criteria for the trial (e.g., when you find that some subjects' characteristics are associated with efficacy and others are not).

Since sample size and inclusion/exclusion should, as a general rule, be determined before the trial begins, you can imagine that these options are not often applied and are nontrivial statistically. I discuss some of the methods for addressing these issues in the following.

Adjusting Sample Size by Counting Events

All powered trials—trials designed to obtain statistical significance—are based on assumptions. Some of these are not directly related to Treatment-Control differences (effect size) and so may be assessed during the trial with little or no statistical repercussions. For example, suppose you are testing the accuracy of a noninvasive device for detecting Stenosis in cardiac valves. In planning the trial, the statistician determined that at least 80 subjects with Stenosis (as measured by some Reference Standard) are needed to adequately test device sensitivity. In other words, 80 positive subjects are required to have sufficient power to demonstrate acceptable sensitivity. When you planned the study, you assumed that at least 1 in 10 of the subjects of the intended use population had Stenosis. Using this assumption, you planned for 800 subjects, anticipating that this will yield the 80 positives required. If you were right, all is well. But if you overestimated the incidence of Stenosis in the relevant population, you will end up with too few positive subjects. Consequently, your trial will not be sufficiently powered, and your chance of demonstrating adequate sensitivity will be smaller than planned. To ensure that by trial's end you have enough subjects for the required power, you may wish to count the number of positive subjects (by Reference Standard) as you go along. This can be done without actually testing whether or not you have diagnosed them correctly with your device. As such, this counting has little or no potential for biasing the study results.

Counting events is, for example, also done in trials meant to demonstrate that Treatment increases survival. To demonstrate efficacy on survival, at least some subjects must, alas, die during the trial; if no subjects die in either Treatment or Control, you have no power to show superiority of the former. In this sort of trial you will have calculated the minimum number of deaths needed to sufficiently power your trial to demonstrate efficacy. You will then count the number deaths as you go along in both Treatment and Control during the trial. Here, too, you will not test efficacy—that is, you will not compare the number of events between Treatment and Control. Rather, you will count the event of interest over all subjects. You will then end the trial only after having achieved the requisite number of events of interest (in this case, death). This will not guarantee that you will demonstrate T > R, but it will guarantee that your power to do so, assuming an effective treatment, is acceptable.

Adaptive Trials

As noted, sample sizes of powered trials are based on assumptions, the most central of which relate to effect size—the degree to which Treatment differs from a comparator. In most cases one can come up with reasonable estimates of effect size from various sources (previous studies, literature, reasonable guesses, etc.). But in some cases trial planners are pretty much in the dark; while they have some idea of effect size, they are not very confident about it. This circumstance might, for example, arise when a novel medication for a hitherto untreated disease is being tested in humans for the first time. In this case you will want to obtain a reasonable estimate of effect size based on interim results.

In the circumstances described it would be especially useful to look at the data as you go along and, based on results obtained, determine the final sample size for the trial. But while it is useful, it can also lead to inflated Type I Error rates. There are several options to deal with such situations, none of which is straightforward statistically or logistically. These include **adaptive designs** and **Bayesian designs**.

In classic adaptive design, interim results are assessed at planned time points. Observed results are then compared to those assumed before the trial began. Then, based on the disparity, decisions are made on the trial's future. In this scenario, initial assumptions relating to T-R differences remain, as does the trial's design, including upper bound of sample size. "Adaptation" typically relates to the ability to stop or continue the trial along the way one or more times based on the observed-assumed comparison noted. Bayesian designs are more flexible in that they enable updating initial trial assumptions using results observed at the interim. Here too data are evaluated at planned time points. But once assumptions are updated with accumulated data, they can be used for "redesigning" the remainder of the trial. In many instances such designs are not realistic options for logistical reasons. But to know whether this is the case, you will need to consult with the statistician and others on your staff. Statistical Principles in Clinical Trials states the following:[15]

> An interim analysis is any analysis intended to compare treatment arms with respect to efficacy or safety at any time prior to formal completion of a trial. Because the number, methods and consequences of these

---

[15] International Conference on Harmonization (ICH). (1998).

comparisons affect the interpretation of the trial, all interim analyses should be carefully planned in advance and described in the protocol. Special circumstances may dictate the need for an interim analysis that was not defined at the start of a trial. In these cases, a protocol amendment describing the interim analysis should be completed prior to unblinded access to treatment comparison data.

In conclusion, looking at data along the way is certainly permitted. But because it has nontrivial implications, it must also be planned correctly. Ideally, the process and the decision-making options implied will be specified in the trial's protocol. Where an unanticipated need for interim analysis arises during the trial, the protocol can be amended accordingly. Specifically, you will need to justify why you wish to conduct these analyses and how you will ensure that they will neither bias the trial nor inflate Type I Error beyond the level allowed.

SUMMARY

Developing a solid trial design depends on numerous factors. Your first step must always be precise delineation of study aims and the audience for which results are intended. Once done, you can proceed with designing the trial correctly with or without interim analyses.

Virtually all designs involve compromises, and there is rarely such a thing as a perfect trial. Your challenge in designing a clinical study is to come up with an optimal configuration given the goals, circumstances, and constraints.

To maximize the likelihood that trial conclusions will be correct, you should, where possible, incorporate various elements into it. These include random assignment, blinding, specification of a Control group, avoidance of interim analyses, and, in general, avoidance of multiple testing. But in real life not all of these may be possible. Virtually every trial configuration is unique and must be approached as such.

Thus, I cannot emphasize enough that solid study design depends on using your head; formal principles will get you only so far, since exceptions are as common as rules.

Clearly, you can do no better than your best when designing a trial under real-world constraints. Sadly, however, there are situations where your best is simply not good enough. It is thus critical to emphasize that *you should not undertake a trial that does not have a reasonable likelihood of providing the information required correctly.* If your best cannot do this, then do not do the trial; a bad trial is worse than no trial at all.

However designed, clinical studies aim to produce information that will guide the future of your product. And this information is encapsulated in the trial's endpoints, which is the topic of the following chapter.

CHAPTER 13

Endpoints

CONTENTS

- The father of artificial organs
- Defining endpoints
- Bias and random error in endpoints
- The process of selecting endpoints in kidney transplantation
- How varying endpoints provide varying pictures of reality
- Uniformity in endpoint measurement
- Dealing with multiple endpoints—choosing among them and identifying those most central
- The relationship between proliferation of endpoints and clear scientific thinking
- Prioritizing endpoints—necessity and difficulty of specifying primary and secondary endpoints
- Surrogate endpoints—examples from oncology, cardiology, nephrology, and infectious disease
- Validity and validation of endpoints
- Repeatability and reproducibility
- Composite endpoints
- Measuring endpoints with scales: categorical, ordinal, interval, and ratio
- Responder analysis
- On the different approaches to safety and efficacy endpoints

Strategy and Statistics in Clinical Trials

203

INTRODUCTION: A HUMANITARIAN AND HIS MACHINE

Reminiscing in his later years, Willem Kolff recalled having been an average student. And though not lacking in human friendship, some of the best days of his youth were spent with animals. There had been rabbits and guinea pigs, pheasants, pigeons, and even sheep. There was a time, he said, when he dreamed of managing a zoo but his father had pointed out that there were only three zoos in The Netherlands. (Fathers, I suppose, will do that.) And so the young boy's dream became the sort of passing phase we might today smile benevolently upon. But there may have been a time—long in the past, no doubt—when we might have shed a tear or two over some unrequited youthful dream.

After completing gymnasium in his hometown of Leiden, Kolff followed in his father's footsteps and attended medical school at the university there. He completed his studies in 1938 and went on to postgraduate studies at the University of Groningen where Polak Daniels, who was to become his mentor, was head of the medical department. Kollf recalls:[1]

> Professor Daniels had one quality which I think is very important. There are some professors who want their students to do exactly what the professor is interested in. This man was different. He set us free, and when I wanted to pursue a certain thing, he would study it and help. All my life I've tried to follow that example and, where possible, allow my students to follow their interest.

In May 1940 the Germans invaded The Netherlands. The Daniels family, who were Jewish, committed suicide. Rather than cooperate with Nazi sympathizers put in charge at Groningen, Kolff moved to a small hospital in Kampen on the Zuider Zee (now called the Ijsselmeer).[2]

The ancient town of Kampan in southwest Netherlands can trace its history well into the Dark Ages. Built by a river, the town had been a major trading center for hundreds of years, but by the time of Kolff's arrival, its trading importance had been long replaced by Amsterdam. In Kampen the young doctor joined the local Resistance, where he saved hundreds of lives "simulating diseases" on individuals in danger of being arrested by the occupying German forces.[3] But his fame would derive from his "other" activity at Kampen: developing an

---

[1] Academy of Achievement. (2008). Willem Kolff interview. *Pioneer of artificial organs*. Washington, D.C. http://www.achievement.org/autodoc/page/kol0int-1.

[2] Blakeslee, S. (2009). Willem Kolff, doctor who invented kidney and heart machines, dies at 97. *New York Times*. http://www.nytimes.com/2009/02/13/health/13kolff.html.

[3] Academy of Achievement. (2008). Willem Kolff interview. *Pioneer of artificial organs*. Washington, D.C. http://www.achievement.org/autodoc/page/kol0int-1.

artificial kidney. "The exciting thing," he would say of the machine he developed, "is to see someone who is doomed to die, live and be happy."[4] He might have been referring to both of his wartime activities.

Kolff constructed the first dialysis machine with what odds and ends he could scrounge in his wartorn country. These included laundry tubs, sausage casings, and an automobile water pump. He treated his first patient with the machine in 1943, but it was only two years and 16 patients later that he experienced his first success. The year was 1945, and The Netherlands had just been liberated. The woman treated was in jail for being a Nazi sympathizer, where she fell into a coma from failed kidneys. The first thing she said upon waking up was that she would divorce her nonsympathizing husband. She went on to live seven more years to age 74.

In the United States alone there are today about 200,000 people on dialysis treatment—individuals who owe their lives to "direct descendants" of Kolff's ramshackle machine. Since his first triumph on September 11, 1945, more than 20 million lives have been saved by the procedure.

Five years after the war Dr. Willem Kolff moved to Cleveland, Ohio. His first years were devoted to improving his English, retaking his medical exams, and becoming a citizen. He would then develop the first completely artificial heart, which he transplanted into a dog in 1957. Some 25 years later at the University of Utah, the artificial heart he had invented was transplanted into a human subject. Kolff received numerous awards for his work and a great deal of international recognition. He was known, and still is, as the "father of artificial organs." Professor Willem Kollf died in 2009, three days before his ninety-seventh birthday.

CHOICES

Humans cannot live with failed kidneys, and dialysis replaces the organ's most important functions to the degree possible. For many dialysis patients the device is a temporary solution—a stopgap until such time that a donor kidney can be found for them.

Kidney transplantation has progressed a great deal since its first, failed instance in 1950 and subsequent successes in Paris and Boston in 1954. Yet despite great improvements and as with medical interventions in general, the procedure fails occasionally. Estimates of permanent kidney failure during the first year postsurgery are as high as 20%, depending on numerous factors. These

---

[4] From the presentation of the Vladimir K. Zworkin Award for outstanding research contributions in the field of medical and biological engineering.

include the organ's source (live donor or cadaver), surgical complications, storage quality of the explanted kidney, and the recipient's health factors. Thus, in some populations, the kidney transplant survival rate is as low as 80% during the first year and is even lower when considering longer periods. But despite difficulties and occasional setbacks, the procedure's rate of success has steadily increased over the past decades. Today, there are large subgroups of patients for whom the first-year Kidney Survival Rate is well over 90%.

To this point, I have implied that efficacy of transplantation can be measured by the amount of time a transplanted kidney remains functioning after surgery—a "Kidney Survival" parameter that seems to make sense for describing the procedure's outcome. Yet the utility of any parameter in capturing the relevant clinical experience of kidney transplantation—or any other procedure, for that matter—should be determined by clinicians rather than statisticians. Still, statistics *does* have some points to make about developing and selecting variables for describing clinical trial results. I shall mention a few of these here.

Before going on, I should note that this chapter deals primarily with measures of efficacy—those parameters with which we mean to demonstrate a trial's efficacy objectives. As examples they are the simplest for me, and they are often central to statisticians' activities in clinical studies. Yet, I should also emphasize that:

1. Assessing outcome in clinical trials is critical for aspects other than efficacy. As noted in Chapter 3, there can be a variety of attributes measured in any particular study, including safety, performance, and pharmacokinetics.
2. In many cases the distinction between efficacy and safety is somewhat blurred. For instance, transplanted kidney failure clearly has implications for subject safety as well. To take another example, the safety of an insulin delivery system can be measured by the rates of hypo- and hyperglycemia episodes associated with it. But these very same rates are also measures of the device's efficacy.
3. Most issues relating to measures of efficacy are relevant for other attributes as well. At the same time, and depending on the circumstances, there can be important differences among the statistical treatment of measures relating to different attributes. Examples of these will be provided later in this chapter.

Getting back to the issue at hand, and as you can imagine, there is more than one informative parameter when it comes to evaluating the efficacy of kidney transplantation. For example, even successfully transplanted kidneys will differ in level of function; some will simply work better than others. One of these functions, for example, is the degree to which the organs are able to clear blood **plasma** of **urea**. Urea is a waste product of protein metabolism that can be measured by the blood urea nitrogen (BUN) test. Another important test of kidney function is creatinine clearance (CCr), which calculates the amount of blood cleared of **creatinine** per unit of time. Creatinine is waste excreted into the blood by muscle activity.

Now choosing efficacy parameters for assessing Treatment outcome is useful in general and is particularly important in clinical trials. Recall that the typical clinical study compares between Treatments and so must have measures for it. We call these measures endpoints, which are usually quantitative values describing the outcome. The National Cancer Institute (NCI) defines an endpoint as follows:

> An event or outcome that can be measured objectively to determine whether the intervention being studied is beneficial. The endpoints of a clinical trial are usually included in the study objectives. Some examples of endpoints are survival, improvements in quality of life, relief of symptoms, and disappearance of the tumor.[5]

RECALLING STUDY DESIGN

The National Cancer Institute writes that we should select endpoints "that can be measured objectively." I should, however, point out that the Institute's statement refers to the *method* of measurement rather than to its *content*. Allow me to explain with an example: Unlike X-rays, **ELISA kits**, and tape measures, Quality of Life (QoL) questionnaires are self-report measures and, thus, subjective. Yet this is how it should be, since when evaluating QoL we wish to know how subjects *feel*; when evaluating these endpoints, we are actually *seeking* the subjective view.

Thus when NCI instructs us to measure endpoints objectively, it does not mean to rule out the use of subjective measures. Indeed, two of the measures it notes—"improvement in quality of life" and "relief of symptoms"—are usually self-reported and subjective in nature. Rather, NCI is suggesting that whichever endpoints we choose to evaluate—be they objective *or* subjective—we do so objectively; that is, we should measure them as accurately and without bias as possible. But really, this should not be a new idea for you. As described in Chapter 12, we measure accurately by eliminating elements in our design that may contribute to error. Recall that in statistics we classify error into two types: random error and bias, the latter generally having greater potential for undermining a clinical investigation than the former.

In the preceding chapter I also pointed out that blinding patients and physicians will go a long way toward eliminating bias. Thus if a patient does not know which Treatment she receives, her answers to a QoL questionnaire cannot be affected (biased) by this knowledge; she will answer without knowing what she is "supposed" to say. (And actually, what she is supposed to say is the truth as she sees it and nothing else.)

You should also keep in mind that blinding is only one of several methods designed for eliminating potential bias in the assessment process. Another common source of bias can be the measurement tool itself. Thus, an inventory including "leading questions" is likely to bias study results as well (e.g., "On a scale of 1 to 10, with 10 being most favorable, how well do you feel now that you've been treated by our world-renowned experts?"). Similarly, a tape measure that has inches marked a bit longer than they should be will regularly provide lengths that are longer than they ought to be. Clearly, the topic of measurement inaccuracy (random error and bias) is crucial when considering endpoint assessment. I have discussed this issue in preceding chapters and will dig no deeper here. Besides, I have already written about it in another book[6] and am not the only one to have done so.

Continued

[5] National Cancer Institute (NCI). *Dictionary of cancer terms.* http://www.cancer.gov/dictionary/.

RECALLING STUDY DESIGN—CONT'D

I should also add that the issue of "subjectivity in measurement" resulting from nonblinding (i.e., bias) arises when assessing apparently objective measures as well. For example, while X-ray machines are neither for nor against any particular result—and in this sense are objective—the individuals operating them and interpreting their outcomes may not be. Consequently, objective endpoints are equally prone to "subjectivity," which can be circumvented by rigorous study design that includes blinding and other safeguards. These may include, for instance, applying procedures to correctly calibrate measurement instruments and designing trials in a way that reduces subject dropout.

So, once again, we encounter the reality that in clinical trials "everything is connected to everything else." In this particular instance we must consider a study's design while we specify endpoints to evaluate its outcome.

[6] *Tal, J. (2000).* Reading between the Numbers: Statistical Thinking in Everyday Life. *New York: McGraw-Hill.*

NCI's definition of endpoints naturally focuses on those relevant to oncology trials—measures, for example, relating to the disappearance of a malignant tumor. But the principle of "measuring to evaluate outcome"—the idea that we must record endpoints if we are to assess Treatment—is the same for trials in all indications.

Using two of the parameters enumerated by NCI and adding the others already noted, I now have five endpoints for assessing transplantation success:

- Survival Time of transplanted kidney
- Survival Time of patient
- Kidney Function measured by BUN
- Kidney Function measured by CCr
- Patient Quality of Life

It may well be that these endpoints are sufficient for capturing the clinically relevant experience of kidney transplantation. Indeed, they may be more than enough. Nevertheless, allow me to introduce yet another endpoint into the mix. And for this particular measure I shall need to present some background first.

When transplanting a kidney—or most other biological organs for that matter—the patient's immune system will recognize the implant as foreign and attack it. The system's assault may be sufficiently effective to cause irreparable damage to the transplanted body part, causing permanent failure. To minimize this reaction, transplanted patients are usually given medications of which the function is to suppress those parts of the immune system that might damage the newly introduced organ. While these compounds are usually effective in the middle and long term, they often cannot prevent episodes of *acute rejection* early on. A single acute rejection episode in kidney transplantation will not usually lead to permanent failure. But it will not help. And multiple acute rejections, which are most common soon after surgery but can happen at other times as well, increase the likelihood for permanent failure.

Perico and colleagues[7] write, "Delayed graft function [DGF] is a form of acute renal failure resulting in … risk of acute rejection episodes and decreased long-term survival [of the transplanted kidney]." They add, "Several new drugs show promise in animal studies in preventing or ameliorating … delayed graft function, but definitive clinical trials are lacking." Thus DGF is yet another endpoint for assessing transplantation success. It is, however, problematic because its definition can vary across medical centers, patients, and physicians. As a result, DGF may not be a precise enough measure for determining outcome in clinical trials. For the moment—but for the moment only—I shall put aside this issue and define DGF as the need for dialysis treatment following kidney transplantation. Adding this parameter to those already enumerated, we now have a total of six endpoints for evaluating transplantation outcome. How, then, do we choose among them?

UNIFORMITY IN MEASURING ENDPOINTS

Efficacy endpoints in clinical trials are designed to evaluate Treatment outcome.[8] As such, they describe different Treatments' successes and are used to compare among them. It is thus imperative that they be measured uniformly across centers, investigators, patients, and so on. If a parameter is evaluated differently under varying circumstances, any group differences on it may be due to factors other than Treatment; and absence of group differences may be due to inconsistent measurement rather than to lack of efficacy. Thus, it stands to reason that an endpoint measured inconsistently should not be used for describing outcome of medical interventions in a clinical study. And while the principle is obvious enough, it is sometimes difficult to apply in practice.

Let us take the example of DGF, which we defined as the need for dialysis after kidney transplantation. It turns out that the word "need" is open to interpretation, with some physicians quicker to the "dialysis trigger" than others. Thus, a conservative physician may order dialysis based on early signs of a kidney's weakening function, while one less conservative may give the transplanted kidney more time to recover before making a final decision on dialysis. Now some of these differences in clinical practice among physicians are due to personality

or erroneous reading of guidelines and so can be made uniform with suitable action. For example, you might convene a meeting of all participating investigators in the trial to reach consensus on the circumstances in which posttransplantation dialysis is "needed." If you obtain consensus, DGF will be defined and measured uniformly throughout the study. As such, it will also be a suitable endpoint for your trial.

Now all this is well and good when disagreements among physicians can be bridged. But this is not always the case, since such differences are often attributable to dissimilarities in clinical experience and/or deeply held opinions. And when this is the case, it is unrealistic to expect all physicians to agree to the same criteria for any particular intervention. In DGF there can be several solutions to the problem, including the following:

- Seek consensus as described.
- Allow to participate in the trial only those physicians who are willing to accept endpoint definitions as written in the protocol.

[8] This, of course, is also the case for safety endpoints, performance endpoints, and those measuring other aspects of Treatment outcome.

Continued

[7] Perico, N., Cattaneo, D., Sayegh, M. H., & Remuzzi, G. (2004). Delayed graft function in kidney transplantation. *Lancet*, 364(9447), 1814–1827.

UNIFORMITY IN MEASURING ENDPOINTS–CONT'D

- Discard the endpoint altogether and, as a possible alternative, define transplanted kidney failure using laboratory tests assessing kidney function (e.g., BUN and/or CCr).
- Record the endpoint despite lack of uniformity and relegate it to a minor role in statistical testing and consequent conclusions. When doing so, you essentially state that the parameter in question:
  - Is sufficiently interesting to assess, and
  - Cannot be measured accurately enough for reaching definitive conclusions with it.

When designing a clinical trial, you can choose any of the preceding, but choose you must.

Considering the specific case of DGF, I described the difficulty and presented several solutions for it. Similar solutions apply in other indications. Yet, there is no universal answer for nonuniformity in measuring endpoints because there is none for dealing with measurement error in general. Indications differ, as do physicians, endpoints, and clinical trials. So at the end of the day you will need to tailor your approach to the study at hand, its logistics, endpoints, and personnel.

Be that as it may, measuring endpoints precisely—with minimal error and bias—is critical in clinical trials. So critical, in fact, that if you cannot do it properly, your trial will likely fail to meet its objectives.

MULTIPLE TESTING REVISITED

Your Company has developed NG-12 for countering organ rejection in kidney transplantation. Having read the preceding section, you know there are at least six alternatives for describing your results and thus six endpoints for comparing T (NG-12) to some standard of care R. Which do you choose?

Now this might seem like an odd question. Why, in fact, pick among endpoints when you can choose *all* of them? Well, this may not be a bad idea. But it is probably not a good one either. First, you cannot usually expect an experimental method to be superior to standard of care on every single parameter measured. Thus, staking your study's success on demonstrating T > R on all endpoints measured seems much too risky. Second, even if T is truly superior to R on every conceivable efficacy measure in the population, there is always the chance of failing by chance on one or two of them in a given trial (i.e., a sample). So even if you have an outstanding molecule, conducting multiple tests with the expectation of success on all of them is risky and should be avoided. Be that as it may, NG-12's future will depend a great deal on the endpoints you choose to test it with. So you had better think them out carefully before making a final decision.

I wrote in Chapter 12 that conducting numerous statistical tests increases the likelihood of succeeding by chance—of obtaining favorable results when you do not really "deserve" them. Not surprisingly, you can also fail by chance. The more statistical tests you perform—the more endpoints you compare—the greater the probability for erroneous results *in either direction*. In statistics the issue is known as *multiplicity* or *multiple testing* (see Chapter 10).

In the preceding chapter I noted that every time you conduct a statistical test you have some chance of getting erroneously lucky—of rejecting the Null when you should not—that is, of concluding the drug is effective when it is not. We call this Type I Error. The flip side is *not* rejecting H_0 when you should—of not saying T > R when this statement is actually correct. This is termed Type II Error and will be dealt with at length in Chapter 14 in the context of sample size determination. For the moment it is enough to know that the more tests you conduct, the greater your chance for erring.

One solution for this particular problem is to simply measure fewer endpoints, which will naturally yield fewer statistical tests. This is definitely legitimate but should only be used if the endpoints excluded are expendable—when the information they provide is relatively unimportant. But this is not the case here, where eliminating one or more of the six to reduce the number of statistical tests would be a sort of scientific "Don't ask, don't tell." To one less subtle this might be construed as scientific dishonesty.

It seems, then, that you are now between a commercial rock and a scientific hard place:

- Commercially you want your trial to succeed, and one way of doing this is by limiting the number of statistical tests for showing success, which in turn suggests reducing the number of endpoints measured.
- Scientifically you would like to measure all trial endpoints that can contribute to your understanding of differences between T and R.

This is a common quandary in clinical trials.

Virtually every study requires that you choose between what will and will not be measured. One generally cannot measure *all* endpoints *always*, since the number of potentially informative endpoints is typically prohibitive. Thus in most clinical trials there is no question of *not* leaving endpoints out. The more relevant issue is which to include. I will address this and several other pertinent topics in the following sections.

SELECTING ENDPOINTS TO INCLUDE IN YOUR TRIAL: PART I

When fearing failure due to multiplicity, selecting few endpoints for your trial may solve the problem. But this is an ill-advised strategy if it leads to excluding useful information. There is in fact an alternative that is practical and commonly used. I shall soon discuss it. But for the moment I would like to remain with this "paring down of endpoints," which I believe goes to the heart of what it means to perform good clinical research.

In this book I have generally approached clinical trials as a commercial enterprise. They often are, but sometimes they are not. Yet be they commercial or academic, they are scientific endeavors as well. And whatever your motive for a clinical study, you should be doing good science rather than bad.

Now the term *good science* is sufficiently sweeping that describing it would require a book of its own. Indeed many have been written on the topic but this is not one of them. In the current context, the concept encompasses a long list of elements of which the correct application yields replicable results—that is, results that will be repeated when a trial is repeated. One central element of good science is *clear thinking*, itself an elusive idea. This is not a formal term in clinical trials, and I do not have a good definition for it either. But well defined or not, the concept is vital to much of what we do in clinical trials (and elsewhere).

When I encounter a long list of endpoints in a study's protocol, a warning light will come on. Experience has taught me that researchers will often attempt to disguise an ill-conceived study with a plethora of endpoints; they try to cover up a study's weaknesses by measuring and then measuring some more. It as if the researcher is saying, "I'm not quite sure what I want to show or even what I *can* show, so I'll measure everything under the sun and something good will surely turn up." I have already noted that this can introduce statistical complications. But this is not the half of it.

Clinical trials must be well thought out. They should be done well or not at all. Merely conducting a study with good intentions and great hopes is unlikely to yield meaningful results. The most prominent statistician of the previous century, Sir Ronald Fisher, wrote, "To call in the statistician after the experiment is done may be no more than asking him to perform a postmortem examination: he may be able to say what the experiment died of."[9] So if you want your trial to achieve its goals you must design it right, which includes selecting its endpoints well.

Now there are certainly instances where you require multiple endpoints to properly describe the Treatment in question. Indeed, virtually every clinical trial collects information on numerous parameters and this is perfectly acceptable. On the other hand, researchers will often specify many endpoints because they have not done their homework—have shirked the intellectual effort of thinking clearly. And this is a recipe for failure.

In NCI's definition, endpoints are selected to demonstrate that "the intervention being studied is beneficial." In other words, endpoints must be closely tied to a Treatment's benefit; they are, as explained in Chapter 4, a direct translation of study objectives into measurable parameters. Now in early stages of trial planning it is often the case that neither objectives nor endpoints are clearly defined. This is fine. Yet if you are to do good science, a clearer picture must

---

[9] Quoted in *Nature Drug Discovery*. http://www.nature.com/drugdisc/news/articles/424610a.html.

eventually emerge. And choosing endpoints for your trial is part and parcel of this clarification process. In other words, the *process of endpoint selection can also be that of clarifying your thinking* about the trial at hand.

When study objectives are well defined, endpoints will pretty much "select themselves." But when they are not, you can apply the process in reverse. Thus if you have some difficulty defining study objectives precisely, make a list of all those parameters you believe are potentially useful. Once done, review the list and evaluate the degree to which each endpoint is useful in describing your product's performance. You will then select those that best serve your purpose, which in turn will assist you to better define the trial's objectives.

In the following section I use our running example and some others to show this. I also describe the more standard alternative for dealing with multiple endpoints.

SELECTING ENDPOINTS TO INCLUDE IN YOUR TRIAL: PART II

Select multiple endpoints and require success on all of them, and you have built a self-destruct mechanism into your trial. In the preceding section I noted one solution for this, which is specifying fewer endpoints. When appropriate, there is a good deal to be said for this route, including the following:

- Forcing you to think clearly about the study at hand.
- Reducing your chances of obtaining results by chance alone.
- Reducing the burden of data collection on both subjects and investigators.
- Decreasing costs.

Yet paring down the number of endpoints to a bare minimum is not always an option. Often, a relatively large number of variables must be measured to thoroughly comprehend the effect of Treatment, and there is no way around it.

I will now return to NG-12, where all six efficacy endpoints were deemed useful and should be retained. Here, as in most studies, the best way to deal with difficulties arising from multiplicity is *prioritizing* the endpoints by importance. Allow me to explain: Even when all measures considered are informative, some are typically more so than others. Indeed, in most trials you will be able to identify a single endpoint that best reflects your study's efficacy objective.[10] This is called the study's **primary endpoint**. Once identified, your first priority becomes demonstrating success on this parameter. It is the measure on which you stake your trial's success: Show that T is superior to R on the primary

---

[10] A reminder: Primary endpoints can, of course, refer to objectives other than efficacy. Keep in mind that for the sake of simplicity I focus here on efficacy and will add a few words about other endpoint types later in this chapter.

endpoint, and you win. Otherwise, you lose. And this is independent of results on other, secondary endpoints.

By specifying a primary efficacy endpoint, you will have addressed all the salient issues discussed:

1. Eliminated multiplicity, since you are staking success on a single statistical test only.
2. Retained all scientifically meaningful measures and relegated all but one to "less than primary" status.
3. Increased your chance for success.
4. Identified which measure is most intimately associated with your efficacy objective and in the process defined your trial's objective precisely.

Thus, in the majority of clinical studies assessing efficacy, you should choose a single endpoint (in some cases two, but rarely more) for demonstrating the trial's main efficacy objective. This single measure will be your trial's principal parameter for determining "whether the intervention being studied is beneficial."

The ICH guidelines state the following:[11]

> The primary variable ("target" variable, primary endpoint) should be the variable capable of providing the most clinically relevant and convincing evidence directly related to the primary objective of the trial.
>
> Secondary variables are either supportive measurements related to the primary objective or measurements of effects related to the secondary objectives.... The number of secondary variables should be limited and should be related to the limited number of questions to be answered in the trial.

As you can see, the solution for multiplicity can be straightforward: Select as many endpoints for study as you feel necessary, but make sure to specify which is primary and which is not. At the same time this does not absolve you of thinking carefully about your choice of endpoints in general—both primary and others. As the guidelines point out:

a. The primary variable should provide "the most convincing evidence directly related to the primary objective."
b. "The number of secondary endpoints should be limited."

---

[11] International Conference on Harmonization (ICH). (1998). *Note for Guidance on Statistical Principles for Clinical Trials.*

Let us now apply our newly gained knowledge to assessing NG-12 for kidney transplantation. Recall that I enumerated six measures for this trial. These can be grouped conceptually as follows:

1. Kidney function (DGF, CCr, BUN)
2. Survival (subject and kidney)
3. Subjective feeling (QoL)

Since all relate to efficacy of kidney transplantation, they are correlated conceptually and probably statistically as well. In this sense it is somewhat artificial to group them separately. Yet this categorization serves my purpose, and I shall keep to it for the moment.

Of the categories enumerated, the second seems most informative clinically. After all, surgeons transplant kidneys to function properly and, perhaps, to increase life expectancy as well. Thus, if "importance in general" were the criterion for choosing endpoints, you would likely choose Kidney or Overall Survival. But this is not necessarily the case since, as the guidelines point out, your primary endpoint should be that which best addresses your study's objectives. Now recall that the aim of NG-12 is to reduce harmful immune reactions to the transplanted organ. Using the reasoning presented, it would seem that your primary endpoint should relate directly to immune response rather than, say, to Kidney Survival. Perico and colleagues write, "Delayed graft function [DGF] is a form of acute renal failure resulting in ... risk of acute rejection episodes and decreased long-term survival [of the transplanted kidney]." In other words, acute rejection (which NG-12 aims to avoid) leads to both DGF and shortened Kidney Survival.

Following Perico and colleagues and the logic presented for selecting primary endpoints, we seem to have narrowed down our choice to two endpoints: DGF and Kidney Survival. And of these, DGF is most directly related to immune response. Perhaps, then, we have our primary endpoint? Well, maybe.

PRECEDENT

I have been discussing the intricacies of an issue that can nonetheless be straightforward. As I shall point out in the next section, there are instances where a study's primary efficacy objective is sufficiently clear and simple that the primary endpoint all but selects itself. Then there are also those occasions where your life is made easier by *precedent*.

As you might expect, in most instances you will not have been the first to investigate a particular clinical phenomenon.

And when this happens and past designs and objectives are sufficiently similar to yours, the path for selecting a primary endpoint may be clear. Then, depending on your opinion of the quality and appropriateness of earlier research, you may decide to conform to it or come up with your own endpoint even so. Often, however, the choice will depend on factors beyond your control like company preference and regulatory policy. As much as one wishes to do as good science as

Continued

SELECTING ENDPOINTS TO INCLUDE IN YOUR TRIAL: PART III

If a drug is meant to reduce fever, then Temperature should likely be the primary endpoint in a trial assessing efficacy with it. And if a diagnostic test aims to detect some disease, then Accuracy (quantified by Sensitivity, Specificity, and the like) is your natural choice. At times determining primary endpoints can, in fact, be fairly straightforward.

Suppose, however, that you wish to evaluate the efficacy of a cardiac **stent**, a kind of mesh tube inserted into clogged arteries for widening and keeping them open. A reasonable measure of success is Change in Stenosis—of abnormal narrowing in the blood vessel—before and after the procedure. You might also assess Change in Blood Flow through the artery. But while both these parameters relate to the stent's local physiological effects, neither describes the general *clinical benefit* to the patient. This might be better characterized by parameters such as future occurrence of Myocardial Infarction (MI) and Survival, which are further in both time and concept from Change in Stenosis and Blood Flow.

Recall that NG-12 is designed to reduce damaging immune reactions in kidney transplantation. As such, its most direct measure of efficacy is the Immune Reaction itself. The DGF endpoint, while associated with such reactions, is not a direct measure of them. Further down the timeline, we have Kidney Survival, which is likely most meaningful to both patients and nephrologists.

Each of the preceding endpoints for NG-12—Immune Reaction, DGF, and Kidney Survival—is a link in a chain for describing NG-12 efficacy. If you wish you can add even more links to gain a deeper understanding of the phenomena in question. This is perfectly legitimate. But of these, which should be your primary endpoint? When you have "more direct" and "more clinically meaningful," which one should you choose?

I do not have a definitive answer for you. First, I am a statistician and can only advise on endpoint selection, since it is for the investigator to make the final determination on this. I am not shirking responsibility here but merely conceding a meager understanding of biological/clinical processes, which are required for specifying endpoints in a particular indication. As an aside, even investigators who possess both the knowledge and experience sometimes find it difficult to prioritize endpoints on a scale of "primaryness." Yet, this does not absolve me from presenting the principles involved, which I shall proceed to do.

As trivial as it may seem, you should keep in mind that *medical interventions are designed to provide clinical benefits for patients*. It makes little sense to widen arteries when this does not ease Climbing Stairs, increase Survival, and/or provide other tangible results for patients. Similarly, a cancer drug that reduces Tumor Size but does nothing for Survival or QoL is unhelpful. Indeed, the NCI suggests this when writing that endpoints must be capable of demonstrating that "the intervention being studied is beneficial." We can safely assume that "beneficial" refers to the patient as a whole rather than to some local physiological outcome unrelated to patient health and well-being. The ICH states this as well when writing that a primary endpoint "should be the variable capable of providing the most *clinically relevant* [emphasis added] and convincing evidence directly related to the primary objective of the trial." Here you can generally substitute "clinically relevant" with "beneficial to patient."

CLINICAL UTILITY AND THE BENEFIT TO THE PATIENT

I said before that you can generally substitute "clinically relevant" with "beneficial to patient," and this is true. At the same time, "generally" is not "always," and the relationship between clinical and patient benefit is sometimes complex. For example, a relatively toxic drug for some terminal disease might increase Survival while substantially reducing the quality of the patient's remaining days. Should you be developing this sort of drug at all? And once developed, should you ask the patient to decide whether she wants to take it? Perhaps it is the patient's physician and/or family who should decide. These have been important questions for many years now, and I suspect they will become even more important as life spans increase and medical technology advances. But with your permission I shall leave this for medical ethics books and will remain with the (generally true) statement that clinical and patient benefit are positively correlated.

As a general rule, not without its exceptions, our most important endpoints should measure the effect our medical product has on patients' lives. While direct physiological measures, like blood pressure and Stenosis, are informative, they are often less useful than information on how a patient *feels*.

Now all this would be simple when considering endpoints that are "direct but clinically meaningless." But there are very few such animals. In most instances direct measures of an intervention are correlated to some degree or another with clinical outcomes. Thus, for example, you can expect at least some relationship between Change in Stenosis and QoL. Similarly, Change in Number of Bacteria in the blood before and after antibiotic treatment is highly correlated with Fever and other clinical parameters of bacterial infections. And since both Stenosis and Bacteria are predictive of clinical phenomena, they provide clinically meaningful information as well. To take an extreme example, if a nonclinical endpoint X perfectly predicts a clinical endpoint Y, the two are equally informative. When this is the case, either X or Y can be selected, with the choice determined by cost and convenience. This, then, is another important issue underlying our discussion of endpoint selection: Direct (and less than perfectly clinically meaningful) measures are typically easier and cheaper to obtain than clinical ones. Thus, you will usually prefer the former for cost and the latter for information. And here, as in many other instances in clinical trials, you will need to optimize your choices in a manner that is acceptable to your target audience, be they scientists, regulators, and/or others.

To this point I have used the words "direct" and "indirect." Getting nearer the language of clinical trials, the National Institutes of Health defines a **surrogate endpoint** as follows:

> A biomarker intended to substitute for a clinical endpoint. A surrogate endpoint is expected to predict clinical benefit (or harm, or lack of benefit or harm).[12]

To some degree or another, I have in fact been dealing in this section with the "surrogateness" of endpoints—the degree to which nonclinical endpoints can be used as substitutes for clinically informative ones. And I have presented the principle, not without its exceptions, that primary efficacy endpoints should be clinically meaningful. But I have also pointed out that it is often cheaper and more convenient to obtain surrogate endpoints. The choice is yours and should ultimately depend on your study's context. In early R&D you often seek little more than "hints of efficacy," in which case surrogates might do. Conversely, in later stages of development you will require more definitive proof of clinical benefit. And if your study is pivotal, a clinically meaningful primary endpoint will almost always be required.

VALIDITY, RELIABILITY, AND BIAS

Although I have not specifically used the term, much of this chapter has been addressing the **validity** of endpoints—the degree to which they describe meaningful, real-world product attributes. For example, Presence of Stenosis (yes/no) is a valid endpoint for a diagnostic test designed to detect clogged arteries, while DGF provides valid information in kidney transplantation; both of these endpoints are said to describe what the products they relate to *do*. White Blood

---

[12] Biomarkers Definition Working Group. (2001). Biomarkers and surrogate endpoints: Preferred definitions and conceptual framework. *Clin Pharma Col Ther*, 69, 89–95.

Cell Count (WBC), on the other hand, is not relevant for assessing efficacy of a sleeping pill. Yet, it may still be valid for assessing safety, since such a pill should be affecting sleep while causing no change on parameters such as WBC (and others). Thus, in general:

- Only valid endpoints can definitively demonstrate product attributes such as efficacy and safety.
- Validity is adjudged in a context, so a measure that is informative in one circumstance may not be so in another.
- An endpoint cannot be said to be valid in *any* context until it is demonstrated as such. The process of validation is often complex and cumbersome. It is also beyond the scope of this book.
- Because validation is usually a project unto itself, you should, to the degree possible, avoid selecting study measures that must first be validated.

Now it makes perfect sense that a study's endpoints should be meaningful for it. At the same time you cannot justify an endpoint simply because it *seems* to be meaningful to you. We are doing science here and a variable is valid only after having been *shown* to be so.

Still, investigators are often tempted to use nonvalidated measures for demonstrating primary and secondary objectives. A common reason is the knowledge-based conviction that there exists no valid endpoint to aptly describe the phenomenon investigated. When this is indeed the case, there are several approaches for dealing with the problem, including the following:

- Select a validated endpoint that may be less than ideal under the circumstances but is "good enough"—one that is sufficiently correlated with the phenomenon of interest to provide a reasonable measure of it.
- Take the long route by developing a new endpoint and validating it. While this will no doubt require both effort and expense, there is sometimes no way around this.
- Change the trial's design so an existing validated endpoint will be adequate for it. While this is a sort of tail-wagging-the-dog solution—adapting a trial to an endpoint rather than the reverse—producing evidence based on validated endpoints is *that* important.
- Develop an endpoint that "makes sense" and use it as is. This is not a good solution even if the measure appears well defined and meaningful.

Another reason for considering nonvalidated endpoints is associated with statistical power—with the ability of your trial to result in (correct) rejection of the Null Hypothesis.

Suppose your company has decided to move ahead with NG-12, and the initial plan is for DGF to be the planned trial's primary endpoint. Unfortunately the resources allotted are limited, and no more than 40 subjects can take part in the study—20 per group. Having done your homework, you know that the rate of DGF in your population when using standard procedures is about 25%. Thus you expect that in your trial about 5 placebo subjects will experience DGF. Given a very optimistic drug effect, you estimate that there will be only 2 subjects experiencing DGF in NG-12. In other words, under the best of circumstances you anticipate rates of 25% and 8% in T and R, respectively. Now these are impressive numbers and if they were to accurately represent the truth in the population, you have yourself a powerful drug. Unfortunately your planned trial will have a small sample size, and the actual frequencies associated with these rates will not suffice for achieving statistical significance. So instead you seek an alternative endpoint of which the event rate is likely to be higher.

After much thought and discussion with the investigator, you come up with an endpoint termed "Early Transplantation Outcome," which is scored as follows:

- Success = 1: If *both* of the following occur:
  - No DGF within 30 days of transplantation *and*
  - Recovery of at least 80% of normal Creatinine Clearance function by 72 hours postsurgery.
- Failure = 0: Either of the above not occurring.

You anticipate that scoring primary efficacy using this **composite endpoint**—one combining multiple variables—will substantially increase the primary endpoint event rate, giving you a fighting chance for statistical significance despite the small sample. But while your composite might make clinical sense—and may be validated in the future—it has yet to be used and must be assumed invalid. Selecting an endpoint that will provide sufficient event rates for reasonable power is a good idea; choosing an unsubstantiated primary endpoint is not.

All of this does not mean that yet-to-be-validated endpoints should be excluded from clinical trials. After all, if you do not incorporate such measures into studies, they cannot be validated. But you should not use them for formal proof of product attributes.

A valid endpoint must also be capable of providing accurate results consistently; it should be without **bias** and have **reliability**. By definition, a reliable measure yields similar results when it should; in other words, it displays little variation when measuring the same thing repeatedly. In clinical trials we typically distinguish two types of reliability:

1. **Repeatability** is the variation obtained when measuring under very similar circumstances—for example, when assessing WBC in two **aliquots** from the same blood sample, using the same instrument and lab technician on the same day.

2. **Reproducibility** is the variation obtained when measuring the same thing under less similar circumstances—for example, assessing WBC of two aliquots from the same blood sample on different days and/or using different lab technicians.

Both repeatability and reproducibility assess variation where there should be none. At the same time we must remember that in the real world there is no such thing as perfect measurement; *all measurement is unreliable to some degree.* So instead of aspiring to perfectly reliable endpoints, we must set our sights more modestly on those that can provide enough consistency. Now "enough" is another one of those bothersome words that should be defined more precisely. To keep things simple, I will just mention here that this implies "enough to serve our purposes." And in clinical trials this usually means giving your trial a reasonable chance to achieve its objectives.

At the same time I should point out that reliability does not ensure accuracy; a measure can be both consistent and biased at the same time. A simple example is a tape measure that yields outcomes that are generally off by a couple of inches. If I used this measure repeatedly on the same object, I might get very similar results each time. Yet even so my outcomes will be biased by 2 inches on average.

When the extent of bias is known, it can be corrected, and the measure can be made good. For example, in the preceding case, all I need to do is subtract 2 inches from any outcome obtained to eliminate bias. Yet in many cases we suspect bias but have no adequate method for estimating it. Consequently, one should make every effort to apply methods that are likely to be unbiased. In the preceding chapter I described two of the more powerful methods for this: blinding and randomization.

In sum, for an endpoint to be useful I must ensure that it be measured both reliably and without bias. But while this is a prerequisite for validity, it does not guarantee it. For example, a consistently precise measure of Height is of little use in assessing the efficacy of an antibiotic. In other words, reliability and lack of bias are necessary but not sufficient conditions for validity.

MEASUREMENT PROPERTIES OF ENDPOINTS

In statistics we distinguish several kinds of measurement scales by the information they provide. The three-value "Gold," "Silver," and "Bronze" scale used in competition informs on placement or *order*. With it, I know who came before whom but cannot know the actual *distance* between the top finishers. Not surprisingly, we call this an **ordinal scale**.

Ordinal scales abound in clinical research, where one survey of 175 published studies found that 70% used them.[13] Well-known examples include the New York Heart Association (NYHA) classification of Heart Failure (1 to 4),[14] general Cancer Staging (usually 1 to 4), and the Ritchie Index for scoring joint tenderness (0 to 3).[15] Since actual arithmetic distance is not meaningful on any of these scales, they need not use numbers. For example, the distance between cancer stages 1 and 2 is not equivalent to that between stages 2 and 3. At the same time these scales provide information on order, so their categories are usually labeled with numbers or letters. And as you have seen, colors will sometimes do as well.

Stenosis (narrowing of a blood vessel) is often reported in percentage terms. Thus, an artery can be said to have 22% narrowing and 45% Stenosis or any other number between 0 and 100% (the latter indicating complete blockage—narrowing to the point blood cannot flow through). Like Temperature and Blood Pressure, Stenosis is measured on a **ratio scale**, which has the following characteristics:

1. The *order* of values is meaningful. Thus, 45% Stenosis is higher than 26%, which in turn is higher than 10% and so on.
2. The *distance* between values is numerically meaningful. For example, the difference between 40% and 60% is numerically equivalent to that between 60% and 80%. However, I use the phrase "numerically equivalent" advisedly here, since it does not necessarily imply "clinical equivalence." For example, the therapeutic implications for 20% and 40% Stenosis may be similar; a physician will often treat patients with either similarly. This is not the case for 40% and 60%, where the latter is much more likely than the former to undergo intervention (e.g., placement of stent). Quantitative values do not necessarily have one-to-one relationships with clinical information, a topic I shall deal with in greater detail in the following.
3. *Ratios* of scale values are interpretable. For example, it makes sense to say that 80% is twice 40%, as is the case with 20% and 10%. At the same time, as in the case of distances, we should remember that identical ratios may have different clinical meanings, depending on the numbers they were derived from.

---

[13] Forrest, M., & Andersen, B. (1986). Ordinal scales and statistics in medical research. *British Medical Journal (Clin Res Ed)*, 292, 537–538.

[14] The Criteria Committee of the New York Heart Association. (1994). *Nomenclature and Criteria for Diagnosis of Diseases of the Great and Great Vessels*, 9th ed. Boston: Little, Brown & Co.

[15] Richie, D. M., et al. (1968). Clinical studies with an articular index for the assessment of joint tenderness in patients with rheumatoid arthritis. *Q J Med*, 37, 393–406.

Ratio scales provide information on order and then some. This reflects the general rule that higher-level numerical scales provide additional information to that of lower ones. For example, if you "un-transform" Gold, Silver, and Bronze back to Time (in, say, seconds), you will have information on both distance and order.

Why then would anyone convert a higher-level scale into a lower one? Some reasons for this will become apparent soon. At this point I suggest you try coming up with one of your own, beginning with the assumption that the International Olympic Committee has chosen their ratio-to-ordinal transformation for good reason.

When discussing measurement on a ratio scale I pointed to the arithmetic operations subtraction and division. These cannot be done with the values Gold, Silver, and Bronze, which points to another characteristic distinguishing scales: the arithmetic operations permissible with them. For example, it makes perfect sense to describe Stenosis in a group of individuals by computing their average. But this is not the case for, say, the dichotomous Healthy/Sick scale that is best described by count and percent—that is, by number and proportion of each category in the group.

Let us now examine a less refined scale of Stenosis that can take on three values only:

> 0—Between 0% and 50%: Low Stenosis and risk; no need for invasive intervention
> 1—Between 50% and 70%: Moderate Stenosis and risk; invasive intervention indicated but not urgent
> 2—Between 70% and 100%: High Stenosis and risk: immediate invasive intervention indicated

Now, most interventional cardiologists would protest that this scale is rather simplistic in that both risk and treatment are determined by a great deal more than Stenosis. I offer my humble apologies, but I shall remain with this scale because it will serve for a statistical example. Indeed as far as many physicians are concerned, statisticians have a great deal to apologize for, regardless. Let the record show that I am willing to take on this burden if only to get on with it, which I am about to do.

Having transformed the continuous 0% to 100% Stenosis scale into three classes, I have converted my ratio scale into an ordinal one and so reduced the numerical information. At the same time I have described clinical implications more directly, which is a natural way for clinicians to approach data.

In the preceding example I chose to transform a ratio scale into an ordinal one. At times, however, I have no choice. For example, the modified Rankin Scale (mRS)[16] is designed to assess functioning of patients who have experienced stroke. The scale has seven values:

> 0—No symptoms at all
> 1—No significant disability despite symptoms; able to carry out all usual duties and activities
> 2—Slight disability; unable to carry out all previous activities, but able to after own affairs without assistance
> 3—Moderate disability; requiring some help, but able to walk without assistance
> 4—Moderately severe disability; unable to walk without assistance and unable to attend to own bodily needs without assistance
> 5—Severe disability; bedridden, incontinent, and requiring constant nursing care and attention
> 6—Dead

While the mRS uses the numbers 1 to 6, their meaning is not of the sort we learned about in school. We cannot, for example, say that the difference between 6 and 5 is equal to that between 3 and 2, nor can we say that 4 is twice 2 (well, I suppose we *can* say it if we really want to). It seems then that some ordinal scales are naturally that, while others result from transformations of higher-level numerical scales.

Yet even mRS, a naturally ordinal scale, can be further transformed for clinical purposes. For example, in a study investigating a treatment for stroke, I may wish to know how many patients reached 0 or 1 at the end of the trial. The question implies a two-category scale where 0 to 1 on the original scale comprise one category and 2 to 6 another. In other words, my 0 to 6 scale has become a two-point scale where the lower value indicates a good outcome (Success) and the higher an inferior outcome (Failure). Once again, I have transformed a scale to indicate meaningful clinical information at the expense of greater statistical resolution.

Dichotomous, 0/1 scales are often termed *qualitative*, as in the Food and Drug Administration's guidance on reporting diagnostic test results.[17] The agency writes as follows:

> Diagnostic results (outcomes) are usually classified as either
> quantitative or qualitative. A quantitative result is a numerical amount

---

[16] Bonita R., & Beaglehole, R. (1988). Modification of Rankin scale: Recovery of motor function after stroke. *Stroke*, 19(12), 1497–1500.

[17] Food and Drug Administration. (2007). *Guidance for Industry and FDA Staff: Statistical Guidance on Reporting Results from Studies Evaluating Diagnostic Tests*. Rockville, MD: Food and Drug Administration.

or level, while a qualitative result usually consists of one of only two possible responses—for example, diseased or nondiseased, positive or negative, yes or no.

At the same time, it is important to note that not all "qualitative" scales are created equal. There are those like success/failure and diseased/nondiseased that are ordinal in that we can meaningfully point to "better" and "worse" outcomes. This is not the case for other parameters such as Gender, Race, and Hospital Center, the values of which have no self-evident ordering.[18]

Over the years it has become generally, though not universally, accepted that the most clinically meaningful outcome on the seven-point mRS is a reduction from some high value to 0 or 1. Thus, while a reduction from 4 to 3 is certainly useful, only an outcome at the lower end of the scale can be considered "success" when evaluating Treatment. Using this classification, I can say that patients reaching 0 or 1 are *responders*, while those remaining at 2 are *nonresponders*. Thus, coding Success or Failure based on whether or not a subject achieved one of the lower mRS values, I am describing response. This transformation allows for **responder analysis**, where I compute the rate (in one or more groups) of those achieving success—that is, compute the proportion responding.

Responder analysis involves two steps:

1. Determining a success criterion at the subject level and labeling a subject who reached the criterion "Responder" and others "Nonresponders."
2. Computing the proportion of Responders in a group.

Throughout this section I have pointed out that statistical and clinical meanings do not necessarily correspond. Responder analysis allows bridging this gap and, in many circumstances, is an optimal interleaving of statistical data and clinical implications. This is best shown with an example, for which I once again return to Stenosis. Suppose I have catheterized a group of subjects whose average Stenosis was 70%, my goal being that each patient be reduced to below 50%. Suppose further that at the end of my trial I find that average Stenosis is 40%. On the face of it I have achieved success. After all, the procedure reduced average Stenosis from 70% by 30 percentage points. At the same time, these numbers do not tell me how many subjects Responded—how many achieved a level below 50%. Depending on actual outcomes, I might have succeeded with more subjects or less. The latter would occur when the average reduction of 30% achieved is due mostly to large reductions in a small number of

---

[18] Hospital centers can, for example, be ordered from smaller to larger. But this is only possible after adding in ratio scale values of size. Given the labels only ("Children's Hospital," "St. Luke's," etc.), there is no natural ordering.

subjects (and small reductions in others). Responder analysis solves this problem in that it provides success/failure information at the subject level. In this case I would code each subject as follows:

> 0—Postprocedure Stenosis ≥ 50% (Failure)
> 1—Postprocedure Stenosis < 50% (Success)

I would then compute the proportion of subjects scored "Success" of the total sample size.

A formal classification of all possible scale types is not necessary for our purposes. It is enough to know that endpoints should be optimally measured and reported. Statistically, ratio scales are most informative and should be used where possible. At the same time, a clinical trial is designed to provide meaningful clinical information, so your choice of measurement, and the manner in which you report it, must take this into account as well.

A note on arithmetic manipulation and statistical testing: I noted that different scales enable different arithmetic manipulations. For example, I can provide average Weight and median Survival Time but neither statistic is particularly useful on a two-value Responder scale. Going one step further, different types of scale values must be tested with different statistical procedures. For example, a t-test compares means, so it is not appropriately applied to ordinal data. Conversely, ordinal data provide information on counts and percentages, which are often analyzed using a Fisher's Exact Test (or a Chi-square test). Thus when conducting statistical tests, statisticians must first determine the type of data they are dealing with. To summarize:

- Scales differ on the amount of numerical (statistical) and clinical information they provide.
- The types of arithmetic manipulations possible with data depend on the measurement scale used, which in turn has implications for statistical testing.
- No scale can be said to be superior to others in all circumstances. Rather, in any particular situation we should select the scale that optimizes both clinical and statistical information.

SAFETY ENDPOINTS

I mentioned early on that most of this chapter deals with efficacy endpoints—endpoints with which you plan to demonstrate a study's efficacy objective(s). This was done for convenience, since the issues I wanted to address were best demonstrated in the context of efficacy. At the same time, many other attributes are measured in clinical trials, the most common of which relate to safety.

In most confirmatory trials the Null and Alternative hypotheses concern efficacy. To avoid problems associated with multiplicity, we specify, where possible, a single confirmatory efficacy endpoint (to be analyzed once). If we wish to test multiple efficacy endpoints and/or want to analyze a single endpoint several times, we must make statistical allowance for it. This is not usually the case for safety, which is not generally tested using a confirmatory strategy. Instead, safety endpoints are typically analyzed descriptively—by providing descriptive statistics of results and assessing whether or not safety profiles are acceptable.

But even when safety *is* tested using a confirmatory strategy, the approach will need to differ from efficacy. This is because safety data must be analyzed continuously throughout the trial. After all, it would not be ethical to wait for the end of the trial to find out whether my yet-to-be-tested treatment is safe. Consequently, dealing with the issue of multiplicity in safety can differ markedly from that of efficacy. With your permission, I shall leave this for another book. Regardless, you should be aware that approaches to selecting and testing endpoints can differ as a function of the attributes these endpoints relate to.

SUMMARY

In this chapter I addressed some of the major issues associated with clinical trial endpoints: selecting them, deciding which is primary and which not, making sure they do their job properly, ensuring that they are measured reliably and without bias, and making sure they are valid. Then there is the issue of measurement type (ordinal, ratio, etc.), which is dealt with by selecting scales that are useful statistically *and* clinically.

I noted that the process of determining endpoints can be straightforward, particularly if your study resembles well-designed trials conducted by others. Defining study goals precisely will also enhance the process of endpoint selection. Yet even then complexities will arise if, after defining your objectives, you find there are no validated endpoints for them. When this happens you will need to find a less-than-perfect-but-satisfactory endpoint (recommended) or validate a new one yourself (to be avoided). Alternatively, you might redesign your trial so that existing validated endpoints are a perfect fit for it.

The greatest difficulty in selecting endpoints will arise when you have not precisely defined your study's objectives. Unfortunately, this is not an uncommon occurrence even in experienced organizations. At the same time, you can often leverage this difficulty to your advantage. Specifically, the process of endpoint selection can go a long way to assisting company staff in honing in on study objectives. In other words, endpoint selection can and should be used to clarify what you wish to achieve with your trial.

Clinical trials are costly affairs, and you should feel free to measure as many endpoints as you think are useful. Yet you must also make sure to do the following:

- Measure only as much as the "market can bear." If your data collection becomes burdensome for clinicians and/or subjects, you are liable to end up with bad data; in other words, you will increase your chances of getting missing, unreliable, and biased data, and will generally make a mess of things.
- Address the issue of multiplicity in the confirmatory portion of your trial.
- Specify a limited number of primary and secondary endpoints from the many you have chosen to measure. This will:
    - Show to both yourself and others that you have defined your study objectives well—that you know what you want from the trial, and
    - Provide greater credibility to significant results should they emerge.

So now you have designed your study, selected your endpoints, and specified which is primary and which is secondary. All that remains is for the statistician to tell you how many subjects your trial should include for meeting its objectives. Onward, then, to the next chapter.

CHAPTER 14

Sample Size

CONTENTS

- Defining power intuitively
- Elements of study design affecting power:
  - effect size
  - sampling error
  - measurement Error
  - study design
  - stratification
- The "mechanics" of computing sample size: a simulation for computing sample size in rheumatoid arthritis
- Determining sample size for equivalence and non-inferiority
- Why a nonsignificance difference is *not* equivalence
- Ethics and sample size

INTRODUCTION: A SIMPLE STUDY

When blood alcohol content (BAC) is below 0.03%, the average person will seem normal. When it is 0.0%, this will often happen as well. Now it is generally recognized that driving and alcohol should not mix, and most countries have some laws to that effect. The United States, for example, permits a blood alcohol level of up to 0.08%, and in Japan it is 0.03%. In Germany the law is more involved, with experienced drivers allowed 0.05% and inexperienced none. Other variants abound.

Say you are from Missouri and you want to conduct a confirmatory trial assessing the effects of drink on driving. These are the trial's hypotheses:

H_0: Ingesting alcohol does not affect driving
H_1: Ingesting alcohol affects driving

To test these, you will need to define an endpoint—some parameter to measure "affect" by. I dealt with the issue in preceding chapters and will do so here as well. But before I do, I shall first address study design.

Having defined your objective, you set up a simple trial where each subject will be randomly assigned to either Alcohol or Placebo. Alcohol will be mixed with quinine water (T), and Placebo will be Quinine only (R). About half an hour after ingesting one of the liquids, each subject will undergo testing on a driving simulator. Subjects will be exposed to several simulated challenges and their behavior recorded. Once the trial is completed, you will compare the average performance in T and R on the parameters of interest.

While this is about as straightforward as a controlled trial can be, there are numerous details you must work out before moving forward. The following should be central on your list:

1. Number of subjects per group
2. Target BAC level in the Alcohol group
3. Simulator model

Translating these into our own language, we have:

1. Sample size
2. Effect size
3. Measurement

I will now deal with each, beginning with sample size.

THE (BIG) IDEA

In this chapter I mostly describe trials of which the objective is to show that treatments differ—studies aimed to demonstrate superiority or inferiority. To keep things simple, I will mention superiority almost exclusively; inferiority is merely the flip side of it and the statistical approach to both is the same. Further on I will apply these principles to non-inferiority and equivalence trials, which you will find are not all that different in terms of sample size determination. Be that as it may, *in a confirmatory trial of any kind you must specify a sample that is large enough to provide a reasonable chance for rejecting the Null* (when it should be rejected).

In the typical superiority trial you begin by assuming treatments are equal and conduct a study to show that this is not the case. Once done, you will analyze the data and either:

- Reject the Null, concluding a difference.

or

- Fail to reject the Null and conclude you cannot conclude.

In preceding chapters I noted the possibility of making a Type I Error—of mistakenly rejecting the Null Hypothesis. We label this probability Alpha (α). Here I deal primarily with Type II Error, which is mistakenly failing to reject the Null. For example, if T truly differs from R and your trial did not yield a significant difference between them, you have made a Type II Error—you have not rejected the Null when it should have been rejected.

Clinical research is meant to reveal the truth in the population. In the current BAC trial, *T and R truly differ or not, which has nothing to do with the study*; there is some "inconvertible truth out there" that we aim to discover, and whether or not we do has no effect on it. So while a particular study will not influence the truth,[1] its characteristics will determine our chance to detect it. And a central one of the characteristics is sample size (**N**)—the number of trial participants. So when comparing two groups, *the truth is either of the following and no other*:

- T and R are equal.

or

- T and R differ.

In a superiority trial your objective is to detect the latter when this is indeed the truth.

I chose the BAC example to begin with, since it is generally accepted (by the sober) that alcohol impairs driving. This implies that in this trial you *should* obtain a significant result. This is not a typical trial in the sense that research is generally done to discover novel phenomena rather than to verify known ones. Yet this suits my purpose of discussing statistical power, which here quantifies the chance for detecting a difference when one exists. Clearly, one does not wish to obtain significance when T and R do not differ. So to summarize the case at hand:

- T and R differ in the population. This is the truth.
- Having conducted the trial, you will either:
  a. Reject the Null and conclude that T and R differ (correct), or
  b. Fail to reject the Null (incorrect; commit a Type II Error).

In statistics, we label the chances of making a Type II Error, Beta (β); β is the probability of failing to show that T and R differ when they actually do. If you recall that the probability of making a Type I Error is α, you begin to grasp the imaginative powers of statisticians.

---

[1] With your permission, I shall leave for others the intriguing issue relating to our affecting reality in the process of observing it.

ONE-SIDED AND TWO-SIDED TESTS

In most superiority studies your practical objective is to show T > R (or R > T) rather than T ≠ R. In other words, you aim to show that T differs from R in a certain direction and reject the Null that this is not the case. Discovering the opposite effect—for example, that your drug is inferior to the competitor—is of no commercial interest. In statistics this implies stating **one-sided hypotheses** that yield **one-sided tests**. Conversely, T ≠ R leads to a **two-sided hypothesis** because you will reject the Null hypothesis if T is either superior *or* inferior to R.

These two possibilities—aiming to show difference in a specific direction or in either direction—have some very definite statistical implications. I will not address them here because, importantly, *virtually all clinical trials aiming to show superiority state a two-sided hypothesis regardless*. This is typically the regulator's requirement, as well as that of research presented in scientific journals. In our current example this implies the following hypotheses:

H$_0$: T = R (Driving ability is the same under the influence and not.)

H$_1$: T ≠ R (Driving ability differs between those having consumed alcohol and those not. This leaves open the possibility of rejecting the Null if driving under the influence is worse *or* better than driving over it.)

Having stated these hypotheses you will, at the conclusion of this trial, conduct a two-sided test. A significant result in the hoped-for direction will spell success. If you obtain a significant difference in the opposite direction, you will reject the Null as well, but you will do so grudgingly.

Thus, while the issue of one- and two-sided tests is, theoretically, both interesting and important, I will mostly assume two-sided tests and limit my discussion to them.

Since there are only two possible conclusions in this trial and the likelihood of erring is β, the likelihood of correctly rejecting the Null is 1 – β. Statisticians know how to compute this probability. And while I will describe one example for this, I suggest that you generally leave the mathematical particulars to them. The point is this: *In a superiority trial your chance of concluding that there is a difference when one truly exists is 1 – β*. This is the power of your study to achieve its objective.

To this point I have described a circumstance in which T and R truly differ and you conduct a trial hoping to show this. But if the two indeed differ, why should your study *ever* fail to show it? Well, there can be many reasons for it. I will deal primarily with one of these: *bad luck*.

I shall now return to my running example and explore how one (you, actually) might get unlucky. Suppose that your randomization misfired and that those assigned to the Alcohol group happened to be more experienced drivers than those to Placebo. The formers' performance on the simulator in the trial was indeed diminished by a bit of alcohol but not enough for them to differ from Placebo. In short, alcohol detrimentally affects driving (truly), and your unlucky randomization did not allow you to discover this.

It seems I have hit a couple of nails on the head here and, to mix my metaphors, I did not call them by name. I first mentioned getting "unlucky" and then said that the subjects in T received "a bit of alcohol." Well, it is time to name names.

SAMPLING ERROR

Random samples do not perfectly represent populations, but if done correctly, they are usually close enough. Still, there are times you can get unlucky, and in the preceding section I showed how this might happen in our running example. Specifically, I described how you might obtain large, chance differences at baseline. When this occurs, the study's eventual results will likely misrepresent the truth. We call this particular form of lack of luck "sampling error."

So when I used the word "unlucky" in this context, I am referring to a lack of luck in sampling, which may affect the results down the line. Now there are numerous other ways of getting unlucky in clinical trials; it would not be a human endeavor otherwise. But for the moment I will remain with this particular problematic circumstance, since it is of central importance in the context of statistical power—that is, of the relationship between a study's N and its probability for yielding rejection of the Null (when it should be rejected).

Clearly we would like to avoid sampling error. And while we cannot completely ensure this—indeed, we can be certain that sampling error *will* occur—there is much we can do to reduce it. One central method for reducing sampling error is increasing N. On average, larger samples are more likely to represent the population accurately than smaller ones.[2] In other words, increasing N will, on average, reduce sampling error. This will reduce your chance for getting unlucky, which in turn will increase your chance for discovering the truth.

Keeping with our simple and simplistic example:

- You plan for the drink-and-drive trial with three subjects per group.
- Having randomly selected six subjects from the population, you proceed to randomly assign each to T or R.
- There is natural variation in driving ability in the population, so your six subjects can be ranked in ability from 1 to 6, with 1 being the best and 6 the worst.
- Randomly assigning each to one of the groups, your chance for ending up with the top three drivers in the Alcohol group is 5%; the probability of having at least two of the three top drivers in the Alcohol group is almost 50%.

In short, when there are only six subjects in the trial, your chance of getting a relatively large difference in ability between the groups *before* applying your intervention is high. This will then increase your chances of failing to reject the Null despite the truth that alcohol impairs driving.

---

[2] Provided the sampling is done correctly—without bias.

But if, for example, you plan to include 10 subjects in each of the study groups T and R, your chance of randomly obtaining a great imbalance between them at baseline is much smaller. Here, the chance of the five best drivers ending up in the Alcohol group is near zero. Enlarging your sample per group further—say, randomly assigning 100 subjects to each—you will increase your chances further of:

a. Obtaining a representative sample of the population in each group, and thus
b. Obtaining two groups that are similar in terms of driving ability.

And when treatment arms are similar to begin with, you are pretty much assured that any differences between them at the end of the trial can be attributed to the trial's manipulation—to the difference in Treatment between the two.

Statisticians know the mathematical relationship between the size of N and the degree to which samples represent populations. One example of this is described by the central limit theorem, which is worth looking up.

SAMPLING SCHEMES TO REDUCE SAMPLING ERROR

I have described a study where each of six subjects was randomly assigned to each of two groups. I then pointed out that there is a 5% chance that the best three drivers will end up in T and almost a 50% chance that at least two of the three will be in this Alcohol group. I then noted that increasing N will reduce the likelihood of such imbalances occurring. Well, we can take care of this problem even without increasing the number of participants in the trial.

Suppose that before assigning subjects to Alcohol or Tonic Water Only, you test them on your simulator. Having done this, you can now rank them in driving ability from 1 to 6. You then divide them into three Ability *strata*: the best two drivers in A, the second ability-pair in B, and the remaining in C. You then randomly assign subjects to T and R by strata—that is, you conduct **stratified assignment**. You might, for example, flip a coin to decide which of the two drivers in strata A will be assigned to the Alcohol condition and assign the other to Tonic Water Only. Repeat this for the other two pairs, and you will have reduced the likelihood of a consequential imbalance.

Stratified randomization aims to ensure that subjects in the different treatment groups are similar. Stratified sampling—where one samples specific proportions of individuals from various subpopulations (strata) in the larger population—

is meant to ensure that the subjects selected will be representative of the population of interest. There are various other sampling schemes aimed at increasing the likelihood that treatment groups will be "about equal" at baseline. Depending on the trial, some methods may be more essential than others, though all will typically complicate trial logistics. Here too you would do well to consult with your statistician. I should add the following:

- Stratification of any kind should be used for those parameters that are related to outcome only. For example, cardiology trials often yield different results for men and women. It is thus advisable to ensure that the male–female proportions are about the same in T and R, which can be ensured by stratifying on Gender. Yet, it would make little sense to stratify by variables that are unrelated to the outcome, such as Shoe Size or Eye Color. While subjects do truly differ on them, I suspect that having an imbalance between T and R on, say, Shoe Size will have little or no effect on study results.
- The moral of this story is as simple as it is important: Increasing N is not the only way to reduce your chance of getting unlucky. A well-designed study, which includes a good sampling plan, will increase a study's power independent of sample size.

EFFECT SIZE

One of the more critical decisions you will need to make in the trial described is just how much alcohol to give to the subjects in T. This will greatly affect the expected difference between the groups and, with it, other important trial parameters. By deciding on the BAC level in T, you will influence **effect size**—the degree to which the groups differ when one is given alcohol and the other not.

When BAC is at 0.03% or less, most people will behave normally so that the Treatment effect of alcohol on driving will be subtle; it may only be picked up by a sophisticated simulator and, even then, just barely. But when BAC is, say, 0.12%, its effect on driving will be sufficiently apparent that even an imbalanced assignment of subjects or a crude simulator will detect them. In other words, a large effect size may get you significant differences—may enable you to discover the truth—even in the presence of nontrivial sampling error and/or less-than-optimal measurements.

Effect size refers to the strength of the relationship between two populations. In this case, it is the quantification of the difference in Driving Ability between those receiving alcohol and those not. For example, you might expect those in R to perform 20% better than those in T on a simulator. Alternatively, you might say that subjects in R will react 0.3 seconds faster to a simulated barrier relative to those in T. In these examples, expected effect sizes are 20% and 0.3 seconds, respectively. Effect sizes can be defined in many ways, and it is the statistician's task to define the specific form relevant to the study at hand.

Since large effect sizes are easier to detect than small ones, the former will require smaller sample sizes for rejecting the Null. Thus, even a sample of 3 in each group is likely to demonstrate differences between subjects with BAC = 0.12% and those with BAC = 0.00%. But when BAC in the Alcohol group is low, you will need a larger sample to obtain reasonable power. Thus we have another important principle:

The larger the expected effect size, the smaller the sample required to detect it.

It should now be clear why the statistician will ask you for the expected effect of your trial's manipulation when you ask him to determine N. It simply makes no sense to compute the number of subjects needed in a study without some idea of what you are looking for. If you are looking for the elephant in the room, one look should be enough. But if it is a bacterium you are hoping to detect, you should be using a microscope. Indeed, samples are to statisticians what microscopes are to life scientists. When the expected phenomenon is very large, a crude instrument—a small sample size, a weak microscope, or even the naked eye—is sufficient. But a small effect will only be detected with a powerful tool—a large sample size or a powerful microscope.

Now while it is perfectly logical for the statistician to want an estimate effect for planning a trial, it seems a bit silly as well. After all, one typically conducts a trial to discover an effect that is thus far unknown. And here the statistician is asking you for an estimate of this effect *before* a study begins. Being that an estimate of effect size is needed to compute N, and that this effect cannot be known without a trial, it would appear impossible to compute sample size properly.

Well there is often a difference between theory and practice and so it is here. In reality it is a rare researcher who does not have some idea of what to expect in a study; typically there are known results from animals and humans, in addition to scientific publications related to phenomena under study.

And on those (usually rare) occasions when effect size cannot be estimated intelligently, the alternative is specifying the minimal *clinically meaningful effect*—that is, the effect clinicians require for considering the intervention useful for patients. You would then ask the statistician to specify the N required to have sufficient power to discover this effect or one larger. If the true effect is smaller than this minimum, your N will likely not be sufficient to detect a difference between the groups. At the same time you typically have little interest in detecting an effect that is not commercially viable.

In fact, even when you have a good estimate of effect size, you should ask, "What is the minimal effect that interests me?" and then plan your trial accordingly. More often than not, it will be a waste of resources running a trial to detect a commercially uninteresting effect. Bottom line, regardless of how you estimate T's effect, you have to do it. And, practically speaking, this is not usually a very difficult task.

ON INDUSTRY, SCIENCE, AND SCIENCE IN INDUSTRY

Discovering a commercially uninteresting difference between treatments can be interesting when doing basic science. Thus, a molecule may only slightly affect the body, but the fact that it does may reveal a useful biological mechanism. Indeed, scientists may find meaning where entrepreneurs will not, which is more the rule than the exception. At the same time, commercial organizations—especially those with large, well-funded R&D departments—may be interested in real, though noncommercial, effects as well. This is because detecting weak effects may, with additional research, lead to the discovery of stronger effects. The moral of this particular story is that pharma and biotech companies often ask different questions than basic scientists. But not always.

MEASUREMENT

In the first section of this chapter I noted that stating hypotheses and later testing them require translating a trial's objectives into measurable parameters. We call these parameters *endpoints*, and in our drink-and-drive trial there are many options to choose from, including the following:

- Reaction Time to a simulated obstacle on the road.
- Number of Times per minute subject uses rearview mirror.
- Degree to which subject obeys speed limit.
- Number of attempts needed for successful parking in a tight space.

Depending on trial objectives, you will select one or more of these or some other parameter and collect data from subjects while on the simulator. At the end of the trial you will compare T and R on confirmatory endpoints and will either reject or fail to reject the Null.

In the preceding chapter I noted that endpoints should be measured with precision and without bias. And having endpoints thus measured will increase your trail's power independent of sample size.

AN INTERIM SUMMARY

We have seen that your study's power—its ability to detect true differences of interest—depends on Trial Design, Effect Size, and Sample Size (N). You should not compute N without obtaining information on the other two. In the case of the drink-and-drive trial, you can control effect size by giving smaller or larger quantities of alcohol to subjects in T. But this is not usually the case in clinical trials, where you are pretty much stuck with a given product that has a specific effect size in the intended use population. So of these three factors affecting power, you typically have the least control over effect size. But in most clinical trials you *will* have some control over "quality of measurement." For example, you might employ more accurate instruments than less and make sure that those using them are adequately trained.

Throughout this book I emphasized that everything is connected to everything else. So it is here, where:

- Larger effect sizes are easier to detect than smaller ones.
- Larger N's are more likely to detect effects than smaller ones.
- Accurate measures are more likely to detect effects than less accurate measures.

Part and parcel of your job is to optimize these factors to obtain the required power.

To this point I have discussed factors affecting statistical power but have not indicated what "adequate" power is. Clearly, the greater your power, the better; after all, you conduct a trial to succeed and will have little chance of doing that with weak power. But is 70% power enough or even 80%? Either of these would likely do in Las Vegas, but what about the clinic? As usual, situations vary, and the optimal choice in one study may be less than optimal for another. Still, there is "convention" to consider. The ICH guidelines say the following:

> The probability of type II error is conventionally set at 10% to 20%; it is in the sponsor's interest to keep this figure as low as feasible, especially in the case of trials that are difficult or impossible to repeat.[3]

Keeping in mind that Type II Error is β and power is $1 - \beta$, power is "conventionally set" at 80% to 90%.

HOW IT ACTUALLY WORKS

There are many methods for computing the number of subjects needed for a study. Off-the-shelf programs will suffice for most trial designs, while others are sufficiently unique to require running power simulations for them. While the simulation route is less standard—though certainly common enough—I feel it is more intuitive than theoretical approaches and will use it here for illustrating the process.

Say you are conducting a trial in rheumatoid arthritis (RA) comparing two **monoclonal antibodies**, T and R. Each of these medications is designed to bind to and inhibit Tumor Necrosis Factor α (TNF $-\alpha$), a protein secreted by the immune system. TNF $-\alpha$ is involved in several biologically important pathways, including inflammation. Blocking TNF $-\alpha$ in RA patients aims to reduce inflammation and disease activity. In the best of cases it will induce remission.

There are various continuous scales for measuring RA activity, each with cutoffs for categorizing disease activity. One of these is the DAS-28 (4), of which the cutoffs divide patients into those with "high" or "moderate" activity or "remission." The scale's score is computed by taking into account the following:

- Number of swollen joints of the 28 measured (swollen joint count; SJC).
- Number of tender joints of the 28 measured (tender joint count; TJC).
- Level of C-reactive protein (CRP), a protein found in blood that rises in response to inflammation.
- Pain as measured by the visual analogue scale (VAS; 0 = "no pain," 100 = "unbearable pain").[4]

Your planned trial will include subjects with at least moderate disease activity defined by DAS-28(4) ≥ 3.8. Its objective is assessing the degree to which your monoclonal antibody T induces remission relative to R. Remission is achieved

---

[3] International Conference on Harmonization (ICH). (1998). *Statistical Principles for Clinical Trials.*

[4] The formula combining these variables is DAS28-28(4) = $0.56 \times$ SQRT(TJC28) + $0.28 \times$ SQRT(SJC28) + $0.36 \times \ln(\text{CRP} + 1) + 0.014 \times \text{VAS} + 0.96$.

by reaching DAS-28(4) ≤ 2.3. Thus, at the end of the trial each subject will be classified dichotomously as follows:

"Failure" = 0 = DAS-28(4) > 2.3
"Success" = 1 = DAS-28(4) ≤ 2.3

At trial's end you will compare Proportion Success in T to Proportion Success in R, using a Fisher's Exact Test, a standard method for testing differences in proportions.

Before initiating the study, you wish to determine N if you are to have a reasonable chance of showing that T is superior to R (if indeed it is). Specifically, you want to have at least 80% power to obtain a significant result in favor of T. After discussions with your clinician and statistician, you come up with the following relevant information:

- The sample in your trial will be drawn from a population similar to that used in past studies. The database available at your Company includes about 1,400 subjects, more than half of whom had DAS-28(4) ≥ 3.8 at baseline in their respective study. These subjects are available for your simulation.
- The effect of R in this population is generally known and estimated to be about a 30% reduction in DAS, with a standard deviation of 17%. Thus, the *distribution of R effect sizes is* 30% ± 17%.
- Your estimate for T's effect is 50% in this population, with a standard deviation of 26%. Thus the *distribution of T effect sizes is* 50% ± 26%.
- At the end of your trial you will compare Proportion Remission in two groups, using a Fisher's Exact Test.

You are now ready to program the simulation as follows:

1. "Create" an R group of, say, 50 subjects by:
   a. Randomly selecting 50 subjects with DAS-28(4) > 3.8 from those in your database.[5]
   b. For each subject, determine "success" or "failure" in the R group by:
      i. Randomly selecting an effect of R from a distribution of effects (the mean and standard deviation of which are 30% and 17%, respectively).[6]
      ii. Multiply the subject's DAS-28(4) by the sampled effect, obtaining his or her simulated score at the end of the trial.

---

[5] Sampling will be done "with replacement"—that is, after randomly selecting a subject, he is "returned" to the pool and is available for further sampling. This is because the population of RA sufferers is infinite and, you assume, represented by the patients in your database. Thus, each individual subject in this database represents an infinite number of subjects like him. "Replacing" a subject—returning the subject to the data set, thus making him available for future sampling—maintains the database's representativeness of the infinite population of RA sufferers you wish to include in your trial.
[6] For the sake of simplicity, we will assume that the distribution of effects is normally distributed. Thus, you are asking the computer to randomly select an effect from a normal distribution with mean = 30 and standard deviation = 17.

iii. Recode the resultant score as follows: if above 2.3, subject is classified "failure"; if 2.3 or less, subject is a "success."

iv. Repeat these steps for each of the 50 subjects.

Here is an example for a single subject:

- Subject selected for simulation has DAS-28(4) = 3.6.
- Effect randomly selected from assumed distribution of effects is a reduction of 42% in DAS-28(4).
- Given the subject and effect sampled, score at the end of the trial = $3.6 - 3.6 \times 0.42 = 2.1$.
- Observing 2.1, you find it is below 2.3, which classifies the subject a success.

Repeating the process 50 times yields 50 simulated subjects and a Proportion of Success in the sample. The process is then repeated for T, where the only change is a different hypothesized effect; for each subject an effect is randomly selected from a distribution with a mean of 50% and a standard deviation of 26.

We are almost there! At the end of the simulation described, you have two groups of 50 subjects each: one "treated" with R that yields some Proportion of Success and another "treated" with T that has another Proportion of Success. You then compare the two groups using Fisher's Exact Test and obtain an outcome that is either significant or not. In sum, each individual simulated study will have one of the following two outcomes:

1. T is significantly superior to R (reject Null).
2. T is not significantly superior to R (fail to reject Null).

Having conducted the test, you record the result and save it for future use. You then repeat the process with another sample of 50 subjects per group and obtain another outcome (reject the Null or not).

Now the simulation described can be repeated as many times as you wish. Suppose you repeated it 10,000 times and find that on 28% of occasions T is significantly superior to R–that is, 2,800 times T was significantly superior to R, while 7,200 times it was not. Your conclusion from this simulation is thus: "Given the assumption enumerated, a sample of 50 subjects per group will provide a 0.28 chance of demonstrating T > R"–that is, a sample of 50 subjects will provide 28% power. Since you wish to have power of at least 80%, you repeat this process with a larger sample size. The sample size that yields the required power—typically somewhere between 80% and 90%—is the one specified for the trial. So to summarize:

1. Specify assumptions for the effect of T and R, along with associated standard deviations.
2. Find (or generate) typical baseline data for the subjects you will recruit in the trial.

3. Create samples of varying size (N) for T and R using baseline data and assumed effects.
4. Statistically compare each pair of samples obtained and repeat the process many times (e.g., 10,000).
5. Count the number of times you obtain significant results in the hoped-for direction. The proportion of times this happens is your power for the N used in the simulation.
6. Vary N upward and/or downward until you obtain significant results in 80% to 90% of simulated trials.

Keep in mind that the process described involves simulation with a random selection of the subjects' baseline values and a random selection of effect size. As such, it will produce slightly different results on different occasions. However, if you repeat the process enough times—and in this case, 10,000 is more than enough—the result you get will be reliable: it will be stable. Be that as it may, dealing with the issue of variation in simulation results—as, of course, the simulation itself—is best left to the statistician.

EQUIVALENCE AND NON-INFERIORITY

You have produced a generic equivalent to an ethical drug for which the patent has expired. To have your drug approved, you must show that its pharmacokinetics are similar to the original drug. For example, you will be expected to demonstrate that your drug is equivalent to the original on **C-max**, which is the maximum concentration reached in the blood after taking the drug.

C-max is estimated by giving the subjects the drug, drawing blood at regular intervals, and evaluating the amount of the drug in the samples on each occasion. Typically, the crossover design will be used, where every subject first gets one drug and then the other, and the two results are compared. Half of the subjects will receive T and then R, and half will receive R and then T.

I have often noted that it is pretty much impossible to demonstrate that two products are identical, and so it is here. So instead you will be asked to show that your generic drug's C-max is within 20% of the original. Specifically, for each subject you will compute:

$$Ratio = \frac{C\text{-}max_{generic}}{C\text{-}max_{original}}$$

and be expected to show that this ratio is between 0.80 and 1.25. This translates into the following Null and Alternative hypotheses:

H_0: Ratio > 1.25 or Ratio < 0.80
H_1: 1.25 ≥ Ratio ≥ 0.80

One way of approaching statistical testing is comparing the Ratio obtained to each of the relevant values. Specifically, you will want to show that the Ratio is superior to 0.80 and that it is inferior to 1.25. In other words, our equivalence problem has been transformed into separate statistical tests that we know how to deal with. As such, sample size in equivalence can be computed similarly to that in superiority.

In a non-inferiority trial you want to show that your product R is no worse than T minus some non-inferiority delta. When, for example, the statistic of interest is a Proportion of Success (P), this translates into testing the following hypotheses:

$$H_0: P_T < P_R - \Delta$$
$$H_0: P_T \geq P_R - \Delta$$

where:

P_T—Proportion of Success obtained with the new Test product
P_R—Proportion of Success obtained with the established Reference
Δ—amount by which P_T can be smaller than P_R and still be considered "no worse"

Once again, we essentially have a "superiority scenario."[7] But instead of having to show $T > R$, we are asked to show that T is superior to some value smaller than R. I should note that when $\Delta = 0$, this scenario becomes a standard superiority test where you wish to show $P_T > P_R$.[8]

As in superiority, the required sample size will depend in great measure on the effect size. Effect size here is the expected difference between T and R to begin with (e.g., T − R) and "tacking on" the non-inferiority delta, Δ. Thus, the sample size needed will depend on the following:

- The expected difference between T and R as described in the preceding section. For example, the larger the difference in favor of T, the smaller the sample size needed to show a significant difference.

and

- The size of Δ—the larger the non-inferiority delta, the more we "enlarge" the effect size that needs to be detected and the smaller the sample required.

---

[7] I write "essentially" and this is so. At the same time, the actual statistical approach to sample size determination in superiority and non-inferiority differ. This is a very technical issue having to do with variance estimations and, as you can imagine, is primarily of interest to statisticians. It is certainly beyond both scope and interest of this book.
[8] While "non-inferiority" has been here appropriately restated in "superiority" terms, there are, nevertheless, intricacies relating to sample size computation best left to the statistician.

EQUIVALENCE AND NONSIGNIFICANCE

Suppose you compare T to R and find no difference. Does this mean that T and R are equivalent? Well, it can, but not necessarily. There are many ways to obtain nonsignificant results, and one way of doing this is using a small N—that is, designing a study that has little power to detect a difference even if one exists. When doing this, your nonsignificant result may be due to a lack of power rather than to a similarity between T and R. Consequently, failing to detect a statistical difference between T and R cannot by itself be evidence of equivalence or non-inferiority. It is for this reason that equivalence and non-inferiority designs specify hypotheses such as those described. Specifically, you set up your tests that equivalence or non-inferiority can only be obtained by getting a significant result. In short, *nonsignificant differences cannot provide proof of equivalence*.

A WORD ON ETHICS

Conducting a clinical trial entails exposing participants to new treatments. And being new, we can never be completely certain they are also safe, so, inevitably, clinical trials must be concerned with subject safety. In any clinical study the concern for subject safety is paramount and must precede all other considerations. To quote the World Medical Association Declaration of Helsinki:

> The Declaration of Geneva of the World Medical Association binds the physician with the words, "The health of my patient will be my first consideration," and the International Code of Medical Ethics declares that, "A physician shall act only in the patient's interest when providing medical care which might have the effect of weakening the physical and mental condition of the patient."

> In medical research on human subjects, considerations related to the well-being of the human subject should take precedence over the interests of science and society.

I have to this point avoided the moral and philosophical issues associated with clinical trials; it is a subject unto itself and not the subject of this book. Still, it is necessary to point out that society has accepted clinical trials as both necessary and moral, and that the justification for exposing subjects to new treatments is the potential for scientific and therapeutic gain. Citing the Declaration of Helsinki once more:

> Medical progress is based on research which ultimately must rest in part on experimentation involving human subjects.

> Medical research is only justified if there is a reasonable likelihood that the populations in which the research is carried out stand to benefit from the results of the research.

Thus, whether a trial is more rigorous or less, it must always be justified by the information it has the potential to provide. Consequently, you must be convinced, and be able to convince others, that the study's potential benefits outweigh its potential risks. This in fact is the central consideration of the ethics committee[9] that will need to approve your research before it can be implemented. Following are some implications of this for study design:

- Even less rigorous trials (e.g., exploratory studies) must have the potential to provide useful information—information that is sufficiently useful to outweigh the risks involved.
- Shoddy trials are not only bad policy, but they are also unethical. Given the resources available, you must plan the most scientifically sound trial possible.
- The number of patients participating in a trial—the trial's sample size—must be optimal. If it is too small, the information provided will be negligible and not justify the risk. And if N is too large, you will have unnecessarily exposed more subjects to a new treatment than scientific rigor requires.

SUMMARY

Many factors affect a trial's ability to detect differences between T and R, including the following:

- Sample size—the larger the sample size, the greater the likelihood for detecting an effect when it exists.
- Measurement—the more accurate the measurement, the greater the likelihood for significant results.
- Trial design—the more efficient the design, the greater the chance for significant results.

There are many other factors, for example, the intended use population. Clearly, selecting subjects that are more likely to be helped by your drug will increase your chances of success. Whatever the pertinent factors in your particular trial, it is essential that you not consider them in isolation. Thus, for example, more accurate measurement will reduce the required sample size relative to less accurate measurement. And the same holds true for more efficient design, which will reduce required N as well. That is why when computing N for your trial you will need to conduct extensive discussions with the statistician, as well as with others. With them you will determine key study aspects such as these:

- Trial design, including the endpoints to be measured in the trial.
- Intended use population.
- Minimal therapeutic effect to be detected.

---

[9] Often called **internal review boards** (IRBs).

CHAPTER 15

Concluding Remarks

CONTENTS

- A story with a moral. Maybe.

Some time ago I received a phone call from an unhappy client. He was careful with his words, but the upshot was that he did not appreciate my overzealousness. "When I ask for numbers," he said at some point, "that's exactly what I want."

His request had involved a straightforward statistical task that I had completed and to which I had added an unsolicited opinion. Truth be told, his call caught me off guard and all through it I remained mostly silent. Hanging up the phone, I wondered whether I had done right. I wonder still.

For almost a year I had been working with this client on a diagnostic kit that his company was developing. The kit had been completed a few months before, and investigators had begun collecting data with it. At some point there seemed to be a problem with batch-to-batch stability, and there was talk of modifying the product. The kit was kept as is, and development moved forward.

The product in question is a blood test designed to detect some disease. Its advantage relative to the gold standard is speed and cost; it can be done in most laboratories on sampled blood. The gold standard, on the other hand, requires complex diagnostic equipment and a specialist to interpret its results. So the kit's disadvantage is that it is not a gold standard and never will be. In short, the new test is less accurate but much more accessible than the gold standard.

For several months the Company had been collecting data and had obtained about 300 gold standard negative samples and 40 positive. As is often the case in these indications, negative cases are easier to obtain than positive.

While the Company had collected numerous endpoints, two were of primary interest. The first was Diagnosis of the disease by the gold standard scored dichotomously (Negative or Positive), and the second was a continuous Score produced by the kit. Most values on Score are between 0 and 600, with higher values indicating greater likelihood of the disease.

My first task was to determine the optimal cutoff on Score for determining Positive and Negative. That is, I was asked to find a point on the Score scale below which a subject would be labeled Negative and above which Positive. This would transform Score into a dichotomous scale and provide information in the same form as the gold standard. It would also allow for a direct comparison between the two methods. Once the diagnoses from both the gold standard and the predicate are similarly identified, each subject can be labeled as being one of the following:

- True-positive (TP): Both predicate and gold standard diagnose Positive.
- False-positive (FP): Predicate diagnosis is Positive, while gold standard is Negative.
- True-negative (TN): Both predicate and gold standard diagnose Negative.
- False-negative (FN): Predicate diagnosis is Negative, while gold standard is Positive.

I should note that there is a relatively standard methodology for determining the cutoff X, which I used. At the same time, there can be more than one solution for the problem, depending on Company preferences. Specifically, the choice of X depends in part on which of the two correct diagnoses (TP or TN) interest the Company most and which type of errors (FP or FN) it wishes most to avoid. Be that as it may, I computed X and included it in my brief report. I also provided the resulting level of agreement between gold standard and predicate using statistics such as Sensitivity and Specificity.

My second task was to tell the Company how many subjects would be required for the pivotal trial. Here this meant determining the number of gold standard Positive and Negative subjects to demonstrate some minimal accuracy of the predicate. This too involves standard methodology. Having done the computations, I added my sample size recommendations to the report. I wrote also that there was some flexibility on both cutoff and sample size based on various assumptions, which I suggested we discuss. So far, so good.

I have noted that the analyses required of me were standard. In fact, I had done dozens of similar projects in the past. Where difficulties arose, they were fairly typical as well. As it turned out, all through my computations I felt uncomfortable with the results obtained. I felt they were not sufficiently robust. Here this meant that the cutoff X found, along with the accuracy it yields, may not generalize to a new sample—one that had not been used to determine cutoff and accuracy.

Now you can expect that a cutoff optimized on a specific data set will not work as efficiently on a different data set. But if the first sample was large enough, or the separation provided by X between Positive and Negative on Score clear enough, the results obtained should more or less apply to other data as well. But this was not the case here, where the separation was unimpressive and the number of positive cases used for determining X was small. On top of all this, there was the issue of the kit's relative instability that had not been addressed.

Estimates are by definition estimates, and you can never truly *know* the extent to which they represent the population. As such, you cannot be sure of the degree to which results obtained with one sample will replicate in another. But based on experience, statistics, and intuition, I can gauge the degree to which I can trust my results. And in this case I did not. I felt that using the outcomes I had generated for planning the pivotal trial could easily result in failure of the latter.

So in addition to presenting my results to the client, I described my discomfort and provided some tables and graphs to back up my position. I then recommended extending the learning phase of the study—the phase used for determining X. Specifically, I suggested that at least 50 additional positive cases be obtained and tested before moving on to the pivotal trial. And, recall, positive samples are particularly hard to come by. I wrote that this would provide more robust results and increase the Company's chance to plan the pivotal trial correctly. So while I gave the client what he asked for, I had also—in his view, at least—exceeded my mandate.

The particular individual I was working with is CEO of a small start-up. He is intelligent, experienced, and knows his job well. I had met with him several times, and on two occasions also met with his regulatory and scientific consultants. I felt I knew enough to make the statements I did. At the same time, it was also clear to me that were the Company to follow my recommendation, development would be slowed and costs would rise.

While I had provided my suggestions based on solid statistical principles, I had little knowledge of the Company's overall strategy and the funds available to it. The CEO gently pointed this out to me in our conversation. He then added that the resources available to the Company could cover a pivotal trial but little more. The route I was recommending was simply impossible. In sum, he said, I had been asked to provide sample size requirements based on available data and should have stuck to what I was being paid to do. What he left unsaid is that I had put down my thoughts in a report for everyone to see.

Throughout this book I have suggested that statisticians and other clinical trial professionals often stick their noses into areas outside their immediate expertise. As a general rule, I firmly believe the projects will benefit by it. But rules have exceptions, and this may have been one of them. While my brief report to the CEO was statistically sound, it had major implications for the Company as a whole—implications that had not been asked about.

Now you can imagine that I have no definite formula for correct behavior in such situations, which can often arise when working with start-up organizations. I might, for example, have taken any one of a number of alternative routes, including these:

- Keeping to the task at hand and no more.
- Providing my "additional and less-than-welcome" opinion over the phone. Being more informal in this way, my suggestions may have been more palatable.
- Asking the CEO for a meeting with both him and one or two of the Company's directors to explain my position. This would have allowed him to decide who should be made aware of the information I was to impart.

Any of these might have worked, but, then again, they may not have. Unlike well-designed clinical trials, there are no control groups in life.

Glossary

Note: Italicized terms in definitions indicate that the term appears in the Glossary.

Adaptive testing   In a clinical trial, a design that enables adjustments to a trial design based on accumulating results.

Adverse event (AE)   Unfavorable and unintended sign occurring to a subject in a clinical trial.

Aliquot   In blood tests, refers to a portion of the blood taken. For example, dividing the sampled blood into four aliquots enables four different tests on it.

Alpha (α)   In statistical testing, the probability of Type I Error—that is, of rejecting the *Null Hypothesis* erroneously.

Alternative Hypothesis   In hypothesis testing, the alternative statement to the *Null Hypothesis*.

Analysis of covariance   An *analysis of variance* in which a *covariate*—an extraneous variable to those of interest—is included to reduce expected bias associated with the covariate.

Analysis of variance (ANOVA)   An inferential statistical technique for comparing between means of different groups.

Analysis Population   *See analysis set.*

Analysis set   In clinical trial data, a set of data to be analyzed. In a clinical trial there are often several such sets—for example, the set of all observed values, the set that includes *imputed* data as well, *intent to treat*, and so on.

Animal model   An animal with a disease—naturally occurring or induced—that is either the same as or like a disease in humans. The animal is meant to serve as a (research) model for the human disease.

Anticipated adverse events   An adverse event that is anticipated given the nature of the product/investigation.

Anticoagulant   A substance meant to prevent blood from clotting.

Arm   A group in a clinical trial—for example, "treatment arm," "control arm," and so on.

Autoimmune disease   Disorders in which the body's immune system attacks healthy cells (as opposed to its normal function to protect from potentially harmful foreign substances).

Autologous cell therapy   A procedure where the patient's own cells are removed and manipulated, and then returned to the patient for therapeutic purposes.

Bayesian design   A type of *adaptive design* based on updating trial assumptions based on accumulating results.

Bench testing   Testing in a simulated, nonhuman (virtual) environment—for example, applying specified pressure on a device to assess the amount of pressure it can withstand.

Beta in (hypothesis testing)   In statistical testing, the probability of not rejecting the *Null Hypothesis* when it should be rejected. Also termed *Type II Error*.

Bias (in measurement)	Having systematic error—for example, a thermometer that systematically overestimates temperature or a clinical trial aiming to assess the general population that includes young subjects only.
Biased estimate	An estimate having *bias*.
Binary	See *dichotomous*.
Blinding	In a clinical trial, hiding information from participants to reduce the possibility for bias. See also *double blind*.
Brand-name drug	A drug marketed under a specific manufacturer-selected brand name, often under patent protection (as opposed to a generic drug that is typically sold under the common name for a drug).
Case research form (CRF)	Paper and/or electronic forms used for recording clinical trial data.
Central limit theorem	In probability, a theorem describing the relationship between the sample mean and population mean.
Central tendency	The tendency of quantitative data to cluster around some central value (like mean and median, which are measures of central tendency).
Claim (label claim)	A description in the medical product's labeling of what it can do (e.g., treat disease "X" with side effects "Y").
Clinical meaningfulness	Having clinical (medical) utility.
Clinical research associate (CRA)	Individuals responsible for trial monitoring and other administrative aspects of a clinical trial (e.g., instructing trial staff on study procedures).
Clinical significance	See *clinical meaningfulness*.
Cluster analysis	A statistical technique for discovering grouping (clusters) in data.
C-max	The maximum concentration of a drug in the body (measured by pharmacokinetic analysis).
Coefficient of determination	See *Explained variance; R-square*.
Comparator	In a clinical trial, the product the investigational drug is compared to.
Compliance	Used in various contexts to describe the degree to which instructions are followed—for example, the degree to which a patient complies with the drug regimen prescribed.
Composite endpoint	A single *endpoint* made up of a combination of two or more components—for example, some "overall score" computed from several relevant clinical endpoints.
Confidence interval	A range within which a specific population parameter is to be with a specified degree of confidence (probability).
Confirmatory trial	A controlled trial in which hypotheses are stated in advance and tested after data have been collected.
Confounding	In a clinical trial, an extraneous variable that may affect the outcome and lead to erroneous conclusions (e.g., initial, baseline difference in Age between two groups in a trial).
Control group	In clinical trials, a group used for comparison to the *Treatment group*—for example, a group receiving no Treatment for comparison to that receiving an experimental Treatment.
Correlation	In statistics, a quantitative index for the relationship between variables.
Covariate	In the context of clinical trials, variables other than Treatment that affect clinical outcome.

Creatinine	The broken-down (and no longer useful) form of creatine, an acid produced by the liver and providing some of the energy used by muscles. It is a waste product and is cleared by the kidneys.
Crossover design	A longitudinal study in which the subject receives different treatments in sequence.
Cross-validation	Testing a model/algorithm on the portion of a data set that was not used to construct the model/algorithm.
Data monitoring committee (DMC)	An independent group of experts that monitors accumulated clinical trial data, usually for the purpose of assessing trial safety. The precise responsibilities of a DMC are determined on a trial-by-trial basis and specified in the committee's charter. Also termed data safety monitoring board (DSMB).
Dependent variable	A variable that is determined by *independent* (or explanatory) *variables*.
Descriptive statistics	The area of statistics concerned with describing data quantitatively (e.g., *mean, standard deviation*) and graphically (e.g., histogram, scatterplot).
Development plan	An overall blueprint (plan) for developing a product—for example, a drug development plan.
Dichotomous (variable)	Taking on two values—for example, a diagnostic outcome that can take on either "positive" or "negative."
Dispersion (of data)	In descriptive statistics, the variation in measurements in a *sample* or *population*.
Distribution	A collection of values.
Dose-response	Relationship between the quantities of a treatment given (e.g., dose of a drug) and biological response to them.
Double blind	In a clinical trial, where neither the individual providing the treatment nor the person receiving it knows which of the study treatments it is.
Dropout	In a clinical trial, an individual who drops out of the trial and so does not complete it.
Drug product	The final form of the drug in packaging intended for marketing (includes both the active and inactive ingredients).
Drug substance	The active ingredient in a drug.
Due diligence	The process of evaluating the performance of a product, typically for investment purposes.
Dynamic randomization	A randomization scheme that allows for (dynamic) adjustment during the trial to ensure equality of groups on characteristics of interest.
Effect size	In statistics, a measure of the strength of the relationship between two variables—for example, the difference in effect between new and standard treatment or the ratio of their cure rates.
Efficacy	In clinical trials, the capacity of a product to produce the desired effect—for example, a pill for fever possesses efficacy if it reduces temperature.
ELISA (enzyme-linked immunosorbent assay)	A biochemical technique primarily used to detect an antibody or antigen in (human) liquid samples.
EMEA	European Medicines Agency.
Endpoint	In a clinical trial, a measure of an outcome of interest. For example, (duration of) "survival" is an outcome of interest in many cancer trials.

Enriched population	A population in which there is overrepresentation of a group of interest. For example, in evaluating a diagnostic test, one may conduct a trial with more positive cases than are generally found in the population. This is typically done when positive cases are rare and a representative sample of a given size will yield to few positive cases for investigation.
Equivalence (trial)	A trial with the primary objective of showing that the response to two or more treatments differs by an amount that is clinically unimportant.[1]
Equivalence margins	Upper and lower margins (bounds) around a comparator, within which the new product must be to claim equivalence to the former.
Error of estimation	See *estimation error*.
Estimation	Using a *sample statistic* to estimate the true *population parameter* (which cannot be known precisely).
Estimation error	The inaccuracy associated with estimating the value of a variable (e.g., cure rate of a disease, accuracy of a diagnostic method).
Ethical drug	A drug dispensed only upon written instructions from a medical professional. When used in clinical trials, the term often refers to a branded drug that is under patent protection (as opposed to a *generic* drug).
Ethics committee	See *internal review board* (IRB).
Evidence-based medicine	Application of the best available scientific evidence to medical decision making.
Evolutionary cul-de-sac	Evolutionary development to the point of perfect or near perfect fit to a specific environment. This is hypothesized to yield a small variation of genes in the population, which will not enable the population to survive changes to the environment.
Exclusion criteria	Conditions that preclude an individual's participation in a clinical trial.
Explained variance	The proportion of variation in a variable (or variables) that is explained via mathematical modeling by another variable or variables.
Explanatory variable	See *independent variable*.
Exploratory trial	A study designed to explore a phenomenon more than it is designed to test specific, well-defined hypotheses about it.
FDA	Food and Drug Administration.
First-line treatment	Recommended initial therapy.
Formulation	Pharmacologic substance prepared according to a formula.
Full analysis set	The *analysis set* that is nearest that of *intent to treat* (ITT) given the circumstances.
General linear model	A mathematical model that assumes a linear relationship between variables. It is the basis for a large number of frequently used inferential statistical methods such as *analysis of variance*.
Generalize, generalization (in a clinical trial)	The extent to which the findings of a clinical trial can be reliably extrapolated from the subjects who participated in the trial to a broader patient population and a broader range of clinical settings.[2]
Generic	See *generic drug*.
Generic drug	A drug typically sold under the common name for the drug rather than a brand name. Generic drugs have no patent protection as opposed to the branded drugs of which the effects they are meant to mimic.

---

[1] ICH E9. (1998). *Statistical Principles for Clinical Trials.*
[2] ICH E9. (1998). *Statistical Principles in Clinical Trials.*

Gold standard	The accepted standard. For example, in diagnostic tests, it is typically the most accurate measure in use.
Helsinki committee	See *internal review board*.
Histogram	A graphical technique in descriptive statistics presenting a frequency distribution with the aid of bars.
Hypothesis testing	A statistical method for making decisions about populations from sample data. The method provides information on the likelihood that the observed patterns in the data reflect the truth in the (unknowable) population.
ICH	International Conference on Harmonization.
Imperfect gold standard	A *gold standard* measurement that is nevertheless relatively inaccurate (for a gold standard).
Impute	In data analysis, the process of replacing missing measurements with estimates.
Inclusion criteria	Condition for an individual's participation in a clinical trial.
Independent groups design	A study in which different and unrelated subjects receive different treatments (as opposed to, say, a *paired design*).
Independent variable	A variable of which the value determines that of other variables.
Inferential statistics	The branch of statistics concerned with making conclusions about populations from samples.
Intended use population	The *population* of all those for whom a medical product is intended (i.e., designed for).
Intent to treat (ITT)	The *analysis set* that "includes all randomized patients in the groups to which they were randomly assigned, regardless of their adherence with entry criteria, regardless of the treatment they actually received, and regardless of the subsequent withdrawal from treatment or deviation from the protocol."[3]
Intercept	In linear regression, the point on the y-axis that the regression line crosses.
Interim analysis	Any analysis intended to compare treatment arms with respect to efficacy or safety at any time prior to the formal completion of a trial.[4]
Internal review board (IRB)	A committee (typically internal to a hospital or clinic) that is responsible for deciding whether a clinical trial as described in the trial's protocol is ethical and, if so, can be conducted. Decisions are made in accordance with the declaration of Helsinki.
Interval estimate	An interval within which the true value of a population value is said to be (with a specified probability).
In vitro	An artificial environment outside of living organisms. For example, in vitro fertilization refers to fertilization taking place outside the body.
Ischemic stroke	A condition in which the blood supply to the brain is cut off.
Kurtosis	Degree of "peakedness" of a distribution of numbers.
Laboratory parameters	Typically refers to the parameters obtained from blood tests, such as red and white cell counts, liver enzymes, and so on.
Last observation carried forward (LOCF)	A method to *impute* missing data by replacing a missing value with the last observed quantity measured on the variable in question.
Marginals	In a frequency table, the sums of each of the rows and columns.

---

[3] Fisher, L. D., et al. (1990). Intention to treat in clinical trials. In Peace, K. E. (Ed.) (1991). *Statistical Issues in Drug Research and Development*, pp. 331–350. New York: Marcel Dekker.
[4] ICH E9. (1998). *Statistical Principles for Clinical Trials*.

Mean	Arithmetic average (summing all values and dividing by the number of values).
Measurement error	The difference between the true value of a quantity (e.g., height) and that obtained by measurement.
Mechanism of action (MOA)	The specific interaction with the body through which a medical product produces its effect.
Median	The point in distribution above which and below which are located half the values in the distribution. The 50th percentile.
Model	A description or mathematical statement used to represent reality more simply, such as a *regression* line representing the relationship between height and weight.
Monitoring (clinical trial monitoring)	Oversight activities for monitoring a clinical trial's conduct—for example, ensuring patient rights or ensuring data quality. Such monitoring is typically done by a *clinical research associate* (CRA).
Monoclonal antibodies	Proteins made in the laboratory from a single clone of a B cell, the type of cells of the immune system that make antibodies.
Multiple testing	Conducting more than one statistical test on a set of data, thus increasing the chance for *Type I Error*.
Multiple-arm trial	A clinical trial with more than one *arm*—that is, with at least two treatments tested.
Multiplicity	See *multiple testing*.
N	Letter used to signify a trial's sample size (or that of a group/arm in it).
Natural history (of a disease)	The course a particular disease usually takes.
Neurodegenerative	Loss of neuronal (nerve cell) function or structure due to cells' death. Parkinson's disease and multiple sclerosis are examples of neurodegenerative diseases.
Neuron	A cell of the nervous system found in the brain, spinal cord, and ganglia and nerves of peripheral nervous system.
Neuroprotection	A mechanism or mechanisms that protect nerve cells from degeneration and/or death.
Neuroprotective	Providing *neuroprotection*.
New drug application (NDA)	The vehicle through which drug sponsors formally propose that the FDA approve a new pharmaceutical for sale and marketing in the United States.[5]
Non-inferiority	No worse than a comparator or, more accurately, no worse than a comparator minus some margin (termed *non-inferiority margin*).
Non-inferiority delta	See *non-inferiority margin*.
Non-inferiority margin	The margin (delta) by which a product must be shown to be no worse than the comparator in a non-inferiority trial.
Non-inferiority trial	A trial of which the aim is to show that a product is no worse than a comparator by a pre-specified amount, termed *non-inferiority margin*.
Normal distribution	A theoretical frequency distribution of data that is bell shaped and symmetrical about the mean and median.
Null Hypothesis	In hypothesis testing, the initial stated belief about the value of a population parameter.
Objective performance criterion (OPC)	In a clinical trial, a quantitative criterion that the tested product must meet or exceed. The criterion is computed from a historical database, after matching cases from the historical database to those in the current trial.

---

[5] FDA. http://www.fda.gov/Drugs/DevelopmentApprovalProcess/HowDrugsareDevelopedandApproved/ApprovalApplications/NewDrugApplicationNDA/default.htm.

One-sided hypothesis	A hypothesis that states a departure from the *Null Hypothesis* in a particular direction (in contrast to a *two-side hypothesis* specifying that the departure can be in either direction).
One-sided test	See *one-sided hypothesis*.
Ordinal scale	A scale of measurement that provides information on rank (e.g., first, second, third) but does not provide quantitatively meaningful distances between the ranks.
Outlier	A value in a *distribution* that is numerically distant from the rest of the values.
Overfitting	Fitting a model too closely to a set of data and thus modeling the error in it as well.
P	See *P-value*.
P-value	In *statistical testing*, the probability of obtaining the result observed by chance alone.
Paired design	An experimental design in which (1) the same subjects receive more than one treatment or (2) the subjects receiving different treatments are paired based on relevant characteristics (e.g., Age, Disease History, etc.).
Pairing	See *paired design*.
Partially randomized patient preference design	A clinical trial design in which subjects with strong preferences are allocated to their treatment of choice, while those with no strong preference are randomized in the usual manner.
Performance	The ability of a product to perform as intended. The term is used in various contexts—for example, the ability of a catheter to do as intended when used by the appropriate professional or the accuracy of a diagnostic test.
Pharmacogenomics	An area of pharmacology dealing with the effect of genetic makeup on response to drugs.
Performance Goal	In a clinical trial, a quantitative performance criterion that the tested product must meet or exceed. Performance Goals are often obtained from the scientific literature.
Phase I clinical trial	First stage of clinical testing in humans. A Phase I trial typically includes relatively few subjects and is primarily concerned with assessing a product's safety.
Phase IIa clinical trial	A term used in practice—but not officially defined—to describe an early Phase II trial. A trial that is generally more limited in scope than Phase II (or Phase IIb).
Phase II clinical trial	Controlled clinical studies conducted to evaluate the effectiveness of the drug for a particular indication or indications in patients with the disease or condition under study and to determine the common short-term side effects and risks.[6]
Phase III clinical trial	A large clinical trial of a product that has been shown to be safe and effective in earlier trials. Also termed a *pivotal trial* because it often determines whether the product will receive approval for marketing.
Pilot study	A relatively small, preliminary study conducted in preparation for the main research. It is designed to provide data for planning the main research.
Pipeline	A set of molecules, devices, or other (potential) medical products that a company has under development at a given point in time.
Pivotal trial	Trial from which data will be used to make significant claims. For example, *Phase III trials* are pivotal trials.
Placebo	A dummy medical treatment—that is, a pill that looks, feels, and swallows like one with an active ingredient but contains no such ingredient.

---

[6] Food and Drug Administration (2010). *ClinicalTrials.gov protocol data element definitions (draft)*. http://prsinfo.clinicaltrials.gov/definitions.html.

Placebo effect	An improvement in outcome due to patient's expectation that the treatment is effective, rather than to the treatment itself.
Plasma (blood plasma)	A component of the blood; the fluid in which blood cells are suspended.
Point estimate	A specific, single value obtained from a sample to estimate this value in the population. For example, the sample mean is one's best point estimate for the population mean.
Population	(1) A collection of elements (e.g., people, animals, data) that have at least one characteristic in common (e.g., all are diabetics). (2) All units we wish to understand. For example, the population of all U.S. Type I diabetics includes all those in the United States who suffer from Type I diabetes.
Population parameter	The value of a parameter such as the mean in the population. This can generally not be known precisely and is estimated from a sample.
Post hoc analysis	Unplanned analyses; analyses decided on after the data have been collected.
Power	See *statistical power*.
Power analysis	A statistical technique used for determining the number of subjects needed to detect a phenomenon of interest (e.g., a difference between *Treatment group* and *Control group*).
Preclinical	In clinical trials, relating to the stage of nonhuman research (e.g., animal studies). Despite the term's apparent meaning, preclinical research is often also done in parallel with clinical activities.
Predicate	In device development, an existing device similar to the new device, to which the latter can be appropriately compared.
Prevalence (of a disease)	The number of people living with a specific disease in a specified period of time.
Primary efficacy endpoint	An outcome measure (*endpoint*) used for assessing the main desired effect of a medical product.
Primary endpoint	An endpoint in a trial measuring the phenomenon associated with the trial's primary objective.
Prognostic factors	Factors predictive of disease course/outcome. For example, metastasis (yes/no) is often an important prognostic factor in cancer.
Propensity analysis	In data analysis, a method for assigning subjects in different Treatment groups to subgroups for the purpose of comparing similar subgroups in different treatments. The method is aimed at reducing bias associated with comparing groups that are dissimilar on other than the factor of interest (e.g., such as the treatment received).
Proportion of variance explained	A quantitative index of the degree to which one variable is dependent (or can be explained/ predicted) by another.
Protocol (clinical study protocol)	In a clinical trial, the document that describes the study's objectives, methods, procedures, statistical considerations, and so on.
Protocol violation	In a clinical trial, instances where the trial procedures specified in the protocol are not precisely followed or applied.
P-value	The probability of a statistical test having yielded a Type I Error.
Quality of life (QoL)	A measure of the general well-being of an individual (e.g., a subject in a clinical trial).
Random error	Error that results from chance variation and so has an equal chance of being high or low.
Randomization	In a clinical trial, the process of assigning subjects or objects to a study group (e.g., Treatment or Control) on a random basis.

Range	The difference between the lowest and highest values in a distribution.
Ratio scale	A scale of measurement that provides quantitative values of which the computed ratios are meaningful.
Reference	In a clinical trial, the group against which the new treatment/method (*test*) is compared.
Referral bias	In evaluation of a diagnostic method, referral bias occurs when only a certain subset of individuals (rather than a representative sample) undergoes a diagnostic method under investigation. Also termed "spectrum bias."
Regression	In statistics, a method (model) for describing the relationship between variables.
Reimbursement	Method of payment for medical service, usually by a third-party payer (e.g., health maintenance organization, Medicare).
Reliability	In statistics, the degree of consistency of a measure—that is, the degree to which it produces similar results in circumstances where it should. For example, a reliable blood test will return similar results when repeated on the same blood. *Repeatability* and *reproducibility* are two types of reliability.
Reliable	Having *reliability*.
Repeatability	The consistency results when measuring under similar circumstances—for example, measuring the same blood on the same day with the same instrument by the same operator.
Repeatable	Having *repeatability*.
Representative sample	In statistics, a sample of units being studied (e.g., patients) that reflects—is representative of—the *population* of these units.
Reproducibility	The consistency of results when measuring the same object under different conditions—for example, measuring the same blood using different machines from the same production line.
Reproducible	Having *reproducibility*.
Responder analysis	An analysis of data on a scale of measurement coded as "response" or "nonresponse" for each individual. The "responder scale" is *dichotomous*.
Risk analysis	In a medical product, analysis of its relative risks and benefits.
Robust	Relatively insensitive to change in conditions. For example, a robust model is one that fits reasonably well across different samples of data.
Route of administration	A way of administering a drug into the body (e.g., via pill taken orally, subcutaneous administration).
r-square (r^2)	See *explained variance*.
Sample	A subset of the population.
Sample size	The number of units (e.g., animals, subjects) participating in a trial.
Sample statistic	A statistic such as the mean or standard deviation that is computed with data from a sample.
Sampling	The process of selecting units (e.g., subjects, objects) from a population to create a *sample*.
Sampling distribution	Distribution of sample statistics such as the mean.

Sampling error	The error caused by observing a sample rather than the whole of the population.
Scatterplot	A graph of plotted points to show the relationship between two sets of data in two-dimensions (*x*-axis and *y*-axis).
Scientific method	A systematic method of research involving collection of data for theory building and (hypothesis) testing.
Secondary endpoint	Either supportive measurements related to the primary objective of the trial or measurements of effects related to the secondary objectives.[7]
Sensitivity	In a diagnostic test, the proportion of positives that are correctly identified.
Sensitivity analysis	In data analysis, simulation of the degree of which results are *robust* by systematically changing assumptions and repeating statistical analyses under each.
Serious adverse event (SAE)	In a clinical trial, any untoward event that is at least one of the following: leads to death, is life threatening, requires hospitalization or prolongation of hospitalization, results in persistent or significant disability/incapacity, is a congenital anomaly/birth defect, or requires intervention to prevent permanent impairment or damage.[8]
Single-arm trial	A clinical trial in which all subjects receive the same treatment.
Skewness	Degree of symmetry (or lack of) in a distribution of numbers.
Sleep apnea	A disorder characterized by pauses in breathing during sleep.
Specificity	In a diagnostic test, the proportion of negatives that are correctly identified.
Spread (of data)	Dispersion of data (measured by statistics like the *standard deviation*).
Standard deviation	A value computed from data that measures variation, or dispersion, in it. Dispersion is considered relative to the data's mean.
Standard error	The estimated standard deviation of a sample statistic such as the mean.
Standard error of estimate	In regression, a measure of the model's error in prediction. Conversely, the accuracy of the regression model's prediction.
Standard of care	The accepted, most common treatment for a disease.
Statistical analysis plan (SAP)	A document that contains a more technical and detailed elaboration of the principal features of the analysis described in the protocol and includes detailed procedures for executing the statistical analysis of the primary and secondary variables and other data.[9]
Statistically significant	A result that is unlikely to have occurred by chance (i.e., is likely to reflect the truth).
Statistical power (1 − β)	The capability of a test to detect a real phenomenon (e.g., positive effect of a drug). In *hypothesis testing* it is the probability of rejecting the *Null Hypothesis* when it should be rejected.
Statistical testing	See *hypothesis testing*.
Stenosis	A narrowing, typically used in reference to blood vessels.
Stent	A tube inserted into a tubular part of the body (e.g., blood vessel) to provide support. In the case of blood vessels, it is aimed at allowing more unobstructed flow of blood.
Stratified assignment	See *stratified randomization*.

---

[7] ICH E9. (1998). *Statistical Principles for Clinical Trials.*
[8] http://www.fda.gov/safety/medwatch/howtoreport/ucm053087.htm.
[9] ICH E9. (1998). *Statistical Principles for Clinical Trials.*

Stratified randomization	Randomization done separately within two or more subsets based on subject characteristics (strata) aimed at "equalizing" groups/arms so that any subsequent differences can be attributed to treatment.
Subgroup analysis	In data analysis, comparing subsets of subjects in order to identify patterns in the data.
Substantial equivalence	Considered the same. Substantial equivalence of a new product to a comparator is shown by demonstrating similarity on key attributes (e.g., *safety* and *efficacy*).
Superiority	Being better than another. In clinical trials, aiming to show one product (drug, device, etc.) better than a comparator (other product, placebo, etc.) on an attribute of interest (e.g., safety, efficacy).
Surrogate endpoint	A biomarker intended to substitute for a clinical endpoint[10]; for example, in oncology, where Tumor Size is often used as a surrogate for Survival.
Survival analysis	Analyses involving time to event data—for example, time to death, time to ulcer closure.
Test	In a clinical trial, the product being tested (typically versus some *reference*).
Treatment group	In a clinical trial, the group of subjects receiving an investigational treatment.
Trend toward significance	"Near significance" is often defined as outcomes of statistical testing that produce P-values greater than 0.05 and less than or equal to 0.10.
Two-sided hypothesis	A hypothesis that states a departure from the *Null Hypothesis* in two directions (e.g., either higher or lower). In contrast to a *one-sided hypothesis*.
Type I Error	Rejecting the *Null Hypothesis* erroneously.
Type II Error	Not rejecting the *Null Hypothesis* erroneously.
Unbiased	Not having bias. See also *bias*.
Urea	A waste product produced by the body's metabolizing of protein, which is secreted into the blood and removed by the kidneys.
Valid	Having *validity*.
Validate	To demonstrate *validity*.
Validity	In clinical trials, the extent that a measure (or model) measures what it intends to measure; for example, a valid animal model of a disease is one that provides useful information on the human form of the disease.
Variable	An object (person, place, thing, etc.) that can take on more than one value; for example, Diagnosis is a variable that can take on "positive" or "negative."
Variance	A measure of spread. The square of the *standard deviation*.
Verification bias	See *referral bias*.
Vital signs	Measures assessing the most basic body functions, such as body temperature, pulse rate, and respiration rate.
Washout period	Period it takes for a drug to be completely cleared from the body.

---

[10] Biomarkers Definition Working Group (2001). Biomarkers and surrogate endpoints: Preferred definitions and conceptual framework. *Clin Pharma Col Ther*, 69, 89–95.

Index

In this index the use of *b* indicates text found in a box, and *t* indicates a table.

A

"about as good", 48
"as good as", 47
"at least as good", 47
Accommodation, 54–55, 109
Accuracy, 73, 83. *See also* Precision in measurement
Accuracy, factors affecting, 70
Adaptive designs, 201
Adverse event (AE)
    anticipated, 137
    expected, 192
    serious, 68, 156, 192
Aliquot, 220
Alpha (α), 143, 144, 231. *See also* Type I Error
Alternative hypothesis, 107, 109, 115, 142–143, 144, 148, 153*b*, 194, 229, 232*b*, 241
Analysis of covariance (ANCOVA), 175, 183
Analysis of variance (ANOVA), 80*b*
Analysis populations. *See* Analysis sets
Analysis sets, 176, 177
    full set, 177
    intent to treat, 176–178, 184*b*
Animal model, 2–3, 12–13
Anticipated adverse events, 137
Anticoagulants, 42
Antidepressant study, 169–170
Arms, 7
Assimilate, 58
Attributes
    beginnings, 19
    clinical trial aims and attributes, 50, 50*t*, 156*t*
    in clinical trial design, 64, 155, 159
    clinical trial example, 35–51

comparison of, 36
efficacy, 27–28, 32
endpoints and demonstrating, 219, 220
of interest, 155, 159
introduction, 17–24
objectives in conclusions relation to, 40–41, 46
performance, 29–30
pharmacokinetics, 31
in populations, 60, 108–109
quantitative statements about, types of, 72
safety, 28–29, 220, 227
summary overview, 32–34
types of, 206
What attribute to assess and aim to demonstrate?, 27, 32–34
Audiogram, 56–57
Audiometer Hearing Test (AHT), 56
Autoimmune disease, 2
Autologous cell therapy, 101–105
Average. *See* Mean
Average deviation, 164

B

Bayesian design, 201
Bench testing, 30
Beta, 144. *See also* Type II Error
Bias
    defined, 169
    examples, 169–178
    endpoint, 220
    limiting, limitations in, 150*b*
    methods for avoiding, 180–202
    missing data, and, 171–174
    sources of, 207*b*
Biased estimate, 22

B (continued)

Blinding
    to avoid bias, 180, 186, 202, 207*b*, 221
        alternatives to, 182
        general principle, 190
        importance of, 193
    by design
        possibility of, 159
        threats to validity from lack of, 174
    double blind, 148
    to eliminate bias, 180–182, 207*b*
    overview, 169–178
    unblinding, 174
Blood alcohol content (BAC), 229–244
Brand name drugs, 31

C

Cardiac disorder diagnostic device, 118
Cardiac stent, 216
Case research form (CRF), 191*b*
Central limit theorem, 75
Central tendency, 94. *See also* Average; Mean; Median
Certainty, 69–72, 73
Change endpoints, from baseline, 117*b*
Child development theory, 58
Claim, 38
Classification, 53, 109
Clinical meaningfulness, 93
Clinical research associate (CRA), 191*b*
Clinical significance, 93
Clinical studies, 35–36
Clinical trials
    aims and attributes, 156*t*
    attributes in
        comparison of, 36
        efficacy, 27–28
        performance, 29–30
        pharmacokinetics, 31

Clinical trials *(Continued)*
  quantitative statements about,
    types of, 72
  safety, 28–29
cost controls, 10–13
design of clinical trial design, 158,
    180, 234
  study groups, choice of, 175,
    180, 234
  blinding, 157–159, 174, 180,
    182, 186, 190–191, 193, 202,
    207b
  randomization , 157–158, 180,
    182–186, 221, 234b
  control group, 5, 39, 80b, 140b,
    186–190, 202
estimating product performance, 19
ethics in, 243–244
factors affecting accuracy of
    results, 70–72
funding, 22
informational needs, 156
intended audience, 157
introduction, 1–16
long-term studies, 33b
multidisciplinary nature of, 1
process and stages, 27
reports, 29b
standard procedure, 63–64
summary overview, 15–16
Clinical trials, design
  beginning steps, 155–178
  bias, 169–178
  bias, methods for avoiding,
    180–202
  compliance, 174–175
  complications, 161–166
  control groups, 186–190
  interim analysis
    efficacy, 190–191
    reasons for, 197–202
    safety, 192–193
    statistical considerations,
      194–197
  missing data, 171–174
  The principle underlying solid
    design, 166–167
  questions relating to, 158–161
  random error, 167–169
  summary overview, 202
  unblinding, 174
Clinical trials, examples
  cardiac disorders, 118

psoriasis, 161–163
drink-and-drive trial, 229–244
kidney transplantation rejection,
    210–211
Kinitis, 19
Parkinson's, 136
rheumatoid arthritis (RA), 238
sleep apnea device trial, 86–87
stroke, 116–118
sample size requests, 18
Clinical trials, planning questions
  examples, 36
How do I evaluate accuracy to
    assess risk?, 23
How long is the follow-up
    period?, 23
How much should I invest in
    R&R?, 21
What attribute to assess and aim
    to demonstrate?, 27, 32–34
What can my product actually
    do?, 19
What do I want to show and to
    whom?, 24
What is it good for?, 25, 27, 32
What is my trial's goal?, 22
Who is my product intended for?,
    22
Whom do I want to show my
    results to?, 157
Clinicians vs. statisticians, 28b, 58b,
    81, 82b
Cluster analysis, 80b
C-max, 241–242. *See also*
    Pharmacokinetics
Cofounding, 180
Comparator, 38
Complexity in modeling, 130
Compliance, 30, 37, 174–175
Composite endpoint, 220
Conclusions-objectives relation, 46
Confidence interval
  decision making aided by, 76b
  defined, 75
  overlapping, 87np
  sleep apnea device trial, 86–87
  summary overview, 75–76
Confirmatory efficacy endpoint, 227
Confirmatory endpoints, 160
Confirmatory trial, 122, 131–133,
    227, 229, 230
Congestive heart failure (CHF), 26
Constraints, 117b

Control group, 5, 186–190
Correlation, 94–95. *See also*
    Regression
Cost controls, 10–13
Cost-benefit analysis, 153b
Covariate, 99b. *See also* Analysis of
    Covariance
Creatinine, 206–207
Crossover design, 43
Cross-validation, 131

D

Daniels, Polak, 204
Data
  from diaries, 138b
  into information, 56
  missing, 171–174. *See also*
    Descriptive statistics
Data analysis. *See* Descriptive
    Statistics; Statistical Testing
Data analysis scenarios, 138–139,
    148–150
Data monitoring committee (DMC),
    192
Data presentation, 81. *See also*
    Descriptive Statistics;
    Description
Delaunay, Henri, 111
Demonstrating equivalence. *See*
    Equivalence; Equivalence
    studies; Equivalence testing
Dependent variable, 98–99. *See also*
    Modeling
Description, 93–97
Descriptive statistics, 55–60,
    78–89, 109. *See also*
    Data Presentation; Data
    Description; Graphical
    Descriptive Statistics; Mean;
    Standard Error
Development plan, 17b
Diabetes, 47–48
Diagnostic device, 118–119
  types of, 20–24, 26, 32, 39, 56, 235
Diagnostic kit, 19–24. *See also*
    Diagnostic device
Dialysis machine, 205
Diary data, 138b
Dichotomous (variable), 83
Differences between treatment
    groups, 82–89, 102b. *See also*
    Statistical testing; Hypothesis
    testing

Dispersion, 81. *See also* Descriptive statistics; Standard deviation; Standard error; Standard error of estimate

Distribution
  clinical trial example, 239
  of differences, constructing, 142
  hypothetical examples, 79
  normal distribution, 105, 142
  sampling distribution, 141, 142
  symmetrical around zero, 141

Dose-response, 26, 124

Double blind, 148, 180

Drink-and-drive clinical trial
  design, 229–244
  effect size, 235–236
  interim summary, 237–238
  measurement error, 236–237
  sampling error, 233–234

Dropout, clinical trial subjects, 171, 172, 173, 208, 211

Drug development cost-benefit analysis, 17*b*

Drug development, major stages in
  management review, 3, 18
  pre-clinical trial review, 2
  recruitment, 13–14
  sample size determination, 4–15
  trial length determination, 8–10. *See also* Phase I; Phase II; Phase IIa; Phase III; Pivotal Trail; Preclinical Trial

Drug product, 16

Drug substance, 16

Due-diligence, 4

Dynamic randomization, 184–185

E

Effect size
  ALP clinical trial, 6, 12–13
  drink-and-drive trial, 235–236
  overview, 201–202

Efficacy
  ALP clinical trial, 2, 14–15
  attribute related to, 32
  defining (attributes), 27–28
  evaluation time requirements, 29
  interim data analysis, 190–191
  of kidney transplantation, 205–206
  performance's relation to, 30
  safety vs, 206

sleep apnea device trial, 83. *See also* Efficacy Endpoint

Efficacy endpoint, 116
  clinical trial example, 101, 116, 162, 213–214
  complete closure, 102
  confirmatory, 227
  multiple, testing, 227
  primary, 8, 162, 214
  purpose of, 209*b*
  secondary, 116

Efficacy trials, 28*b*

ELISA (enzyme-linked immunosorbent assay) kits, 207*b*

EMEA, 33*b*, 35–36

Endpoint measures
  NCI on, 207*b*
  uniformity in, 209*b*

Endpoints
  for assessing transplantation success, 208
  change endpoints, 117*b*
  composite endpoint, 220
  defined, 207
  efficacy endpoint
    clinical trial example, 116, 162, 213–214
    complete closure, in skin ulcers, 102
    confirmatory, 227
    multiple, testing, 227
    primary, 8, 162, 214
    purpose of, 209*b*
    secondary, 116
  ischemic stroke trial, 117*b*
  measurement properties, 221–226
  primary endpoint, 167, 213–214
  safety, 137, 226–227
  secondary endpoints, 116, 213–214, 228
  selecting, 211–213
  summary overview, 227–228
  surrogate endpoint, 218
  uniformity in measuring, 209*b*
  validity, reliability, and bias, 218–221

Engine size-acceleration model, 120, 129

Enriched population (in diagnostic testing), 23

Equivalence. *See also* Equivalence studies; Equivalence testing

clinical trial aims and attributes, 50*t*, 156*t*
  clinical trial example, 141, 142–143
  as comparison, 38–50
  defined, 41
  demonstrating, 41*b*, 43
  of generics, 44
  margins, 41
  non-inferiority and, 241–242
  nonsignificance and, 243*b*
  overview, 41–45
  in planning clinical trials, 41–45
  situations to use, 45
  statistical testing for, 146–150
  studies, purpose of, 43–45
  substantial equivalence, 50
  testing, 43–44, 146–150
  using non-inferiority vs. superiority, 44

Error of estimation, 39*b*

Estimation
  certainty and, 69–72
  introduction, 67–76
  points and intervals, 72–75
  summary overview, 75–76
  terminology, 68–69

Estimation error, 39*b*

Ethical drug, 31

Ethics, in clinical trials, 243–244
  physicians in clinical trials, 181*b*
  statisticians, 245–248

Ethics committee, 40. *See also* Internal review board

European Football Championship (European Nations Cup), 112

Evidence-based medicine, 82*b*

Evolutionary cul-de-sac, 128–129

Exclusion criteria, 14, 60, 116
  determining, 176, 200

Expected adverse events, 192. *See also* Adverse events

Explained variance, 95. *See also* Explanation; Proportion of variance explained; Statistical explanation

Explanation
  before and after the fact, 111–133
  and inference in clinical trials, 101–105
  quantifying, 100–101
  scientific, partial nature of, 97–99
  statistical, 93–97

Explanatory variable, 98–99
Exploratory trial, 132–133, 145, 196–197

F

FDA, 33b, 35–36. *See also* Food and Drug Administration
Feasibility trial, 15, 62, 62b, 124, 126. *See also* Phase II trial
FIFA (Fédération Internationale de Football Association), 111
First line treatment, 40
Food and Drug Administration (FDA), 224
Formal conclusions-objectives relation, 46
Formalized hypothesis, 89
Formulation, drug, 31
Full analysis set (FAS), 177. *See also* Analysis sets
Futility analysis, 198–199

G

General Linear Model (GLM), 80b. *See also* Analysis of variance; Correlation; Regression; t-test
Generalize/generalization, 64–65
Generic drug, 31, 44, 241–242
Gold-standard, in device testing, 23, 84–85
Graphical descriptive statistics, 56–57. *See also* Descriptive Statistics

H

Hearing aids, implantable, 56
Heart, artificial, 205
Histogram, 78. *See also* Descriptive statistics
Hyperglycemic episode, 48
Hypoglycemic episode, 48
Hypotheses, 115–119. *See also* Hypothesis Testing; Statistical Testing
Hypothesis testing, 55, 144–145, 148–150. *See also* Statistical testing

I

Immunosuppressive agents, 28–29
Imperfect gold standard, in diagnostic device, 84np
Impute, 171, 172. *See also* Missing data
Inclusion criteria, 14, 60, 116

determining, 176, 200
stroke trial, 111, 117, 170
Independent groups design, 163
Independent variable, 98–99
Inference, 101–105, 108–109
Inferential statistics, 93–97, 104, 105–108, 109
Information, data and, 56, 61, 62b. *See also* Descriptive statistics
Insulin-dependent diabetes, 47–48
Intended audience, 157
Intended use, 22, 26. *See also* Intended Use Population
defining, 26
in dose-response studies, 26
kinitis study, 23
in vaccine studies, 33
Intended use population, 14, 62b, 63–66
defining, 14, 63, 160
example, 62b
nonrepresentative subjects, 175
stroke trial, 118
Intent to treat (ITT), 176–178, 184b. *See also* Analysis Sets
Intercept, 121
Interim analysis
adaptive, 201
ALP clinical trial, 7
classic, 199–200
in clinical trial planning, 159
defined, 151, 198
efficacy, 190–191
error increased through, 149
reasons for, 197–202
safety, 192–193
statistical considerations, 194–197
Internal review board (IRB), 244np
International Conference on Harmonization (ICH)
on avoiding bias, 180
on confirmatory trials, 131, 132
on endpoint selection, 214
on intention to treat principle, 176
on interim analysis, 199–200
on probability of type II error, 237–238
purpose of, 35–36
on randomization, 186
Interval estimate, 72–75. *See also* Estimation

Intuition, 131
Invention, 25
Ischemic stroke, 42, 116

K

Kampen, Netherlands, 204–205
Kidney, artificial, 204–205
Kidney failure, 204–205
Kidney Specific Antigen (KSA), 19
Kidney transplantation
historically, 205–206
organ rejection clinical trial, 210–211
success measures, 208
Kinitis, 19–24
Koala, 128
Koestler, A, 128
Koff, Willem, 204
Kubanga Forest, 105
Kurtosis, 81

L

Laboratory parameters, 137
Last observation carried forward (LOCF), 173. *See also* Imputation
L-Dopa, 136
Logic in modeling, 131
Long-term effects, 33b
Lupus (SLE), 28b

M

Mallory, George, 25
Manipulation, 29
Mannheim Working Group Lower Limb Reflex Response Scale (MLRS), 8
Marginals in frequency tables, 84
Market potential, 17b
Mean, 78
accuracy and the, 78–79, 89
clinical trial example, 103t, 140, 141, 163b, 240
computing, 79, 80b, 141
defined, 94
from description to testing, 80b
dispersion of numbers around the, 81
Kubanga Forest example, 105
normal distribution and the, 105
Measurement, 28b, 58, 84–85, 100–101, 103, 138b, 156, 159, 167, 168, 169,

173,203, 207b, 209b, 210, 214, 221–226, 227, 229, 230, 236–237, 244. *See also* Measurement

Measurement error, 138b, 139np, 168, 210, 229, 236–237, 244. *See also* Measurement

Mechanism of action (MOA), 8

Median, 78

Medical product attributes, 25–34

Medicine
evidence-based, 82b
personalizing, 99b

Missing data, 171–174, 176. *See also* Dropout

Modeling
Animal model, 2–3, 12–13
complexity in, 130
dose-response, 124
engine size-acceleration, 120, 129
the human in, 120–128
limitations, 122b
logic in, 131
overview, 105–108
robustness in, 128–131
sample size in post hoc modeling, 130

Modified Rankin Scale (mRS), 223–224

Monitoring, 14

Monoclonal antibodies, 238

Multiple-arm trial, 39

Multiple statistical comparisons. *See* Multiple testing

Multiple testing, 138b, 150, 151, 152–153, 194–197, 210–211
applying, 198
data analysis scenarios, 136, 148–150
defined, 136, 150, 152, 195, 210
difficulties arising from, avoiding, 213–214, 227
example, 151–153
failure due to, 211
overview, 194–197, 210–211
principles, 152
results of, 151
in safety, 227
solving for, 214
type I Error resulting from, 152
uncontrolled, outcomes of, 152–153

Multiplicity. *See* Multiple testing

N

National Cancer Institute (NCI), 207

National Institutes of Health (NIH), 218

Natural history, 2, 17b

Neurodegenerative, 2

Neurodegenerative disorder, 2

Neurons, 2

Neuroprotection, 2

Neuroprotective, 8

Neuroprotein, 2

New drug application (NDA), 161

Noise, 167–168

Nondisclosure agreement (NDA), 21

Non-inferiority, 37, 41–45, 241–242
defined, 37
demonstrating, 45
overview, 45–50
statistical testing for, 146–150

Non-inferiority delta, 49

Non-inferiority margin, 43–44, 46, 49

Non-inferiority testing, 146–150

Non-inferiority trial, 49

Nonrepresentative subjects, 175

Nonsignificance, 102b, 143, 145–146, 148, 164b, 240, 243b

Non-significant outcomes. *See* Nonsignificance

Normal distribution, 105, 142

Null hypothesis
Apparatone drug trial, 144
defined, 107, 144
inability to prove the, 145
proving the, 145
rejecting the, 108, 144, 147, 153b, 194, 219, 231. *See also* Hypothesis testing; Statistical testing

O

Objective performance criterion (OPC), 39

Objectives
conclusions relation to, 46
equivalence, 41–45
non-inferiority, 37, 41–45
superiority, 37, 38–41

One-sided hypothesis, 232b

One-sided test, 232b

Ordinal scale, 221

Outlier, 79

Overfitting, 122–130. *See also* Robustness

P

Paired designs, 162, 163b

Parkinson, James, 136

Parkinson's disease
Apparatone drug trial
data analysis scenarios, 138–139, 148–150
design, 136–138
formalized hypotheses, 144
interpreting nonsignificant results, 145–146. *See also* Nonsignificance
background, 135–153

Partial-confirmatory approach, 122

Performance, 29–30

Performance goal, 39

Personalized medicine, 99b

Pharmacogenomics, 99b

Pharmacokinetics, 31, 43–44, 45. *See also* C-max

Phase I clinical trial, 2

Phase IIa clinical trial, 4–5

Phase III clinical trial, 4–5. *See also* Pivotal trial

Physicians
ethics in clinical trials, 181b
evidence-based medicine practices, 82b
nonrepresentative, 175
statisticians vs, 28b, 58b, 81, 82b

Piaget, Jean, 54, 55, 58, 109

Pilot study, 7

Pipeline, 17b

Pivotal trial, 26, 62b. *See also* Phase III clinical trial

Placebo, 36, 39, 69, 159, 169–170, 174

Placebo effect, 170

Planned vs. post hoc, 130. *See also* Confirmatory trial; Exploratory trial

Plasma (blood plasma), 206–207

Point estimate, 72–75

Population
attributes, 60, 108–109
ALP clinical trial, 14
creating by defining, 61
defined, 61, 78
enriched, 23

Population *(Continued)*
   inference and, 107
   intended use, 14, 62*b*, 63–66,
      160, 175
   point estimate, 72
   statistics, 60–63
   sufficiently large, 65
   target, 62*b*
Population mean, 63
Population parameter, 68–69
Post hoc analysis, 118–119, 124, 127,
      130, 132, 133, 150*b*. *See also*
      Exploratory trial
Power analysis, 5, 12, 13, 153*b*,
      192, 196*b*. *See also* Sample
      size; Statistical power
Practice-science interaction, 39*b*
Precision of measurement, 209,
      213–214, 221, 247
Preclinical trial, 2
Preclinical trial issues, 2
Predicate (P), 83*np*
Prevalence, 13
Primary Efficacy Endpoint, 8, 113–115,
      116, 137, 161, 214, 215*b*, 218,
      220. *See also* Primary endpoint;
      Efficacy; Efficacy endpoint
   clinical trial example, 116, 162, 214
   principle of, 218
Primary endpoint, 213–228. *See also*
      Efficacy; Efficacy endpoint
Problem-solving, 25
Product development, 27
Prognostic factors, 182–183
Propensity analysis, 190
Proportion of variance explained,
      100. *See also* Explained
      variance; Statistical explanation
Protocol (clinical study protocol), 14
Protocol violations, 176, 177, 181*b*
P-value, 93, 143, 145–146

Q

Qualitative scales, 225
Quality of life (QoL), 207*b*
Quantitative endpoints, 207*b*, 222, 224
Quantitative statements, 72

R

R&R (repeatability and
      reproducibility) study, 21
Random error, 167–169, 170–171,
      178, 207*b*

Randomization, 15–16, 157–158,
      182–186
   dynamic, 184–185
   ICH guidelines, 186
   stratified, 183, 234*b*
Range, 78. *See also* Descriptive statistics
Ratio scale, 222
Recruitment, 13–14
Reference, 39
Reference value, 188
Referral bias, 63
Regression, 94–95
Reimbursement, 115
Reliability, 220
   accuracy and, 221
   defined, 220
   in measurement, 221, 228
   MLRS, 8
   noise and, 167–168
   overview, 218–221
   sample size and, 104*b*
   validity and, 221
Reliable, 8
   conclusions, 4, 168
   defined, 220
   information for planning, 7
   measures, 220
   method to asses risk, 27
   MLRS as, 8
   results, 167–168, 220
Repeatability, 21, 71, 220, 221.
      See also Reproducibility
Repeatable, 21, 70
Representative sample, 14
Reproducibility, 21, 221
Reproducible, 70. *See also*
      Repeatability; Reliability
Research objectives, setting, 35–51
Responder analysis, 225
Rheumatoid arthritis, 28–29, 238
Risk, 23, 28–29
Risk analysis, 85
Risk-benefit analysis, 29*b*
Robust, 131
Robustness, 128–131
Route of administration, 115
R-square, 122*b*

S

Safety
   clinical trial design element of,
      28–29, 192–193, 220, 227
   defining (attributes), 28–29

demonstrating non-inferiority
      on, 156
   efficacy vs, 206
   endpoints, 137, 226–227
   formal testing for, 156
   interim analysis of, 192–193
   speed vs, 33*b*
   in testing, 64
Sample, 47, 63–66
Sample mean, 63
Sample size, 12–14. *See also* Power
      analysis
   adapting in interim analysis, 200–201
   certainty's relation to, 71, 73
   computing, example using
      simulation, 238–241
   determining, 4–15, 18, 230,
      241–242
   effect size, and, 210–211, 235
   equivalence, in, 226, 241
   noninferiority, in, 226, 241
   post hoc modeling, in, 130
   random error and, 169
   reliability and, 104*b*
   sampling error, 233–234, 234*b*
Sample statistic, 68–69, 72
Sampling
   biased, 175
   error and, 168
   luck in, 233
   nature of, 47
   overview, 63–66
   with replacement, 239*np*
Sampling distribution, 141, 142
Sampling error, 47, 74, 233–234, 234*b*
   defined, 47, 74
   example, 107–108, 140
   overview, 233–234
   reducing, 74, 112–113, 234*b*
   results of, 104, 107–108, 139, 143,
      168
Scatterplot, 78
Science-practice interaction, 39*b*
Scientific explanation, 97–99
Scientific justification, 17*b*
Scientific method, 80*b*
Secondary endpoint, 116, 213–228.
      See also Endpoints
Sensitivity, 85, 87, 118, 126–127,
      132, 188, 216, 246
Sensitivity analysis, 171
Serious adverse event (SAE), 68, 156,
      192

Shaking Palsy, 135–153
Similarity, 148
Simplification, 79
Single arm trials, 39
Skewness, 81
Sleep apnea, 82–83
Sleep apnea device trial, 82–89
Soccer, 111
Specialization, 128–129
Specificity, 85, 86, 87t, 118, 126–127,
    132, 188, 216, 246
Spread, 94
Standard deviation, 58, 163b
Standard error, 122b, 131, 142
Standard error of estimate, 122b,
    131
Standard-of-Care, 5, 40
Statistical analysis plan (SAP), 116
Statistical decision making, 138b
Statistical explanation, 93–97,
    103, 104
Statistical indicators, 131
Statistical inference, 104
Statistical input into trial design
    Eliminating bias. See Bias,
        methods for avoiding
    recruitment, 13–14
    sample size. See Power analysis;
        Sample size; Statistical power
    trial length, 8–10
Statistical power (1-β), 10, 160–161,
    162, 163b, 196b, 197,
    200–201, 219, 231–233,
    237–238. See also Power
    analysis; Sample size
Statistical significance, 92–109
    clinical significance and, 93
    clinical trial example, 156, 219–220
    description, inference, and testing,
        93–97
    explanation and inference in
        clinical trials, 101–105
    importance of, 104
    nonsignificant results, 145–146
    overview and limitations, 92–109
    quantifying explanation,
        100–101
Statistical testing, hypothesis testing,
    55, 115, 144, 146–150
    equivalence, 41–45
    noninferiority, 37, 41–45
    superiority, 37, 38–41
Statistical thinking, 53–66, 82b

Statisticians
    clinicians vs, 28b, 58b, 81, 82b
    ethical obligations, 40, 227
Statistics
    descriptive, 55–60
    population, 60–63
    samples, 63–66
Stenosis, 216, 222
Stent, 216
Stereotyping, 78, 105
Stratified assignment, 234b
Stratified randomization, 183, 234b
Study Design, 7–9, 160, 161, 175,
    181b, 202, 230, 243–244
Study Objectives, 50, 197, 207, 213,
    227
Subgroup analysis, 117
Subject recruitment. See Recruitment
Substantial equivalence, 50
Sufficiently safe, 68
Summary statistics, 55–56
Superiority, 37, 38–41
    clinical trial aims and attributes,
        50t, 156t
    clinical trial example, 149
    declaring in clinical trials, 115,
        196b
    defined, 37
    non-inferiority trials and, 45
    overview, 38–41
    proving, 195, 200–201, 242
    publishing results and, 157
    sample size and, 242np
    statistical solutions for showing,
        148
    in trial design, 159
    using equivalence vs, 44
Superiority trial, 42, 45, 230
Surrogate endpoint, 218
Survival analysis, 137

T
Target population, 62b. See also
    Intended use; Intended use
    population
Test, 39
Tocqueville, Alexis de, 53, 78–79, 81
Topical drugs, 31
Treatment group, 5
Trend toward significance, 145–146
Trial length, 8–10
T-test, 41, 80b, 164b, 226
Two-sided hypothesis, 232b

Two-sided test, 232b
Type I Error. See also Null hypothesis
    avoiding, 153b
    clinical trial example, 144
    defined, 88, 143, 210–211, 231
    increasing probability of, 199
    inflated, 201
    interim analysis, 194
    from multiplicity, 148–150, 152,
        194–197
    percent chance, determining, 144,
        149–150, 151, 152, 153b
    in practice, 196b
    Type II error relation to, 153b,
        196b
Type II Error, 88. See also Alternative
    hypothesis
    defined, 88, 144, 210–211, 231
    ICH guidelines, 237–238
    Type I Error relation to, 153b, 196b

U
Unblinding, 174
Unreliable, 2, 221
Urea, 206–207
Uterine fibroid removal, 29

V
Valid, 71
Validate, 2–3
Validity, 191, 218–221
Variable, 94–95. See also Endpoints
    dependent, 98–99
    dichotomous, 83
    explanatory, 98–99
    independent, 98–99
Variance, 141
Variance explained, 95–97. See
    also Explanation; Statistical
    explanation; Proportion of
    variance explained
Verification bias, 63
Vital signs, 137
In vitro testing, 2

W
Warfarin, 42
Washout period, 43
Wholly confirmatory, 121
World Medical Association
    Declaration of Helsinki,
        243–244
World War II, 204

Printed and bound by CPI Group (UK) Ltd, Croydon, CR0 4YY
03/10/2024
01040316-0005